Register Now for Online Access to Your Book!

Your print purchase of *Handbook of Spasticity: A Practical Approach to Management,* **includes online access to the contents of your book**—increasing accessibility, portability, and searchability!

Access today at:
http://connect.springerpub.com/content/book/978-0-8261-3975-7
or scan the QR code at the right with your smartphone. Log in or register, then click "Redeem a voucher" and use the code below.

A0WDE2KW

Scan here for quick access.

Having trouble redeeming a voucher code?
Go to https://connect.springerpub.com/redeeming-voucher-code

If you are experiencing problems accessing the digital component of this product, please contact our customer service department at cs@springerpub.com

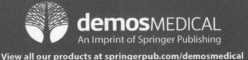

demosMEDICAL
An Imprint of Springer Publishing

View all our products at springerpub.com/demosmedical

HANDBOOK OF SPASTICITY

Handbook of Spasticity

A Practical Approach to Management

Monica Verduzco-Gutierrez, MD
Professor and Chair, Department of Rehabilitation Medicine
Long School of Medicine
University of Texas Health Science Center at San Antonio
San Antonio, Texas

Nicholas C. Ketchum, MD
Associate Professor
Department of Physical Medicine and Rehabilitation
Medical College of Wisconsin
Milwaukee, Wisconsin

Editors

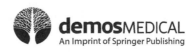

demosMEDICAL
An Imprint of Springer Publishing

Springer Publishing Company, LLC
www.springerpub.com
connect.springerpub.com

Acquisitions Editor: Beth Barry
Compositor: Exeter Premedia Services Private Limited
Production Editor: Joseph Stubenrauch

ISBN: 978-0-8261-3974-0
ebook ISBN: 978-0-8261-3975-7
DOI: 10.1891/9780826139757

SUPPLEMENTS:
Student Materials (Chapter 21 audio/video PowerPoint) ISBN: 978-0-8261-3976-4

23 24 25 26 / 5 4 3 2 1

Medicine is an ever-changing science. Research and clinical experience are continually expanding our knowledge, in particular our understanding of proper treatment and drug therapy. The authors, editors, and publisher have made every effort to ensure that all information in this book is in accordance with the state of knowledge at the time of production of the book. Nevertheless, the authors, editors, and publisher are not responsible for any errors or omissions or for any consequence from application of the information in this book and make no warranty, expressed or implied, with respect to the content of this publication. Every reader should examine carefully the package inserts accompanying each drug and should carefully check whether the dosage schedules therein or the contraindications stated by the manufacturer differ from the statements made in this book. Such examination is particularly important with drugs that are either rarely used or have been newly released on the market. The publisher has no responsibility for the persistence or accuracy of URLs for external or third-party Internet websites referred to in this publication and does not guarantee that any content on such websites is, or will remain, accurate or appropriate.

Library of Congress Control Number: 2023942295

Contact sales@springerpub.com to receive discount rates on bulk purchases.

Publisher's Note: New and used products purchased from third-party sellers are not guaranteed for quality, authenticity, or access to any included digital components.

Printed in the United States of America by Gasch Printing

Contents

Contributors

Harsha Ayyala, MD, Brain Injury Fellow, Department of Physical Medicine and Rehabilitation, Baylor College of Medicine, Houston, Texas

Abana Azariah, MD, Clinical Chief, Disorders of Consciousness Program, Attending Physician, Brain Injury and Stroke Program, TIRR Memorial Hermann; Assistant Professor, Physical Medicine and Rehabilitation, University of Texas McGovern Medical School, Houston, Texas

Laxman Bahroo, DO, FAAN, Professor and Director, Neurology Residency Program, Medstar Georgetown University Hospital, Washington, District of Columbia

Eve Boissonnault, MD, FRCPC, Assistant Clinical Professor, Department of Physical Medicine and Rehabilitation, Centre Hospitalier de l'Université de Montréal, Montreal, Quebec, Canada

Laurie Dabaghian, MD, Clinical Assistant Professor, Hackensack Meridian School of Medicine, Director of Physical Medicine and Rehabilitation Consult Services, Hackensack University Medical Center, Hackensack, New Jersey

Madeline A. Dicks, DO, Spinal Cord Injury Fellow, University of Texas Health Science Center at Houston, Houston, Texas

Steven Escaldi, DO, Medical Director, Spasticity Management Program, Johnson Rehabilitation Institute, JFK University Medical Center, Edison, New Jersey; Clinical Associate Professor, Department of Rehabilitation Medicine, Rutgers Robert Wood Johnson Medical School, Piscataway, New Jersey

Alberto Esquenazi, MD, Professor and Chair and Director, Sheerr Gait and Motion Analysis Laboratory, MossRehab, Department of Physical Medicine and Rehabilitation, MossRehab/Jefferson, Philadelphia, Pennsylvania

Reza Farid, MD, Professor of Clinical Physical Medicine and Rehabilitation, University of Missouri, Columbia, Missouri

Heather Finlayson, MD, FRCPC, Clinical Associate Professor, Division of Physical Medicine and Rehabilitation, Faculty of Medicine, University of British Columbia, Vancouver, British Columbia, Canada

Gerard E. Francisco, MD, The Wulfe Family Chair in Physical Medicine and Rehabilitation, Distinguished Teaching Professor, University of Texas System, Chairman and Professor, Department of Physical Medicine and Rehabilitation, University of Texas Health Science Center at Houston, McGovern Medical School; Chief Medical Officer and Director, Neurorecovery Research Center, TIRR Memorial Hermann, Houston, Texas

Mark Gormley Jr., MD, Clinical Assistant Professor, Department of Physical Medicine and Rehabilitation, University of Minnesota, Minneapolis, Minnesota; Associate Medical Director, Pediatric Rehabilitation Medicine, Gillette Children's Hospital, Saint Paul, Minnesota

William A. Ramos Guasp, MD, Department of Physical Medicine, Rehabilitation and Sports Medicine, University of Puerto Rico School of Medicine, San Juan, Puerto Rico

Shivani Gupta, DO, Attending Physician, Physical Medicine Rehabilitation Medicine, Advocate Christ Medical Center, Oak Lawn, Illinois

Christina K. Hardesty, MD, Associate Professor of Orthopedic Surgery, Rainbow Babies and Children's Hospital; Associate Residency Program Director, Case Western Reserve University, Cleveland, Ohio

Kristen A. Harris, MD, Resident, Physical Medicine and Rehabilitation, University of Pittsburgh Medical Center, Pittsburgh, Pennsylvania

Kimberly Heckert, MD, Director, Spasticity Management Fellowship, Clinical Associate Professor, Rehabilitation Medicine, Sidney Kimmel Medical College, Thomas Jefferson University, Philadelphia, Pennsylvania

Faiza Khan Humayun, MD, Medical Director, Polytrauma Inpatient Rehabilitation, James Haley VA Hospital, Physical Medicine and Rehabilitation Service, Tampa, Florida

Cindy B. Ivanhoe, MD, Director, Spasticity and Associated Syndromes of Movement, TIRR Memorial Hermann; Clinical Professor, Physical Medicine and Rehabilitation, University of Texas McGovern Medical School, Houston, Texas

Jorge Jacinto, MD, Director of Adult Neurorehabilitation Department, Head of Gait Laboratory, Head of Adult Spasticity Clinic, Centro de Medicina de Reabilitação de Alcoitão, Alcabideche, Portugal

Jacob B. Jeffers, MD, Brain Injury Fellow, Department of Physical Medicine and Rehabilitation, University of Texas Health Science Center at Houston, McGovern Medical School, Houston, Texas

Farris Kassam, BSc, MSI 3, Faculty of Medicine, University of British Columbia, Vancouver, British Columbia, Canada

Nicholas C. Ketchum, MD, Associate Professor, Department of Physical Medicine and Rehabilitation, Medical College of Wisconsin, Milwaukee, Wisconsin

Heakyung Kim, MD, Professor and Chair, Department of Physical Medicine and Rehabilitation and Kimberly-Clark Distinguished Chair in Mobility Research, University of Texas Southwestern Medical Center, Dallas, Texas

Blaise Langan, DO, Resident Physician, University of Texas Health Science Center at San Antonio, San Antonio, Texas

Sheng Li, MD, PhD, Professor, Director, Stroke Rehabilitation and Recovery Research, Department of Physical Medicine and Rehabilitation, McGovern Medical School, University of Texas Health Science Center at Houston; Director of Neurorehabilitation Research Lab, TIRR Memorial Hermann, Houston, Texas

Katherine Lin, MD, Medical Director, Polytrauma Outpatient TBI Services, South Texas Veterans Health Care System; Adjoint Assistant Professor, Department of Rehabilitation Medicine, University of Texas Health Science Center at San Antonio, San Antonio, Texas

Manuel F. Mas, MD, Assistant Professor, University of Puerto Rico School of Medicine, Department of Physical Medicine, Rehabilitation and Sports Medicine, Hospital de Trauma de la Administración de Servicios Médicos de Puerto Rico, San Juan, Puerto Rico

Marissa McCarthy, MD, Program Director, Physical Medicine and Rehabilitation Residency, Department of Neurology, Division of Physical Medicine and Rehabilitation, University of South Florida, Tampa, Florida

John McGuire, MD, Professor of Physical Medicine and Rehabilitation, Director, Stroke Rehabilitation and Spasticity Management, Medical College of Wisconsin, Milwaukee, Wisconsin

Selina M. Morgan, PT, DPT, NCS, Assistant Professor, Department of Physical Therapy, University of Texas Health Science Center at San Antonio, San Antonio, Texas

Jessica Mulhern, DO, Physiatrist, Rehabilitation Medicine, Rehabilitation Associates of the Main Line, Paoli, Pennsylvania

Michael C. Munin, MD, Professor, Department of Physical Medicine and Rehabilitation, University of Pittsburgh School of Medicine, Pittsburgh, Pennsylvania

Brian J. Nagle, MD, MPH, Movement Disorders Fellow, Department of Neurology, Medstar Georgetown University Hospital, Washington, District of Columbia

Sindhoori Nalla, DO, MHSA, Clinical Assistant Professor, Department of Rehabilitation Medicine, Sidney Kimmel Medical College, Thomas Jefferson University, Philadelphia, Pennsylvania

Ahmed Z. Obeidat, MD, PhD, Associate Professor, Founding Director, Neuroimmunology and MS Fellowship Program, Department of Neurology, Medical College of Wisconsin, Milwaukee, Wisconsin

Marilyn S. Pacheco, MD, Chief of Rehabilitation Services, Edward Hines Jr. VA Hospital, Hines, Illinois

Shivani Patel, DO, Resident Physician, Department of Physical Medicine and Rehabilitation, Penn State College of Medicine, Penn State Health, Hershey, Pennsylvania

Andrea Paulson, MD, MPH, MBA, Associate Medical Director, Pediatric Rehabilitation Medicine, Gillette Children's Hospital, Saint Paul, Minnesota

Rajiv Reebye, MD, FRCPC, Clinical Associate Professor, Division of Physical Medicine and Rehabilitation, Faculty of Medicine, University of British Columbia, Vancouver, British Columbia, Canada

Natasha L. Romanoski, DO, Associate Professor, Department of Physical Medicine and Rehabilitation, Penn State College of Medicine, Penn State Health, Hershey, Pennsylvania

Mary E. Russell, DO, MS, Assistant Professor, Vice Chair – Quality and Compliance, Department of Physical Medicine and Rehabilitation, University of Texas Health Science Center at Houston, McGovern Medical School, Houston, Texas

Michael Saulino, MD, PhD, Chief, Department of Physical Medicine and Rehabilitation, Cooper University Hospital; Professor and Chair, Cooper Medical School of Rowan University, Camden, New Jersey; Adjucant Asssociate Professor, Department of Rehabilitation Medicine, Sidney Kimmel Medical College, Thomas Jefferson University, Philadelphia, Pennsylvania

Tulsi Shah, MD, Resident, Department of Neurology, Medstar Georgetown University Hospital, Washington, District of Columbia

Anjali Sivaramakrishnan, PT, PhD, Assistant Professor, Department of Physical Therapy, University of Texas Health Science Center at San Antonio, San Antonio, Texas

Sandeep K. Subramanian, PT, PhD, Assistant Professor, Departments of Physical Therapy, Physician Assistant Studies, and Rehabilitation Medicine, University of Texas Health Science Center at San Antonio, San Antonio, Texas

Areerat Suputtitada, MD, Professor, Department of Rehabilitation Medicine, Faculty of Medicine, Chulalongkorn University, and King Chulalongkorn Memorial Hospital, Bangkok, Thailand

Andrea Perrone Toomer, MD, Physical Medicine and Rehabilitation, Culicchia Neurological Clinic, Department of Neurosurgery, Louisiana State University, Health Sciences Center, Marrero, Louisiana

Heather W. Walker, MD, Medical Director, MUSC Rehabilitation Hospital, Encompass Health, Affiliate Associate Professor, Medical University of South Carolina, Department of Neurosciences, Charleston, South Carolina

Thomas Watanabe, MD, Clinical Director, Drucker Brain Injury Center, MossRehab/Einstein Healthcare Network, Elkins Park, Pennsylvania

Matthew David Wilhelm, DO, Resident Physician, Department of Neurology, Division of Physical Medicine and Rehabilitation, University of South Florida, Tampa, Florida

Paul Winston, MD, FRCPC, Department of Physical Medicine and Rehabilitation, University of British Columbia, Victoria General Hospital, Victoria, British Columbia, Canada

ShaEssa L. Wright, DO, MBS, FAAPMR, Assistant Professor, Department of Physical Medicine and Rehabilitation, Department of Pediatrics, Penn State Milton S. Hershey Medical Center, Penn State College of Medicine, Hershey, Pennsylvania

Preface

The concept behind creating this first edition of *Handbook of Spasticity* stemmed from sharing a passion for treatment of spastic hypertonia, because of a devotion to our patients who often improve from treatment of their disabling spasticity. We saw a need to provide information about key concepts in spasticity management more effectively to students, residents, and fellows on rehabilitation or neurology rotations in hopes that they will come to learn and treat spasticity holistically and with a patient-centered approach. Spasticity impacts over 12 million people worldwide and is disabling. Some of these patients may be unable to get out of nursing homes or have more community access due to their disability. Spasticity has also been shown to be undertreated in certain populations and countries. The need to expand our knowledge base both within and outside our specialties is imperative to ensure more access to care. Subsequently, the idea behind providing a clinical resource for trainees grew to encompass all who are involved in taking care of persons impacted by spasticity. This handbook has been created with this focused, yet broader call to convey key clinical information to all clinicians who provide care to persons with spasticity and their rehabilitative needs.

We formatted this handbook with the goal of providing easily accessible key information that is portable; thus, it is provided in a compact print version as well as an online version with some video cases to enhance learning. The most up-to-date information has been organized efficiently in each chapter to the use of combined text and bullet points and tables to allow for rapid access at the bedside, for clinics, or to refer to while studying. The chapters are grouped into four sections that include "What Is Spasticity?" This section is a broad overview and includes definitions, epidemiology, and pathophysiology. The section called "Assessment and Evaluation" focuses on measurement and scales with easy tables for reference, gait assessment, and setting appropriate goals. The section on "Treatment" focuses on both pharmacologic and nonpharmacologic treatments, including emerging technologies. The last section is also quite novel and is called "Disease Management: A Case-Based Approach," which focuses on management of diseases and includes online video content. Our collaborating authors from around the world bring years of experience across numerous subspecialities.

This handbook is intended for medical students; residents in neurology and physical medicine and rehabilitation (PM&R); fellows in specialties that focus on conditions related to spasticity such as neurosurgery, orthopedics, and geriatrics; those in primary care who take care of patients with neurologic disabilities; allied health professionals, including physical, occupational, and speech therapists; and advanced practice providers, nurse practitioners, and rehabilitation nurses. This handbook is necessary for anyone first delving into the world of spasticity management, or as a reference for someone who already treats spasticity (or may have learners with them at the bedside), and for those in practice who strive to improve their spasticity management skills.

We wish to thank our many contributing authors who have lent their precious time, amazing talent, and leading expertise to make this amazing handbook come to fruition. They are a star-studded cast, and we truly appreciate their efforts and input. We also want to thank Hannah Greco and all the editorial staff at Springer Publishing for their guidance throughout this process. We cannot forget to thank our spouses – Leonard Gutierrez (Monica) and Erin McGonigle (Nick) – as well as our children for always supporting our career and love of spasticity. Finally, we dedicate this book to the patients we are lucky to care for. Your resilience through adversity has inspired each page of this handbook. We hope you enjoy this book and remain motivated to improve the lives of persons with spasticity.

Monica Verduzco-Gutierrez, MD
Nicholas C. Ketchum, MD

What Is Spasticity?

I Definition: Spasticity and Upper Motor Neuron Syndrome

Marilyn S. Pacheco

DISTINGUISHING SPASTICITY

Spasticity [spas·tic·i·ty | \spa-'sti-sə-tē] is an abnormal increase in muscle tone or stiffness of muscle. The term *spastic* is from Latin *spasticus* and from Greek *spastikos* that means afflicted with spasms and *spaon* (to draw out, stretch). Hippocrates used the term spasms to describe epileptic fit but the term *spasticity* has only been used in recent literature. Clinically, a person affected with spastic paralysis was first reported around 1838.[1]

In 1980, J. W. Lance presented the most well-known and referenced physiological definition of spasticity.[2,3]

> *"Spasticity is a motor disorder characterized by a velocity-dependent increase in tonic stretch reflexes (muscle tone) with exaggerated tendon jerks, resulting from hyperexcitability of the stretch reflex, as one component of the upper motor neuron syndrome".*

Muscle tone is usually described as "the tension in the relaxed muscle" or "the resistance, felt by the examiner during passive stretching of a joint when the muscles are at rest." Tone is the resistance of resting muscle to passive movements.[4] The meaning of tone is uncertain and vague. Each assessment has inter-rater variability and examination becomes subjective to the examiner as to what is resistance to passive stretch. What is felt by examiner is the change in resistance or force per unit change in length of tissue. However, muscles in a person are never in a completely relaxed state. Muscle tone may reflect a readiness to a movement, and muscle tone is difficult to assess when the person is asked to relax and not to make any movement. Muscle tone is a form of the neuromotor system that reacts to the signals coming from upper levels of movement formation by refining the excitability of the sensory and motor cells for active postural or movement control. This definition makes muscle tone an active contributor to movement and postural tasks.[5]

There are different clinical presentations from spasms to rigidity. In current times, spasticity is one hallmark of an upper motor neuron (UMN) disorder and it represents one of the most important impairments for clinicians who care for patients with central nervous system (CNS) disease. Spasticity is used to describe phenomenon of muscle overactivity that is seen in upper motor neuron syndrome (UMNS), a damage to nerve pathways within the brain or spinal cord that control muscle movement. It can occur in association with spinal cord injury (SCI), multiple sclerosis (MS), cerebral palsy (CP), stroke, brain or head trauma, amyotrophic lateral sclerosis, hereditary spastic paraplegias, and heredodegenerative diseases. Spasticity describes the co-occurrence of involuntary muscle hyperactivity and central paresis.[6]

Spasticity is only one of the many different features of the UMNS. The UMNS can occur following any lesion affecting some or all the descending motor pathways. The UMNS is an unclear valuable concept. Aspects of the UMNS explain for disability and consequences rather than the more narrowly defined spasticity itself[7] Dr. John Hughlings Jackson, a notable 19th century neurologist, was one of the first to recognize that a lesion of the CNS could simultaneously result in the development of positive and negative signs, although he was uncertain that the lesion directly caused the observed signs. In humans, a lesion of the descending corticospinal motor system can produce the negative sign of muscle weakness during voluntary effort and, at the same time and in the same muscle, the positive sign of increased resistance to passive stretch. The combination is the key feature of muscle spasticity, although it is important to recognize that spasticity is one of a number of positive signs that materialize after a UMN lesion. The aggregate of positive and negative signs after a UMN lesion comprises the UMNS.[10]

Table 1.1 gives an overview of UMNS that following a UMN lesion, a combination of sensorimotor signs and symptoms are generally classified as positive, negative, and third phenomenon.[7,8,9]

DEFINING MUSCLE OVERACTIVITY

The phenomenon of presence is the positive findings in UMNS from muscle overactivity.

Table 1.1 Signs and Symptoms of the Upper Motor Neuron Syndrome

Upper Motor Neuron Phenomenon	Clinical Presentation
Positive phenomenon = muscle overactivity or phenomenon of presence	Increase tendon reflexes with radiation of effect Clonus Positive Babinski sign Spasticity Extensor spasms Flexor spasms Positive support reaction Co-contraction Associated reactions (synkinesis) Spastic dystonia
Negative phenomenon = muscle underactivity or phenomenon of absence	Weakness Reduced dexterity Fatigue Impaired motor planning Impaired motor control
Third phenomenon = leading to disability	Stiffness Contracture Pain

Clonus

Clonus is a low-frequency rhythmic oscillation in one or more limb segments that is generated by rapid stretch and hold of muscle group. Clonus sustained for five or more beats is considered as clinically abnormal. Clonus can be elicited during examination and it can be triggered by voluntary movement or by sensory stimulation. On electromyography (FMG), it has repetitive rhythmic burst of short-duration electrical activity (frequencies of 6 to 8 Hz). It can be sustained or non-sustained and can be stopped by repositioning clonic muscles at shorter lengths. Both clonus and spasticity are results of stretch reflex increase in gain, which is a change in neuronal response sensitivity to initial input depending on the secondary input.[9,10]

Co-contraction

Co-contraction is the simultaneous activation of agonist and antagonist muscles during voluntary movement. It can be activated or deactivated at the cortical level and is related to switching mechanism of reciprocal inhibition in the cord. In normal individuals, co-contraction is normal and beneficial as it helps stability of a joint for tasks, such as in walking or in carrying a gallon of milk. When a co-contracting antagonist undergoes stretch and develops superimposed spasticity, the combination is called spastic co-contraction. There is simultaneous contraction of the agonists and antagonist muscles. Clinically, patients with co-contractures have slow effortful movements. This is different from the dysfunctional co-contraction called spastic dystonia.[7,9,10]

Dystonia

In 1911, Oppenheim introduced the term dystonia. Dystonia is defined as sustained or intermittent muscle contractions resulting in abnormal, often repetitive movements, postures, or both. These movements are typically patterned and may be tremulous or twisting and aggravated by voluntary action. Dystonia can be focal, segmental, restricted to one half of the body (hemi dystonia), or generalized. The heterogeneous presentation and the various etiologies ranging from genetic causes to neurodegenerative disorders point to multiple mechanisms that contribute to the pathophysiology of dystonia. In 2013, revised definition was proposed that "dystonia is a movement disorder characterized by sustained or intermittent muscle contractions causing abnormal, often repetitive movements, postures, or both. Dystonic movements are typically patterned, twisting, and may be tremulous. Dystonia is often initiated or worsened by voluntary action and associated with overflow muscle activation."[11]

Dystonia can occur in variety of conditions, but it is the classic study of Denny-Brown wherein spastic dystonia and its fixed postures and attitudes were described after cerebral cortex ablations of monkeys. It is dystonia happening in the presence of spasticity and primarily due to abnormal supraspinal drive, characterized by an inability to inhibit muscle activity despite efforts to do so. It was not dependent of sensory afferent input at the spinal reflexes level. There is continuous muscle contraction caused by cortical damage and not eliminated by dorsal root section. Spastic dystonia is sensitive to stretch, and prolonged stretching can reduce it.

Paratonia

Paratonia, first described by Friedlander in 1828, and later by Dupre in 1910, is described as increased muscle tone in response to passive movement, proportional to the strength of the stimulus applied. The degree of resistance depends upon the speed of movement. It can be faciliatory in the early stages, where the patient actively assists passive movements and becomes oppositional with advancing pathology when the resistance increases with increasing movements. Paratonia is non-velocity dependent and the absence of a catch and the fact that paratonia can be elicited in any direction of movement differentiates it from spasticity.[12,6]

Flexor and Extensor Spasms

Spasms are sudden involuntary movements that often involve multiple muscle groups and joints. They can be repetitive and sustained. These represent an exaggerated reflex withdrawal response to nociceptive stimuli and are mediated by polysynaptic intersegmental spinal cord circuits.[4]

Flexor spasm is a flexor withdrawal reflex that results in flexor muscle contraction when there is activation of the polysynaptic flexor reflex afferents, exciting the flexor and inhibiting extensor motor neurons. The flexor reflex afferents are sensory afferents that convey touch, temperature, pressure, nociceptors, secondary endings, and free nerve endings. Clinically, flexor reflex examples range from Babinski toe response to mass flexor reflex characterized by intense interjoint flexion spread to the abdominals.[9,10]

Extensor spasm is an extensor reflex that is both polysynaptic and interjoint in nature. It can be stimulated by sensory dermatomal stimulation of the groin, buttock, and posterior leg as well as proprioceptive input from the hip.

Both flexor and extensor spasms maybe core substrate for more complex coordinated patterns such as locomotor stepping generators. Both are seen particularly after spinal cord lesions. Excessive flexor withdrawal on ground can lead to impaired stance phase, while excessive flexion during swing phase can mimic steppage and impair advancement or subsequent foot placement. However, extensor posture can sometimes offer a functional advantage in the lower limbs for stability in weightbearing.[9,10]

Associated Reactions

Associated reactions happen when there is a release of postural reactions deprived of voluntary control leading to synkinesis, thus also known as synkinesia. It is an involuntary activity in one limb that is associated with a voluntary movement effort made by the other limb. Flexion of the arm when walking and when yawning and sneezing are associated reactions that can occur due to the disinhibited distribution of voluntary motor activity into the affected limb. It is suggested that unaffected bulbospinal motor pathways may have taken over the role of damage UMN tracts during the transmission of descending voluntary commands.[9,10]

Clasp-Knife Phenomenon

Clasp-knife phenomenon is the description of the sudden release of resistance that happens while passively stretching a muscle. During initial movement, the tone is high due to overactive stretch; thus, there is increase resistance that is felt on passive stretching. On sustained movement with continued stretching, the inverse stretch reflex kicks in, and a sudden release of resistance occurs, relaxing the muscles with a "give away" feel like the resistance of a folding knife blade. In the later stage, as contractures set in, this is replaced by a non-elastic solid resistance.[4,6] It is length dependent. This phenomenon can be seen in spasticity. An example is that of flexion range of motion. Initially, when the knee is bend (quadriceps is short), increased resistance is felt (spasticity is more). However, with continued stretching (quadriceps is lengthening), after reaching a critical length, the resistance suddenly decreases.[6]

Rigidity

Rigidity is not velocity dependent or length dependent. There is resistance to movement in all directions. It equally affects flexors and extensors and gives rise to uniform resistance to passive stretching in all directions known as "lead pipe" phenomenon. Hypertonicity in Parkinson disease (PD) was also noted to be regularly interrupted as a "cogwheel phenomenon" at a 6 to 9 Hz frequency, which is higher than the frequency of rest tremor (4–5 Hz) and postural tremor (5–6 Hz). There can be superimposed tremor, or "an underlying, not yet visible, tremor" results in intermittent increase in tone during the passive movement of a joint and gives rise to "cogwheel" rigidity in PD. Cogwheeling can be present even if there is no overt tremor. Rigidity is one of the cardinal signs of PD. It is present in both the phenotypes of PD ("akinetic-rigid" and "tremor dominant") while more marked in the former phenotype. While appendicular rigidity is generally more than axial rigidity in idiopathic Parkinson disease (IPD), marked axial rigidity indicates atypical parkinsonism like progressive supranuclear palsy (PSP).[6,10]

Gegenhalten

Gegenhalten is also known as counter hold. It is an increase in muscle tone proportional to the force applied. The muscles stiffen in proportion to the force applied when the limb is moved passively. Clinically, it feels that the patient is actively opposing the movement.[4]

Catatonia

Catatonia is a neuropsychiatric syndrome accompanying a wide range of psychiatric, neurologic and medical conditions with motor, behavioral, affective, and autonomic features. The clinical features include abnormal posturing, waxy flexibility, and gegenhalten. In waxy flexibility, patients maintain limbs in positions placed by others for a long time.[4]

DEFINING THE THIRD PHENOMENON

Muscle Contracture

Muscle contracture is one feature of UMN syndrome that leads to disability. A contracture is defined as the loss of full active and passive range of motion in a limb that results from limitations imposed by the joint, muscle, and/or soft tissue. Muscle contracture is the physical shortening of muscle length and is accompanied by fixed shortening of other soft tissues such as fascia, nerves, blood vessels, and skin. Contractures typically occur due to periarticular connective tissue restriction involving muscles, tendons, ligaments, and joint capsule. These types of contractures are not mutually exclusive and frequently occur together. Contracture can occur due to prolonged immobility of the limb and/or a lack of weightbearing in the lower limbs. Generally, any illness with resulting immobility puts a patient at a high risk of developing contracture. Contracture needs physical and surgical methods to undo.[10]

DEFINING SPASTICITY

Spasticity is a common complication of many neurologic conditions affecting UMN. There is a lack of strict definition and variations in the clinical measurement of spasticity.[13]

In 1972, Burke defined spasticity as increased resistance to passive movement due to a lowered threshold of tonic and phasic stretch reflexes. Symptoms may include hypertonicity (increased muscle tone), clonus (a series of rapid muscle contractions), exaggerated deep tendon reflexes, muscle spasms, scissoring (involuntary crossing of the legs), and fixed joints (contractures). The degree of spasticity varies from mild muscle stiffness to severe, painful, and uncontrollable muscle spasms. Spasticity can interfere with rehabilitation in patients with certain disorders and often interferes with daily activities.[14]

Classification of spasticity into various components are (a) intrinsic tonic spasticity (exaggeration of the tonic component of the stretch reflex, manifesting as increased tone), (b) intrinsic phasic spasticity (exaggeration of the phasic component of the stretch reflex, manifesting as tendon hyperreflexia and clonus), and (c) extrinsic spasticity (exaggeration of extrinsic flexion or extension spinal reflexes). Stretch-sensitive and non-stretch-sensitive positive features have been described in UMN. Spasticity is a condition in which stretch reflexes that are normally latent become obvious. The tendon reflexes have a lowered threshold to tap, the response of the tapped muscle is increased, and usually muscles besides the tapped one respond. Tonic stretch reflexes are affected in the same way.[8]

Lance's definition of spasticity identifies that it is one component of the UMN syndrome. This definition makes no mention to how spasticity is conveyed with active movement. It did not account for the stretch of the contracted spastic muscle or the misconduct of a spastic muscle during voluntary contraction of its antagonist. Occasionally, impaired reciprocal inhibition or inappropriate co-contraction can happen, which can be due to abnormal reflex responses and may also be caused by abnormal neural connectivity within the CNS. This means spasticity depends on length of the muscle. Spasticity in the knee extensor (quadriceps) is more when the muscle is short, but in the upper limb flexors (biceps) and ankle extensors (gastrocnemius, soleus), spasticity is more when the muscles are long. Lance's definition also disregards the role of sensory input (discussed later) in spasticity.[2,3] In 2005, the Support Program for Assembly of a Database for Spasticity Measurement (SPASM) proposed that the term spasticity should be used to describe the entire range of signs and symptoms collectively described as the positive features of the UMN syndrome and that tests used to measure individual aspects of spasticity should be validated. The SPASM project redefined spasticity that focuses on the importance of disordered sensory motor control causing involuntary, inappropriate activity of skeletal muscles.

Spasticity has been defined as: [15]

"Disordered sensorimotor control, resulting, resulting from an upper motor neuron lesion (UMN), presenting as an intermittent or sustained involuntary activations of muscles."

In 2018, a consensus of international spasticity experts was organized by IAB–Interdisciplinary Working Group for Movement Disorders to provide a new definition of spasticity based on its various forms of muscle hyperactivity as described in the current movement disorders terminology.

This new definition supported the use of botulinum toxin (BT) therapy for treatment of spasticity.[16]

> *"Spasticity describes involuntary muscle hyperactivity in the presence of central paresis. The involuntary muscle hyperactivity can consist of various forms of muscle hyperactivity: (i) 'Spasticity Sensu Strictu' triggered by rapid passive joint movements, (ii) 'rigidity' triggered by slow passive joint movements, (iii) 'dystonia' when the involuntary muscle hyperactivity is spontaneous and (iv) 'spasms' triggered by sensory or acoustic stimuli. Complications in the form of pain and contractures may occur."*

The group has also proposed an axis-based approach to spasticity where the severity of the muscle hyperactivity can be described by the Modified Ashworth Scale (MAS), Tardieu Scale, and Frequency of Spasms Score. In axis 1, clinical description includes central paresis, muscle hyperactivity, posture, secondary functional deficits, and complications. In axis 2, etiology of spasticity is classified by underlying pathology. In axis 3, localization involves body part affected by spasticity—arm and leg spasticity, hemispasticity, paraspasticity, and tetraspasticity. Dementia, depression, apraxia, and other additional deficits are included in axis 4.[16]

Spasticity can be classified as "phasic" and "tonic" based on the predominant involvement of either the phasic (dynamic) or tonic (static) components of muscle stretch reflexes. After spinal injury, "phasic" spasticity with brisk stretch reflexes and clonus develops in patients who are ambulatory. However, "tonic" spasticity develops in non-ambulatory patients, demonstrated by passive stretch at ankle and vibratory tonic reflex testing.[16]

The consensus also provided clinicians a documentation sheet to record spasticity according to four different axes, which can be found in the referenced paper.

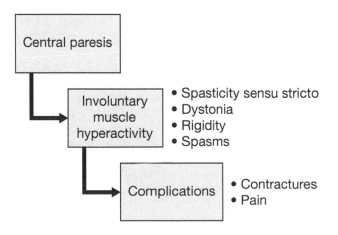

Figure 1.1 New definition of spasticity from IAB consensus.

In 2021, Li, Francisco,[15] and Reymer proposed a new definition of poststroke spasticity. In addition, it was directed that "spasticity manifests only in resting muscles whereas the other related motor impairments arise during activation."

IMPORTANCE OF DEFINING SPASTICITY

The incidence and prevalence of spasticity have different values because of missing proper definition and variations in the clinical measurement of spasticity. Providing an accurate definition can lead to precise epidemiological data.[13] The importance of defining and providing accurate epidemiology of spasticity is due to the third phenomenon of joint contractures and deformities leading to pain and disability that spasticity can cause.

With proper definition such as in the most recent 2018 IAB consensus definition, it allows clinicians to assess components that respond to treatment with BT or not. The documentation into axes provides information for planning treatment with BT or not, with appropriate dosing, and provides goals of treatment. Rigidity, dystonia, spasms, and associated pain can respond to BT therapy. Spasticity sensu stricto may be targeted but can be low in functional significance. BT therapy may not produce relevant functional improvement. Although in some central paresis, if mild, dose adjustments should be made, contractures do not improve with BT therapy as they are based on mechanical alterations unresponsive to BT's paretic effects. However, as contractures are often difficult to distinguish from spastic muscle hyperactivity, probatory BT applications seem justified. Early BT therapy may prevent the formation of contractures. Focusing on treating functional deficits and preventing complications can assist in decision-making of maximal dose usage. Internationally, spasticity due to stroke is usually the only registered indication for use of BT. With this consensus, patients with spasticity due to other CNS diseases may benefit from BT treatment.[16]

REFERENCES

1. Thilmann AF, eds. *Spasticity: Mechanisms and Management, Spasticity: History, Definitions, and Usage of the Term.* Springer-Verlag Berlin' Heidelberg; 1993:1–5 https://doi.org/10.1007/978-3-642-78367-8_1

2. Lance JW. Symposium synopsis. In: Feldman RG, fckLRYoung RR, Koella WP, eds. *Spasticity: Disordered Motor Control.* Chicago, IL; 1980:485–494.

3. Lance JW. The control of muscle tone, reflexes, and movement: Robert Wartenberg Lecture. *Neurology.* 1980;30(12):1303–1313. https://doi.org/10.1212/wnl.30.12.1303

4. Kheder A, Nair KPS. Spasticity: pathophysiology, evaluation and management. *Pract Neurol.* 2012;12(5):289–298. http://doi.org/10.1136/practneurol-2011-000155

5. Ganguly J, Kulshreshtha D, Almotiri M, Jog M. Muscle tone physiology and abnormalities. *Toxins.* 2021;13(4):282. https://doi.org/10.3390/toxins13040282

6. Pandyan AD, Gregoric M, Barnes MP, et al. Spasticity: clinical perceptions, neurological realities and meaningful measurement. *Disabil Rehabil.* 2005;27(1-2):2–6. https://doi.org/10.1080/09638280400014576

7. Barnes MP. An overview of the clinical management of spasticity. In: Barnes MP, Johnson GR, eds. *Upper Neurone Syndrome and Spasticity: Clinical Management and Neurophysiology*. 2nd ed. Cambridge: Cambridge University Press; 2008:1–8.

8. Mayer NH, Esquanazi, A. Muscle overactivity and movement dysfunction in the upper motoneuron syndrome. *Phys Mede Rehabil Clin N Am*. 2003;14(4):855–883. https://doi.org/10.1016/S1047-9651(03)00093 7

9. Segal M. Muscle overactivity in the upper motor neuron syndrome: pathophysiology. *Phys Med Rehabil Clin N Am*. 2018;29(3):427–436. https://doi.org/10.1016/j.pmr.2018.04.005

10. Mayer NH. *Spasticity: Diagnosis and Management*, Brashear and Elovic, ed., 2011, – spasticity and other signs of the upper motor neuron syndrome.

11. Albanese A, Bhatia K, Bressman SB, et al. Phenomenology and classification of dystonia: a consensus update. *Mov Disord*. 2013;28(7):863–873. http://doi.org/10.1002/mds.25475

12. Burridge JH, Wood DE, Hermens HJ, et al. Theoretical and methodological considerations in the measurement of spasticity, *Disabil Rehabil*. 2005;27:(1-2):69–80. https://doi.org/10.1080/09638280400014592

13. Francisco GE, Li S. *Braddom's Physical Medicine and Rehabilitation, 6th edition — Spasticity*. Elsevier, Inc; 2020:447–448.

14. Burke D, Ashby P. Are spinal 'presynaptic' inhibitory mechanisms suppressed in spasticity? *J Neurol Sci*. 1972;15(3):321–326. http://doi.org/10.1016/0022-510x(72)90073-1

15. Li S, Francisco GE, Rymer WZ. A new definition of poststroke spasticity and the interference of spasticity with motor recovery from acute to chronic stages. *Neurorehabil Neural Repair*. 2021;35(7):601–610. http://doi.org/10.1177/15459683211011214. Epub 2021 May 12. PMID: 33978513

16. Dressler D, Bhidayasiri R, Bohlega S, et al. Defining spasticity: a new approach considering current movement disorders terminology and botulinum toxin therapy. *J Neurol*. 2018;265(4):856–862. https://doi.org/10.1007/s00415-018-8759-1

2 Epidemiology of Spasticity

Tulsi Shah, Brian J. Nagle, and Laxman Bahroo

INTRODUCTION

In this chapter, we discuss the prevalence of spasticity across various disease states ranging from stroke to multiple sclerosis (MS), traumatic brain injury (TBI), spinal cord injury (SCI), and cerebral palsy (CP). Each disease state impacts a different population and a specific part of the central nervous system and results in a different pattern of spasticity involving the upper or lower limb such as monoplegia, diplegia, hemiplegia, or quadriplegia (Table 2.1). Furthermore, each disease state results in a unique set of challenges for the patients and caregivers. This chapter discusses the impact of spasticity including disability, patient's quality of life (QOL), and caregiver burden.

Table 2.1 Causes of Spasticity
Stroke
Multiple sclerosis
Traumatic brain injury
Spinal cord injury
Cerebral palsy

STROKE

Spasticity is commonly seen after upper motor neuron lesions, and one of its most common causes is stroke. Each year, approximately 795,000 patients in the United States have a new or recurrent stroke.[1] A stroke is due to the decrease or loss of blood supply to a part of the brain that causes a decrease in oxygen delivery and thus an insult or injury to the brain called infarction. Spasticity can occur with any damage along the pyramidal tract or extrapyramidal fibers and, as a result, can lead to hypertonia.

Spasticity is more common in flexor muscles of the upper extremities with the common pattern of adduction and internal rotation in the shoulder; flexion of the elbow, wrist; and fingers; and pronation in the forearm. In the lower extremities, spasticity is more commonly found in extensor muscles with a typical pattern of adduction in the hip, extension of the hip and knee, and plantar flexion and inward rotation of the foot. Based on many studies, spasticity is more frequently observed in the upper extremities than the lower extremities. Based on the review article by Kuo et al., studies have found that greater severity of paresis, hemi-hyperesthesia, and

13

low Barthel Index score at baseline, which assesses activities of daily living (ADLs) and functional independence in patients with stroke, were all predictors of poststroke spasticity. However, there are no studies that have consistently found that insult in a specific neuroanatomical location in the cerebrum leads to spasticity, and thus more data and larger studies are needed to further characterize if there is an association between the location of the lesion in the brain and poststroke spasticity.[2]

The prevalence of spasticity in stroke survivors ranges from 30% to 80%.[2] Data suggests that poststroke spasticity may occur as early as 3 days after a stroke. Sunnerhagen et al. reviewed seven different studies that collected data on onset and time course of spasticity after a stroke. These studies used the Modified Ashworth Scale (MAS), which is described elsewhere. The results of these studies varied widely. Opheim et al. reviewed data from patients with a first-ever stroke. From 117 patients with impaired arm function, 25% had spasticity in at least one muscle group at day 3, 44% after 4 weeks, 38% at 3 months, and 46% after 12 months. Lundstrom et al. showed that out of 49 patients, 4% had spasticity (MAS score 1) 2–10 days poststroke, 27% at 1 month, and 23% at 6 months. Wisset et al. found spasticity in 25% of their 94 participants 2 weeks after stroke. Although all of these results do vary, this data suggests that poststroke spasticity may occur as early as 3 days after stroke, and at the very least, most patients show evidence of spasticity within the first month after stroke. Based on other studies reviewed by Sunnerhagen et al., spasticity typically remains during the first 3 to 6 months, and typically even 1 year, after stroke. There is not much data that studies the presence of spasticity >12 months after stroke; however, a study by Welmer et al. showed that from 66 patients, 20% had spasticity 18 months after stroke. Though it is assumed that most patients experience reflex-mediated spasticity, some may also experience spasticity due to intrinsic changes in muscle fibers, as evidenced by this study showing that there were four patients who developed spasticity for the first time at their 18-month follow-up.[3] Studies show that the number of patients with severe spasticity seems to increase during

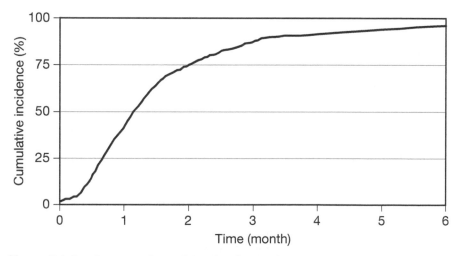

Figure 2.1 Development of spasticity after first stroke.

Source: Nam KE, Lim SH, Kim JS, et al. When does spasticity in the upper limb develop after a first stroke? A nationwide observational study on 861 stroke patients. *J Clin Neurosci.* 2019;66:144-148. https://doi.org/10.1016/j.jocn.2019.04.034.

the first year, with the peak prevalence at 4 weeks after stroke.[4] The review by Kuo et al. suggests that the neuronal components of spasticity peak at 3 months, but the muscular components of spasticity continue to increase with time (Figure 2.1).[2,5]

Symptoms associated with spasticity following stroke include pain, joint contractures, and joint stiffness. A study by Wissel et al. showed that 72% of patients with spasticity experience pain.[2] The severity and progression of spasticity-associated pain may be reduced with early intervention and preventive measures in patients after stroke.[6] Early recognition and management of poststroke spasticity is essential to increase the potential success of rehabilitation and improve QOL. In the long term, spasticity can result in urinary incontinence, limit mobility, and thus affect walking, sitting, and standing, ultimately making it difficult for patients to independently perform ADLs. This in turn can result in increased risk of falls, high caregiver burnout, and eventually patient disability.[2] Based on a 2009 survey, 89% of participants reported total or partial inability to work as a result of their spasticity.[6] A study by Doan et al. demonstrated that higher levels of disability are significantly associated with a decrease in health-related QOL as well as an increase in caregiver burden. This was measured by using the Disability Assessment Scale to measure the patient's disability at baseline (measured by the four domains of hygiene, dressing, limb posture, and pain). The key outcome of health-related QOL was measured by the EQ-5D questionnaire (measures five health status dimensions – mobility, self-care, usual activities, pain and/or discomfort, and anxiety and/or depression) and the SA-SIP30 (questions about eight different domains – body care and movement, mobility, household management, ambulation, social interaction, communication, emotional behavior, and alertness).[3] Early management of poststroke spasticity is important to reduce long-term complications of spasticity and overall improve the function and independence of patients.

MULTIPLE SCLEROSIS

MS is an immune-mediated demyelinating disease of the central nervous system in which destruction of myelin results in a disruption of communication along the central white matter tracts, resulting in nonspecific symptoms such as weakness, numbness, tingling, cognitive changes, and fatigue. A landmark study from 2019 estimated the prevalence of MS in the United States in 2017 to be 913,925.[7] Spasticity is one of the most common symptoms of MS, ranging from 40% to 84%, with its severity often increasing with time and progression of the disease. This can result in stiffness, pain, limited range of motion and mobility, difficulty with personal hygiene, and impairment of QOL.[8,9]

Based on data collected from a registry of 20,969 patients, 16% had no spasticity, 19% mild, 17% moderate (frequently affecting activities), 13% severe (daily activities requiring modification), and 4% total (preventing daily activities). This data also showed that spasticity in patients with multiple sclerosis was more prevalent in patients who were male, disabled, and unemployed, had longer duration of the disease, and had more relapses in the months leading up to the survey.[10]

The most common spasticity patterns in MS are flexor and extensor patterns, with the lower extremities often affected more than the upper extremities or trunk. With flexor spasticity, patients may have involuntary flexion of the hips or knees toward the chest. This usually involves the hamstring muscles. With extensor spasticity, patients may have involuntary extension of the hips and knees with the legs very close together or crossed over at the ankles. This usually involves the quadriceps and adductors of the legs. In patients that experience spasticity in the upper extremities, this can make it difficult to perform ADLs and thus impede QOL.[11]

Several studies have analyzed data on the effects of spasticity in patients with MS and how this translates to their QOL. One such study from Germany, the MOVE 1 study, aimed to collect data to determine the impact of spasticity on QOL and ADLs, in addition to a variety of other factors. From the 414 patients studied, 68.6% had persistent tonic spasticity, 25.8% paroxysmal phasic spasticity, and 5.6% with both types. The symptoms that patients found more disturbing were muscle stiffness (77.4%) and restricted mobility (68.8%), followed by fatigue (50%) and pain (46.2%). This study also found that disability worsened as spasticity worsened. Additionally, 61.1% of patients with severe spasticity reported that spasticity impaired activities daily compared to 16.4% with mild spasticity.[8]

Another study done in the United Kingdom aimed to look at similar measures of QOL in patients with MS-related spasticity. This study used the Leeds Multiple Sclerosis Quality of Life (LMSQOL), an 8-item questionnaire created specifically to measure overall QOL in MS. Approximately 85% of the 701 participants reported some degree of spasticity. The results showed that increasing severity of spasticity is associated with worsening QOL in terms of employment, anxiety, depression, self-esteem, relationships, pain, fatigue, activity limitations, and difficulty with their bladder in addition to other variables such as fatigue, anxiety, and activity limitations.[9]

The CANDLE study in Spain involved 409 participants across 53 neurology clinics. A reduction in QOL was reported on all domains of the SF-12 questionnaire (general health, physical function, role-physical, bodily pain, social function, mental health, role-emotional, vitality, physical component summary, and mental component summary). Spasticity played a greater role in the physical aspect than the mental aspect of QOL.[12]

All of these studies aimed to determine the impact of MS-related spasticity on QOL, and although all of them used different measures to determine if there is a direct role, they all concluded that the greater the spasticity, the worse the QOL. It is vital that physicians recognize the role spasticity has in this population and how it impacts their daily living when proposing management options for treating spasticity.

TRAUMATIC BRAIN INJURY

Traumatic brain injury (TBI) is a broad term used to describe various mechanical cranial injuries, including those involving hemorrhage of varying degrees (i.e., cerebral contusion, subarachnoid hemorrhage, subdural hemorrhage, and epidural hemorrhage), skull fractures, diffuse axonal injury (DAI), cerebral edema, or a combination of these. TBI can be classified in three ways: clinical, radiographic, and mechanistic. Clinical classification divides TBI into three categories based on Glasgow Coma Scale (GCS): mild (GCS 13–15), moderate (GCS 9–12), and severe (GCS ≤8). Radiographic classification is based on description of the findings on imaging (e.g., degree of midline shift). Finally, mechanistic classification separates TBI into categories such as closed head injury, penetrating head trauma, crash or vehicular injury, and blast injury. At a cellular level, damage occurs twofold. The initial impact causes primary injury to the cells, whether this is due to shear forces as in DAI or hemorrhage. Each type of primary pathologic injury can then start a cascade of biochemical effects that lead to various types of secondary injury with the predominant secondary injuries depending on the type of primary insult. Secondary injury can result from oxidative stress and formation of free radicals, calcium-mediated cell damage, inflammation, and increased apoptosis.[13] While the primary and secondary injuries can be severe and lead to death, they also contribute to long-term sequelae, such as spasticity.

Globally, TBI is a leading cause of disability with a worldwide incidence of 369 per 100,000 individuals per year and prevalence of 759 per 100,000 per year.[14] This incidence is an increase from 2005 when incidence was 200 per 100,000 individuals per year, though there was evidence suggesting this was an underestimation given the paucity of data, particularly in developing regions.[15] Data from the Global Burden of Diseases, Injuries, and Risk Factors (GBD) 2016 TBI and SCI Collaborators show an increase in both incidence (3.6%) and prevalence (8.4%) in TBI from 1990 to 2016.[15] However, it appears these increases varied based on sociodemographic index (SDI) with changes in incidence of −9.4% and −10.7% in high and high-middle SDI countries, respectively, compared to 21.8%, 11.1%, and −9.3% in middle, low-middle, and low SDI countries, respectively. Prevalence data followed a similar trend with percentage change of −7.9% and −5.4% in high and high-middle SDI countries, compared to 32.4%, 18.7%, and 3.3% in middle, low-middle, and low SDI countries, respectively.[16] In Europe, a review of descriptive studies of TBI incidence, mortality, or case fatality showed a similar trend among studies with data representing 23 European countries ranging collectively from 1972 to 2012, though with a high degree of variability between studies without standardization of data.[17] The most common mechanisms of these injuries are falls and motor vehicle road accidents.[17,18]

While data suggest higher case-fatality rate in TBI,[18] it is still a major contributor to disability with years of life lived with disability (YLD) increasing 8.5% globally between 1990 and 2016, representing 8.1 million YLD in 2016.[16] Spasticity is one potential sequela that can contribute to disability, through limitation of movement or pain, though data pertaining to spasticity following TBI are sparse and rely on inferences from other mechanisms of injury. A review by Sunnerhagen et al. (2019) found no studies pertaining to predicting spasticity onset and development following TBI up to 12 months after insult and concluded that findings from the seven studies reviewed pertaining to spasticity development following stroke could be applied to TBI, "because the neurobiological background for development of spasticity after a brain injury is similar whether caused by stroke or trauma."[19] However, given the different mechanisms leading to varying primary and subsequent secondary injuries, there may be pathogenic differences between TBI and stroke, and even between different mechanisms of TBI, with regard to the development of spasticity, warranting further research in this area. A small 12-month prospective study by Singer et al. (2004) examined incidence of ankle contracture following moderate to severe TBI (GCS 12 or less on presentation) and demonstrated that plantar flexor and invertor muscle tone was predominantly spastic in 13.3% of individuals, compared to 21.9% with predominantly dystonic tone and 64.7% with normal tone. Over the 12-month study period, no patients with spasticity or normal tone went on to develop ankle contractures, while 74% of those with predominantly dystonic tone developed ankle contracture in the first 16 weeks.[20] Given the lack of epidemiological data pertaining to development of spasticity after TBI, this is an area of study that should be investigated further to better understand the relationship between TBI and spasticity.

SPINAL CORD INJURY

Spinal cord injury (SCI) is a nonspecific term used to describe various mechanical spinal cord injuries. While several classification systems exist, such as describing the mode of primary injury (flexion, extension, axial load, penetrating injuries), the primary injury is always a result of the mechanical force causing persistent or transient cord compression, laceration or transection of the cord, and fractures or displacement of the vertebrae. Like TBI, primary injury of SCI leads to a cascade of secondary injury, which has downstream effects at the cellular and systemic levels. While acute intervention often cannot change the primary insult, therapeutic interventions in the acute period are aimed at preventing further injury from secondary injuries, such as hypoxia, hypoperfusion, disruption of the blood–spinal cord barrier, hemorrhages and thromboses, excitotoxicity, free radicals, calcium-mediated cell damage, and apoptosis. Edema is another secondary injury that tends to peak 3 to 6 days after injury with slow resolution over weeks, at which time further injury persists in the form of inflammation-mediated neurodegeneration. Injury is also frequently classified clinically based on the degree and distribution of weakness into incomplete quadriplegia (accounting for 45% of cases), incomplete paraplegia (22%), complete paraplegia (20%), and complete quadriplegia (13%).[21] Worldwide falls are the most common mode of injury and account for more than 50% of age-standardized incidence in nine GBD-defined regions, followed by road-related injuries.[16] The one region where this did not hold true was in the North Africa and Middle East region, where the most common cause of SCI was conflict and terrorism in 2016.[16] In the United States, motor vehicle accidents are the most common cause of SCI, accounting for 38% of cases, followed by falls (31%), acts of violence (14%), and sports or recreation (9%).[21]

SCI remains a leading cause of disability worldwide with an annual global age-standardized incidence of 13 per 100,000 and prevalence of 368 per 100,000 in 2016. Data from GBD 2016 TBI and SCI Collaborators show no significant overall change globally in incidence (−3.6%) and prevalence (−0.2%) in SCI from 1990 to 2016.[16] However, when comparing countries of different SDI, more significant increases can be seen in middle and low-middle SDI countries in incidence (5.8% and 17.9%, respectively) and prevalence (25.6% and 22.6%, respectively).[16] Despite this, incidence rates remain highest in the high SDI regions of high-income North America and Western Europe (both 26 per 100,000 individuals in 2016), though country-level data demonstrates age-standardized incidence rates in 2016 were highest in Syria (136 per 100,000), followed by Yemen (42 per 100,000) and Afghanistan (37 per 100,000).[16]

Despite a global 10% decrease in YLD between 1990 and 2016 due to SCI, it remains a major cause of disability with 9.5 million YLD globally in 2016.[16] It has been suggested that stratification of the GBD 2016 data further into severity of SCI would better help to delineate this burden of disability.[18] In one study, 65% of patients with SCI were unemployed.[22] Pain and spasticity contribute greatly to disability in people with SCI. Pain has been found to prevent some from returning to work more than even loss of motor function.[23] While reports of pain in SCI are variable, it is likely prevalent in about 66% of patients, 30% of which report severe pain, though no clear predictors of pain have been identified.[23] This may be due in part to lack of a universal classification system for pain in SCI, though some have suggested a model that separates SCI pain into (a) nociceptive pain further divided into musculoskeletal and visceral and (b) neuropathic pain divided into pain above the level, at the level, or below the level of injury.[23] Similarly, spasticity has also been found to be prevalent in 65% to 78% of people at least 1 year from SCI with no association between presence of spasticity and time since primary injury.[24] A cross-sectional survey of patients with SCI in Denmark by Andresen et al. (2016) examined both pain and spasticity in patients with SCI. The sample was predominantly men (77%), mean age of 54.6 ± 14.6 years, and mean time since injury of 18.2 ± 12.8 years. Seventy-three percent of the sample reported continuous or daily recurring pain and 71% reported symptoms of spasticity with 67% and 46% receiving treatment for their pain and spasticity, respectively. Symptoms of neuropathic pain were identified in 60% of those reporting pain, making up 43.6% of the total study sample, and found to have significantly higher rating of their pain compared to those without neuropathic-type pain.[22]

With prevalence of spasticity and pain in SCI so high, it is no wonder that QOL can be greatly affected. One study sample reported "at least moderate influence on their daily life" in 77% of surveyed patients with SCI.[22] Limitations in movement, whether due to weakness or spasticity, affect QOL by making it difficult for one to carry out their ADLs to include ambulation and self-care, leading to increased risk of decubitus ulcers, infections, and inability to participate in rehabilitation. Pain cannot only affect QOL directly, but indirectly through affecting sleep, leading to fatigue. These complications when present also affect the patient's safety as well as increase caregiver needs, which further affects QOL.[24] In a study by Andresen et al., patient's reporting pain were significantly more likely to report SCI impacting their daily life more than those not in pain, and were also found to be significantly older, female, and unemployed and have a greater degree of sleep disturbance. Those suffering from neuropathic pain symptoms not only had significantly lower QOL scores compared to those not in pain but also had lower physical and mental health scores compared to those with non-neuropathic pain. Spasticity was also associated more often with tetraplegia as well as greater impact on daily life, higher unemployment, sleep disturbance, and low satisfaction with physical health compared to those without spasticity. Finally, there was an association between pain and spasticity symptoms in that those with neuropathic pain reported higher frequency of spasms and those with any type of pain reported higher muscle stiffness scores. Other factors identified to affect QOL were females associated with lower mental health scores, QOL scores significantly lower in those reporting high pain interference and shorter time since injury, and lower physical health scores associated with tetraplegia.[22] Of note, there are features of spasticity that may contribute to prevention of further decline in QOL that may be overlooked, including increased muscle bulk and strength to aid in stability while sitting and standing, during transfers, and during performance of some ADLs, as well as preventing osteopenia and increasing venous return, which may hypothetically lower risk of deep venous thrombosis formation.[24]

CEREBRAL PALSY

CP is a permanent congenital movement disorder due to abnormal brain development, often before birth. This typically leads to different motor impairments in childhood affecting posture and motor function, and very commonly, patients are affected by spasticity. One in 500 children suffer from CP. A European network classified CP into four main subtypes: unilateral spastic, bilateral spastic, dyskinetic, and ataxic.[25]

Since many children in the United States obtain healthcare coverage through Medicaid, one study collected data from this specific population of 3,294 children between the ages of 2 and 20 years with CP. Within this group, 69.8% had spasticity, as indicated by coding, suggesting this is likely an underestimation. From the total population, 69.5% of children had further classification of their CP – from these, 20.8% had hemiplegia, 15.6% had diplegia, 32.9% had quadriplegia, and 0.1% had monoplegia.[26] Other papers suggest that the prevalence of spasticity in CP is as much as 90%.[27]

CAREGIVER BURDEN IN PATIENTS WITH SPASTICITY

Reduced QOL for patients with spasticity, regardless of their underlying neurologic disease, has been highlighted several times throughout this chapter. The causes of spasticity discussed earlier can also have a significant economic effect, for instance, expenses related to spinal cord injuries can exceed $1 million in the first year, and lifetime expenses can be upward of $4.5 million.[13] What is often overlooked are the indirect and nonpecuniary costs, such as the increased caregiver burden associated with taking care of such patient populations. One study surveyed 615 participants, of which 427 were patients and 188 were caregivers, receiving botulinum toxin type A injections for treatment for at least 1 year. The study used an internet-based survey with questions regarding the impact of spasticity on patients' ability to work and function, ADLs, QOL, and the impact of botulinum toxin therapy on patients' lives. The caregivers were most often parents (40%) or another family member (27%). The study found that spasticity clearly impacted both patients and caregivers, notably with the ability to work and the cost of the injections. Twenty-nine percent of caregivers reported that being in their role impacted their own professional status with 21% reporting they had to work part-time and 8% not working due to their responsibility as a caregiver. Of note, all respondents of the survey (both patients and caregivers) noted that botulinum toxin treatment improved their lives.[27]

KEY POINTS

- Spasticity is seen early in patients with stroke.
- Severity of spasticity impacts the QOL of patients and caregivers.
- While studies are limited, spasticity is underestimated across the globe.
- Individuals with greater amounts of spasticity or spasticity involving multiple limbs needed more assistance with ADLs and spasticity had higher impact on physical, mental and social needs.

REFERENCES

1. Centers for Disease Control and Prevention. *Stroke Facts*. CDC. Published May 25, 2021. https://www.cdc.gov/stroke/facts.htm
2. Kuo CL, Hu GC. Post-stroke spasticity: a review of epidemiology, pathophysiology, and treatments. *Int J Gerontol*. 2018;12(4):280–284. https://doi.org/10.1016/j.ijge.2018.05.005

3. Doan QV, Brashear A, Gillard PJ, et al. Relationship between disability and health-related quality of life and caregiver burden in patients with upper limb poststroke spasticity. *PM&R*. 2011;4(1):4–10. https://doi.org/10.1016/j.pmrj.2011.10.001

4. Sunnerhagen KS, Opheim A, Alt Murphy M. Onset, time course and prediction of spasticity after stroke or traumatic brain injury. *Ann Phys Rehabil Med*. 62(6):431–434. Published online May 2018. https://doi.org/10.1016/j.rehab.2018.04.004

5. Nam KE, Lim SH, Kim JS, et al. When does spasticity in the upper limb develop after a first stroke? A nationwide observational study on 861 stroke patients. *J Clin Neurosci*. 2019;66:144–148. https://doi.org/10.1016/j.jocn.2019.04.034

6. Ward AB. A literature review of the pathophysiology and onset of post-stroke spasticity. *Eur J Neurol*. 2011;19(1):21–27. https://doi.org/10.1111/j.1468-1331.2011 .03448.x

7. Wallin MT, Culpepper WJ, Campbell JD, et al. The prevalence of MS in the United States. *Neurology*. 2019;92(10):e1029–e1040. https://doi.org/10.1212/wnl.0000000000007035

8. Flachenecker P, Henze T, Zettl UK. Spasticity in patients with multiple sclerosis--clinical characteristics, treatment and quality of life. *Acta Neurol Scand*. 2014;129(3):154–162. https://doi.org/10.1111/ane.12202

9. Milinis K, Tennant A, Young CA. Spasticity in multiple sclerosis: associations with impairments and overall quality of life. *Mult Scler*. 2016;5:34–39. https://doi.org/10.1016/j.msard.2015.10.007

10. Rizzo MA, Hadjimichael OC, Preiningerova J, Vollmer TL. Prevalence and treatment of spasticity reported by multiple sclerosis patients. *Mult Scler J*. 2004;10(5):589–595. https://doi.org/10.1191/1352458504ms1085oa

11. *Managing Spasticity in MS*. 2022. https://www.nationalmssociety.org/ NationalMSSociety/media/MSNationalFiles/Brochures/Brochure-Managing-Spasticity-in-MS.pdf

12. Arroyo R, Massana M, Vila C. Correlation between spasticity and quality of life in patients with multiple sclerosis: the CANDLE study. *Int JNeurosci*. 2013;123(12): 850–858. https://doi.org/10.3109/00207454.2013.812084

13. Robinson CP. Moderate and severe traumatic brain injury. *CONTIN. Lifelong Learn. Neurol*. 2021;27(5):1278. https://doi.org/10.1212/CON.0000000000001036

14. James SL, Theadom A, Ellenbogen RG, et al. Global, regional, and national burden of traumatic brain injury and spinal cord injury, 1990–2016: a systematic analysis for the Global Burden of Disease Study 2016. *The Lancet Neurol*. 2019;18(1):56–87. https://doi.org/10.1016/s1474-4422(18)30415-0

15. Burke D, Wissel J, Donnan GA. Pathophysiology of spasticity in stroke. *Neurology*. 2013;80(3, Supplement 2):S20–S26. https://doi.org/10.1212/wnl.0b013e31827624a7

16. Bryan-Hancock C, Harrison J. The global burden of traumatic brain injury: preliminary results from the Global Burden of Disease Project. *Inj Prev*. 2010;16(Supplement 1):A17–A17. https://doi.org/10.1136/ip.2010.029215.61

17. Brazinova A, Rehorcikova V, Taylor MS, et al. Epidemiology of traumatic brain injury in Europe: a living systematic review. *J Neurotrauma*. 2018;38(10):1411–1440. https://doi.org/10.1089/neu.2015.4126

18. Badhiwala JH, Wilson JR, Fehlings MG. Global burden of traumatic brain and spinal cord injury. *Lancet Neuro*. 2019;18(1):24–25. https://doi.org/10.1016/ s1474-4422(18)30444-7

19. Sunnerhagen KS, Opheim A, Alt Murphy M. Onset, time course and prediction of spasticity after stroke or traumatic brain injury. *Ann Phys and Rehabil Med*. 2018;62(6): 431–434. https://doi.org/10.1016/j.rehab.2018.04.004

20. Singer BJ, Jegasothy GM, Singer KP, Allison GT, Dunne JW. Incidence of ankle contracture after moderate to severe acquired brain injury. *Arch Phys Med Rehabil.* 2004;85(9):1465–1469. https://doi.org/10.1016/j.apmr.2003.08.103

21. Rabinstein AA. Traumatic spinal cord injury. *CONTIN. Lifelong Learn. Neurol.* 2018;24(2):551–566. https://doi.org/10.1212/con.0000000000000581

22. Andresen SR, Biering-Sørensen F, Hagen EM, Nielsen JF, Bach FW, Finnerup NB. Pain, spasticity and quality of life in individuals with traumatic spinal cord injury in Denmark. *Spinal Cord.* 2016;54(11):973–979. https://doi.org/10.1038/sc.2016.46

23. Burchiel KJ, Hsu FP. Pain and spasticity after spinal cord injury: mechanisms and treatment. *Spine.* 2001;26(24 Suppl):S146–S160. https://doi.org/10.1097/00007632-200112151-00024

24. Adams MM, Hicks AL. Spasticity after spinal cord injury. *Spinal Cord.* 2005;43(10):577–586. https://doi.org/10.1038/sj.sc.3101757

25. Cans C, De-la-Cruz J, Mermet MA. Epidemiology of cerebral palsy. *Paediatr and Child Health.* 2008;18(9):393–398.

26. Pulgar S, Bains S, Gooch J, et al. Prevalence, patterns, and cost of care for children with cerebral palsy enrolled in medicaid managed care. *J Manag Care Spec Pharm.* 2019;25(7):817–822. https://doi.org/10.18553/jmcp.2019.25.7.817

27. Patel AT, Wein T, Bahroo LB, Wilczynski O, Rios CD, Murie-Fernández M. Perspective of an international online patient and caregiver community on the burden of spasticity and impact of botulinum neurotoxin therapy: survey study. *JMIR Public Health and Surveillance.* 2020;6(4):e17928. https://doi.org/10.2196/17928

3 Pathophysiology

Sheng Li and Gerard E. Francisco

INTRODUCTION

Spasticity is commonly viewed as a phenomenon associated with hyperreflexia of stretch reflexes. The etiology of stretch reflex hyperreflexia remains poorly understood. In this chapter, a theoretical framework is described to highlight the pathophysiology of spasticity and its interactions with other motor impairments. Clinical implications of this pathophysiological account are further elaborated.

SPASTICITY AS A MANIFESTATION OF MALADAPTIVE PLASTICITY

From a longitudinal view, recovery of muscle strength and motor function commences almost immediately after the onset of a central nervous lesion, while spasticity emerges with a time delay and evolves over time. For instance, a relatively predictable pattern of recovery is reported after a stroke regardless of type (ischemic or hemorrhagic) or location (cortical or subcortical).[1] Brunnstrom[2,3] empirically described the stereotypical stages of motor recovery from flaccidity to full recovery of motor function. As a stroke survivor recovers from one recovery to the next toward recovery of normal movement in an orderly manner in the course of complete motor recovery, spasticity emerges, evolves, decreases, and eventually disappears. However, spasticity may evolve and persist after its emergence if further recovery is arrested.[1,3] Such observations of emergence, evolvement, and disappearance of spasticity imply that spasticity is a reflection of abnormal plasticity. However, the pattern of motor recovery and emergence and disappearance of spasticity may not be the same in different etiologies of the upper motor neuron (UMN) syndrome. What is commonly seen is the observation of a period of "shock" after the initial injury (traumatic or acquired, brain or spinal), which is followed by a gradual return of reflexes, but not a sudden progression to hyperreflexia. This process occurs usually between 1 to 6 weeks after the initial injury and is regarded as an attempt at restoration of function through emergence of novel neuronal circuitry.[4] Plastic rearrangement occurs within the brain and spinal cord (see reviews).[4-10] This process of plastic rearrangement often results in muscle overactivity and hyperreflexia, and thus spasticity.[11] In a longitudinal study that examined the time course of development of spasticity and contractures at the wrist after 6 weeks of stroke, the authors reported that patients who recovered arm function showed signs of spasticity at all assessment points but did not develop contractures. In contrast, patients who did not recover useful arm function had signs of spasticity and contracture tested over a follow-up course of 36 weeks.[12] In the course of motor recovery, spasticity interacts with and amplifies the effects of other impairments, such as weakness, and impaired coordination, thus contributing to limited mobility and participation.[13] For example, weakness tends to cause immobilization in a shortened muscle length and predisposes to contracture and accumulation of extracellular matrix (ECM) deposits and the development of spasticity in the same muscles. In turn, spasticity worsens contracture and muscle stiffness and triggers a vicious cycle.[5,6,14] These numerous abnormalities and interactions produce a dynamic picture of varying clinical presentations after a UMN lesion.[5,6]

Pathophysiology of Spasticity

Spasticity has been defined as a phenomenon of increased resistance to passive stretch mediated by hyperreflexia of spinal stretch reflexes.[7,15–17] The etiology of spinal stretch reflex hyperreflexia remains poorly understood, although some insights have advanced our understanding of the complexity of spasticity. Current understanding of pathophysiology for poststroke spasticity is summarized here.[5,7–9,18–21] As shown in Figure 3.1, a stroke often leads to damages to motor cortex and its descending corticospinal tract (CST). Muscle weakness (usually unilateral) occurs immediately after CST damages, subsequently leading to incoordination and joint immobilization. Due to its anatomic proximity to CST, corticoreticular pathways are damaged as well, resulting in diminished inputs from the dorsolateral reticulospinal (RS) tracts into the spinal motor network. Since the dorsolateral RS tracts provide inhibitory inputs, its impairment makes the descending excitatory inputs

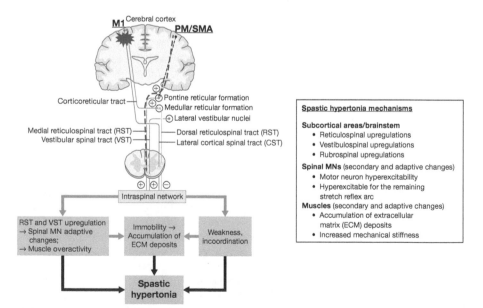

Figure 3.1 Schematic illustration of pathophysiology of spastic hypertonia. See text for details.

unopposed and becomes hyperexcitable over time (Figure 3.1, red dotted line). Such hyperexcitability has been observed in several pathways, including medial RS, vestibulospinal, and rubrospinal tracts.[19,22,23] RS hyperexcitability appears to be the most likely mechanism related to poststroke spasticity. It provides unopposed excitatory descending inputs to spinal stretch reflex circuits, resulting in elevated excitability of spinal motor neurons and spinal reflex circuits.[74] This adaptive change can account for most clinical findings of spasticity, for example, exaggerated stretch reflex, velocity-dependent resistance to stretch, muscle overactivity, or spontaneous firings of motor units. As mentioned above, clinical presentation of spasticity is confounded by concomitant changes in peripheral muscle properties, such as ECM deposition and increased muscle stiffness.[20,25] Taken together, it is thus more appropriate to use "spastic hypertonia" to reflect both reflex and non-reflex-mediated increase in resistance. Three different components have been proposed to account for increased resistance of spastic muscles or spasticity (Figure 3.1). These components are adequately distinguished neither in clinical examinations[26] nor in laboratory settings.[27]

- **Hyperreflexia and reflex stiffness.** It is mediated by hyperexcitability of stretch reflex circuits as a result of unopposed medial RS hyperexcitability.
- **"Active" muscle stiffness (hyaluronan accumulation).** Hyaluronan is the primary component in the ECM and functions to lubricate the muscle fiber gliding system during muscle force transmission.[28] The normal turnover of the ECM decreases after immobilization or paresis, thus increasing its concentration and the molecular weight and macromolecular crowding within and between muscular compartments.[29,30] These changes can increase fluid viscosity[31] and decrease lubrication between muscle fibers and compartments. Such change may be perceived by the stroke survivor as stiffness.[32] Hyaluronidase is an enzyme that hydrolyzes hyaluronan, thus specifically targeting the "active" muscle stiffness component. Raghavan et al.[25] reported that passive resistance was significantly reduced in stroke survivors after hyaluronidase injections.
- **"Passive" muscle stiffness (muscle fiber changes and connective tissue fibrosis).** Due to immobilization, spastic muscle fibers may rest at a shortened length and muscle fibers become more stiff as a result.[33] Furthermore, fibrosis could be developed secondary to the deposition of collagen within and between muscle bundles later on in the chronic phase.[34] These changes increase passive, mechanical stiffness of the muscle.

The above pathophysiology of spastic hypertonia is present after neurologic impairments of different origins. However, clinical characteristics of spasticity vary according to lesion locations. In incomplete spinal cord lesions, both the CST and dorsolateral reticulospinal tract (RST) are often damaged in the dorsolateral cord, while damages to medial pathways (medial RST and vestibulospinal tract (VST)) are less severe. A similar pattern of disinhibition phenomenon is observed, including spasticity, flexor spasms, and hyperreflexia. In complete spinal cord injury (SCI), both excitatory and inhibitory supraspinal descending inputs to spinal interneuronal network are damaged, and thus both stretch reflex and flexor reflex afferents are completely disinhibited. Therefore, a different pattern occurs, including a strong flexor pattern, and paraplegia with predominant flexion features.[9,35]

IMPLICATIONS FOR CLINICAL MANAGEMENT

Advances in understanding the underlying pathophysiology make it easier to understand clinical presentations and to assess spasticity and guide treatment plans. Such clinical presentations are listed in Table 3.1.

Implications for Understanding Clinical Presentations

As illustrated in Figure 3.1, the reflex-mediated presentation of spasticity is mainly attributed to unopposed medial RS hyperexcitability originated from pontine reticular formation as a result of disinhibition. Clinical features of spasticity can be categorized into different groups, based on pathophysiological changes along the neuroaxis from spinal cord to reticular formation and beyond, including (a) altered intraspinal network and hyperexcitable spinal stretch reflex circuits; (b) hyperexcitable RST and diffused, stereotyped activation; and (c) disinhibited reticular formation centers and their interactions with other brainstem centers and cortical areas.

Due to adaptive changes of hyperexcitability of spinal stretch reflex circuits, normal sensory stimuli could trigger exaggerated reflex responses. Such afferent input could be mediated by excitation of velocity-sensitive afferent spindles (group Ia) or muscle length-sensitive afferent fibers (group II) or a combination of two.[36] As such, it is reported that spasticity is both velocity- and muscle length-dependent[16] (Table 3.1A).

Table 3.1 Clinical Features Associated With Spasticity

(A) Associated with hyperexcitable spinal stretch reflex circuits

- Increased resting tone and velocity- and muscle length-dependent resistance
- Exaggerated response to normal stimuli (passive stretch at various speeds) or noxious stimuli (cutaneous and nociceptive)

(B) Associated with diffuse, stereotyped RST activation

- Spastic co-contraction (disordered motor control), e.g., attempt to extend the elbow leads to activation of elbow flexors → co-contraction
- Stereotyped synergy pattern (shoulder adduction, internal rotation, elbow, wrist, and finger flexion)
- Associated reactions (abnormal spread of motor activities)
- Dynamic tone (change with posture)

C) Associated with disinhibited reticular formation occurs and associated interactions with other brainstem centers and cortical areas

- Fluctuating tone (decreased night and during sleep)
- Elevated tone with pain (via connections with reticular formation)
- Elevated tone with emotional changes, such as anxiety and anger (via connections with reticular formation)
- Change with respiratory activities (increased with cough; a flaccid hand opens when a patient with acute stroke yawns)
- Associated with sympathetic symptoms (e.g., CRPS poststroke)
- Associated with other noxious stimuli (e.g., UTI, constipation)

CRPS, complex regional pain syndrome; RST, reticulospinal tract; UTI, urinary tract infection.

Source: Modified from Li S, Francisco GE. New insights into the pathophysiology of poststroke spasticity. *Front Hum Neurosci*. 2015;9:192. https://doi.org.10.3389/fnhum.2015.00192

RS projections are divergent and diffuse to a group of synergistic muscles.[37,38] In the presence of weak CST activation, such RS activation leads to clinical observations of stereotyped synergy pattern, for example, shoulder adduction, internal rotation, and elbow, wrist, and finger flexion; RS also has bilateral projections, although ipsilateral projection is predominant.[37,39] Unilateral voluntary activation on one limb is often accompanied with involuntary activation of spastic muscles on the contralateral side, that is, associated reactions or motor overflow. It is known that changing posture from sitting to standing is associated with activation of RS pathways. This explains why posture-dependent increase in muscle tone is observed, or dynamic tone (Table 3.1B).

The reticular formation has very divergent but well-organized projections to other areas/centers in the brainstem and cortex.[40] Other than motor function and posture, the reticular formation and its projections are involved in the regulation of other basic survival functions, such as breathing, posture, pain, temperature, and mood. RS hyperexcitability could alter interactions among these functions; thus, spasticity is associated with some of these functions. For example, recruitment of both plantar flexor and dorsiflexor muscles was observed in a stroke survivor with spasticity during normal breathing at rest, but with a predominance of plantar flexion during coughing.[5] Similarly, this mechanism could also account for other common clinical observations that spasticity changes with temperature (weather [tighter in winter]), pain, emotion (anxiety, anger), and time (day and night fluctuation). For experienced clinicians, a sudden change in spasticity may result from and is a presenting sign of changes in medical conditions, among which urinary tract infections (UTIs) are commonly observed (Table 3.1C).

Implications for Clinical Assessment

Ashworth Scale and Tardieu Scale and their variations are common clinical scales for spasticity assessment. Passive stretch of a joint is performed in both scales with certain speeds. However, the joint position is not standardized. As discussed in Table 3.1A, spasticity is both velocity- and muscle length-dependent. Change in the initial joint position yields different assessment outcomes (Figure 3.2). Flexor digitorum superficialis (FDS) spasticity changes from 2 on Modified Ashworth Scale (MAS)

FDS: MAS 2   FDS: MAS 0

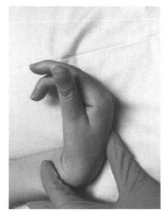

Figure 3.2 Muscle length dependence of finger flexor spasticity.

when the wrist is in the neutral position to 0 when the wrist joint is held in flexion. The muscle length of FDS is shortened when the wrist joint is flexed; thus, FDS has less spasticity. This muscle length (joint position) dependence of spasticity needs to be taken into account in clinical assessment.

The RS hyperexcitability mechanism of spasticity is able to also offer an alternative approach to assess the severity of spasticity. Since RS projections play an important role in maintaining joint position and posture against gravity,[42] its anti-gravitational force effect could lead to a shift in neuromuscular balance favoring anti-gravity muscle groups, for example, upper limb flexors and lower limb extensors. This new balance could be reflected by a change in the resting angle of a joint, that is, the more spastic the muscle is, the more abnormal resting angle the involved joint maintains. The concept of abnormal resting angle is particularly helpful in the clinical assessment of spasticity of small muscles or muscles that are difficult to access (e.g., sternocleidomastoid muscle). The severity of sternocleidomastoid muscle spasticity could be estimated based on abnormality of head posture.

Implications for Spasticity Management

The RS hyperexcitability mechanism of spasticity can also guide pathophysiology-based treatment plans. The monoamines serotonin (5-HT) and norepinephrine (NE) are the primary neurotransmitters that mediate the effects of RS projections. The monoaminergic inputs via unopposed hyperexcitable RST provide powerful neuromodulatory changes of spinal motor neurons, greatly increasing their excitability and facilitating persistent inward currents (PIC).[42-44] The PIC is generated by voltage-activated channels that tend to remain activated, leading to a plateau behavior.[45] PICs are associated with subthreshold depolarization of spinal motor neurons, that is, spinal motor neurons are hyperexcitable, and thus spinal stretch reflexes are hyperactive. Therefore, PICs are possible spinal mechanisms mediating spasticity. Appropriate pharmacologic treatments can be selected or avoided in spasticity management, according to this pathophysiological understanding.[46] For example, serotonergic agents (such as escitalopram) can augment spasticity,[47] while anti-serotonergic agents (cyproheptadine) facilitate relaxation time of spastic muscles.[48] Tizanidine can reduce descending NE drive, thus improving independent joint control in chronic stroke survivors with moderate to severe motor impairments.[49]

As shown in Figure 3.1, paresis (weakness) and spasticity are mediated by different underlying mechanisms. Clinical presentations are a combination of weakness and spasticity. For example, during an attempt to extend fingers in stroke survivors with finger flexor spasticity, their effort results in finger flexion instead, secondary to involuntary activation of spastic finger flexors during such attempt.[50] The inability of voluntary finger extension likely results from (a) weak extensors by diminished voluntary activation secondary to CST damage and (b) co-activation of spastic flexors secondary to hyperexcitable RS activation after loss of inhibition. Understanding of these two separate mechanisms underlying impaired voluntary control of upper limb extensors is critical for management. Essentially, spastic flexors could be "therapeutically weakened" via botulinum toxin injection. As such, residual weak extensors may be able to function adequately, since the primary goal of the extensors is to open the hand or extend the elbow in preparation for functional operation by the flexors in most activities of daily living (ADLs) that do not require significant activation of the extensors.[51] We name it "therapeutic weakness" with the goal of improving motor control of the antagonist. This concept is further supported by another study,[52] where 15 stroke survivors with finger flexor spasticity and residual finger extension received botulinum toxin injection to the finger flexors and electrical stimulation to the finger extensors 4 weeks (5 days per week) after injections. Finger flexor spasticity significantly reduced, and finger extensor strength and active hand function significantly improved 2 and 6 weeks after injections.

It is well documented that botulinum toxin injection effectively reduces spasticity, pain, and positioning, and it unlikely improves active upper extremity function, such as reaching and grasping.[53,54] As discussed previously, better understanding of underlying mechanisms for disordered motor control allows new therapeutic use of botulinum toxin. The finding that "therapeutic weakness" of spastic flexor muscles is associated with functional improvement is important in that it can reshape the goals of using this therapy. In particular, "therapeutic weakness" using botulinum toxins could be considered in stroke survivors who have residual voluntary extension in the upper extremity.

KEY POINTS

- Spasticity is commonly viewed as a phenomenon associated with hyperreflexia of spinal stretch reflexes.
- Spasticity has multidimensional underlying mechanisms, which are not fully understood.
- Hyperexcitability of descending brainstem pathways, especially RS hyperexcitability, is the pathophysiology mediating spasticity.
- Spasticity interacts with other motor impairments and peripheral changes, often presented clinically as spastic hypertonia.
- This theoretical framework helps to better understand clinical features associated with spasticity, assess spasticity, and guide treatment plans.

REFERENCES

1. Twitchell TE. The restoration of motor function following hemiplegia in man. *Brain.* 1951;74(4):443–448. https://doi.org.10.1093/brain/74.4.443
2. Brunnstrom S. Motor testing procedures in hemiplegia: based on sequential recovery stages. *Phys Ther.* 1966;46(4):357–375. https://doi.org.10.1093/ptj/46.4.357
3. Brunnstrom S. *Movement Therapy in Hemiplegia. A Neurophysiological Approach.* New York: Harper & Row; 1970.
4. Balakrishnan S, Ward AB. The diagnosis and management of adults with spasticity. *HandbClinNeurol.*2013;110:145–160.https://doi.org.10.1016/B978-0-444-52901-5.00013-7
5. Gracies JM. Pathophysiology of spastic paresis. II: emergence of muscle overactivity. *Muscle Nerve.* 2005;31(5):552–571. https://doi.org.10.1002/mus.20284
6. Gracies JM. Pathophysiology of spastic paresis. I: paresis and soft tissue changes. *Muscle Nerve.* 2005;31(5):535–551. https://doi.org.10.1002/mus.20284
7. Nielsen JB, Crone C, Hultborn H. The spinal pathophysiology of spasticity - from a basic science point of view. *Acta Physiologica.* 2007;189(2):171–180. https://doi.org.10.1111/j.1748-1716.2006.01652.x

8. Burke D, Wissel J, Donnan GA. Pathophysiology of spasticity in stroke. *Front Neurol.* 2013;80(3 Suppl 2):S20–S26. https://doi.org.10.3389/fnhum.2015.00192

9. Mukherjee A, Chakravarty A. Spasticity mechanisms - for the clinician. *Front Neurol.* 2010;1:149. https://doi.org.10.3389/fneur.2010.00149

10. Nudo RJ. Mechanisms for recovery of motor function following cortical damage. *Curr Opin Neurobiol.* 2006;16(6):638–644. https://doi.org.10.1016/j.conb.2006.10.004

11. Farmer SF, Harrison LM, Ingram DA, Stephens JA. Plasticity of central motor pathways in children with hemiplegic cerebral palsy. *Front Neurol.* 1991;41(9):1505–1510. https://doi.org.10.1212/wnl.41.9.1505

12. Malhotra S, Pandyan AD, Rosewilliam S, Roffe C, Hermens H. Spasticity and contractures at the wrist after stroke: time course of development and their association with functional recovery of the upper limb. *Clin Rehabil.* 2011;25(2):184–191. https://doi.org.10.1177/0269215510381620

13. Mayer NH, Esquenazi A. Muscle overactivity and movement dysfunction in the upper motoneuron syndrome. *Phys Med Rehabil Clin N Am.* 2003;14(4):855–883, vii–viii. https://doi.org.10.1016/s1047-9651(03)00093-7

14. O'Dwyer N, Ada L, Neilson P. Spasticity and muscle contracture following stroke. *Brain.* 1996;119(Pt 5):1737–1749. https://doi.org.10.1093/brain/119.5.

15. Lance JW. Symposium synopsis. In: Feldman RG, Young RR, Koella WP, eds. *Spasticity: Disordered Motor Control.* Chicago: Year Book Medical Publishers; 1980:485–494.

16. Li S, Francisco GE, Rymer WZ. A new definition of poststroke spasticity and the interference of spasticity with motor recovery from acute to chronic stages. *Neurorehabil Neural Repair.* 2021;35(7):601–610. https://doi.org.10.1177/15459683211011214

17. Bose P, Hou J, Thompson FJ. Frontiers in neuroengineering traumatic brain injury (TBI)-induced spasticity: neurobiology, treatment, and rehabilitation. In Kobeissy, F.H., Ed. *Brain Neurotrauma: Molecular, Neuropsychological, and Rehabilitation Aspects.* Boca Raton (FL): CRC Press/Taylor & Francis © 2015 by Taylor & Francis Group, LLC; 2015.

18. Brown P. Pathophysiology of spasticity. *J Neurol Neurosurg Psychiatry.* 1994;57(7):773–777. https://doi.org.10.1046/j.1468-1331.2002.0090s1003.x

19. Li S, Francisco G. New insights into the pathophysiology of post-stroke spasticity. *Front Hum Neurosci.* 2015;9:192. https://doi.org.10.3389/fnhum.2015.00192

20. Stecco A, Stecco C, Raghavan P. Peripheral mechanisms contributing to spasticity and implications for treatment. *Curr Phys Med Rehabil.* 2014;2:121–127. https://doi.org.10.4103/1658-354X.121087

21. Li S. Spasticity, motor recovery, and neural plasticity after stroke. *Frontiers in neurology.* 2017;8:120. https://doi.org.10.3389/fneur.2017.00120

22. Owen M, Ingo C, Dewald JPA. Upper extremity motor impairments and microstructural changes in bulbospinal pathways in chronic hemiparetic stroke. *Front Neurol.* 2017;8:257. https://doi.org.10.3389/fneur.2017.00257

23. Miller DM, Klein CS, Suresh NL, Rymer WZ. Asymmetries in vestibular evoked myogenic potentials in chronic stroke survivors with spastic hypertonia: evidence for a vestibulospinal role. *Clin Neurophysiol.* 2014;125(10):2070–2078. https://doi.org.10.3389/fneur.2017.00257

24. Li S, Francisco GE. New insights into the pathophysiology of post-stroke spasticity. *Front Hum Neurosci.* 2015;9:192. https://doi.org.10.3389/fnhum.2015.00192

25. Raghavan P, Lu Y, Mirchandani M, Stecco A. Human recombinant hyaluronidase injections for upper limb muscle stiffness in individuals with cerebral injury: a case series. *EBioMedicine.* 2016;9:306–313. https://doi.org.10.1016/j.ebiom.2016.05.014

26. Vattanasilp W, Ada L, Crosbie J. Contribution of thixotropy, spasticity, and contracture to ankle stiffness after stroke. *J Neurol Neurosurg Psychiatry.* 2000;69:34–39. https://doi.org.10.1136/jnnp.69.1.34

27. Malhotra S, Pandyan AD, Day CR, Jones PW, Hermens H. Spasticity, an impairment that is poorly defined and poorly measured. *Clin Rehabil.* 2009;23:651–658. https://doi.org.10.1177/0269215508101747

28. Fraser JR, Laurent TC, Laurent UB. Hyaluronan: its nature, distribution, functions and turnover. *J Intern Med.* 1997;242(1):27–33. https://doi.org.10.1046/j.1365-2796.1997.00170.x

29. Nishimura M, Yan W, Mukudai Y, et al. Role of chondroitin sulfate-hyaluronan interactions in the viscoelastic properties of extracellular matrices and fluids. *Biochim Biophys Acta.* 1998;1380(1):1–9. https://doi.org.10.1016/s0304-4165(97)00119-0

30. Cowman MK, Schmidt TA, Raghavan P, Stecco A. Viscoelastic properties of hyaluronan in physiological conditions. *F1000Res.* 2015;4:622. https://doi.org.10.12688/f1000research.6885.1

31. Knepper PA, Covici S, Fadel JR, Mayanil CS, Ritch R. Surface-tension properties of hyaluronic Acid. *J Glaucoma.* 1995;4(3):194–199.

32. Stecco A, Gesi M, Stecco C, Stern R. Fascial components of the myofascial pain syndrome. *Curr Pain Headache Rep.* 2013;17(8):352. https://doi.org.10.1007/s11916-013-0352-9

33. Friden J, Lieber RL. Spastic muscle cells are shorter and stiffer than normal cells. *Muscle Nerve.* 2003;27(2):157–164. https://doi.org.10.1002/mus.10247

34. Booth CM, Cortina-Borja MJ, Theologis TN. Collagen accumulation in muscles of children with cerebral palsy and correlation with severity of spasticity. *Dev Med Child Neurol.* 2001;43(5):314–320. https://doi.org.10.1017/s0012162201000597

35. Sheean G. Neurophysiology of spasticity. In: Barnes MP, Johnson GR, eds. *Upper Motor Neurone Syndrome and Spasticity: Clinical Management and Neurophysiology.* (2nd ed.) Cambridge University Press; 2008:9–63. https://doi.org.10.1136/jnnp.71.6.822d

36. Li S, Kamper DG, Rymer WZ. Effects of changing wrist positions on finger flexor hypertonia in stroke survivors. *Muscle & Nerve.* 2006;33(2):183–190. https://doi.org.10.1002/mus.20453

37. Baker SN. The primate reticulospinal tract, hand function and functional recovery. *J Physiol.* 2011;589(Pt 23):5603–5612. https://doi.org.10.1113/jphysiol.2011.215160

38. Herbert WJ, Powell K, Buford JA. Evidence for a role of the reticulospinal system in recovery of skilled reaching after cortical stroke: initial results from a model of ischemic cortical injury. *Exp Brain Res.* 2015;233(11):3231–3251. https://doi.org.10.1007/s00221-015-4390-x

39. Ortiz-Rosario A, Berrios-Torres I, Adeli H, Buford JA. Combined corticospinal and reticulospinal effects on upper limb muscles. *Neurosci Lett.* 2014;561:30–34. https://doi.org. 10.1016/j.neulet.2013.12.043

40. Ngeles Fernandez-Gil M, Palacios-Bote R, Leo-Barahona M, Mora-Encinas JP. Anatomy of the brainstem: a gaze into the stem of life. *Semin Ultrasound, CT MRI.* 2010;31(3):196–219. https://doi.org.10.1053/j.sult.2010.03.006

41. Drew T, Prentice S, Schepens B. Cortical and brainstem control of locomotion. *Prog Brain Res.* 2004;143:251–261. https://di.org.10.1016/S0079-6123(03)43025-2

42. McPherson JG, Ellis MD, Heckman CJ, Dewald JPA. Evidence for increased activation of persistent inward currents in individuals with chronic hemiparetic stroke. *J Neurophysiol.* 2008;100(6):3236–3243. https://doi.org.10.1152/jn.90563.2008

43. Mottram CJ, Suresh NL, Heckman CJ, Gorassini MA, Rymer WZ. Origins of abnormal excitability in biceps brachii motoneurons of spastic-paretic stroke survivors. *J Neurophysiol.* 2009;102(4):2026–2038. https://doi.org.10.1152/jn.00151.2009

44. Mottram CJ, Wallace CL, Chikando CN, Rymer WZ. Origins of spontaneous firing of motor units in the spastic-paretic biceps brachii muscle of stroke survivors. *J Neurophysiol.* 2010;104(6):3168–3179. https://doi.org.10.1152/jn.00463.2010

45. Heckmann CJ, Gorassini MA, Bennett DJ. Persistent inward currents in motoneuron dendrites: implications for motor output. *Muscle Nerve.* 2005;31(2):135–156. https://doi.org. 10.1002/mus.20261

46. D'Amico JM, Condliffe EG, Martins KJB, Bennett DJ, Gorassini MA. Recovery of neuronal and network excitability after spinal cord injury and implications for spasticity. *Front Integr Neurosci.* 2014;8:36. https://doi.org.10.3389/fnint.2014.00036

47. Gourab K, Schmit BD, Hornby TG. Increased lower limb spasticity but not strength or function following a single-dose serotonin reuptake inhibitor in chronic stroke. *Arch Phys Med Rehabil.* 2015;96(12):2112–2119. https://doi.org.10.1016/j.apmr.2015.08.431

48. Seo NJ, Fischer HW, Bogey RA, Rymer WZ, Kamper DG. Effect of a serotonin antagonist on delay in grip muscle relaxation for persons with chronic hemiparetic stroke. *Clin Neurophysiol.* 2011;122(4):796–802. https://doi.org.10.1016/j.clinph.2010.10.035

49. McPherson JG, Ellis MD, Harden RN, et al. Neuromodulatory inputs to motoneurons contribute to the loss of independent joint control in chronic moderate to severe hemiparetic stroke. *Front Neurol.* 2018;9:470. https://doi.org.10.3389/fneur.2018.00470

50. Kamper DG, Rymer WZ. Impairment of voluntary control of finger motion following stroke: Role of inappropriate muscle coactivation. *Muscle Nerve.* 2001;24(5):673–681. https://doi.org.10.1002/mus.1054

51. Park WH, Li S. Responses of finger flexor and extensor muscles to TMS during isometric force production tasks. *Muscle & Nerve.*2013;48(5):739–44. https://doi.org.10.1002/mus.23804

52. Lee JM, Gracies JM, Park SB, Lee KH, Lee JY, Shin JH. Botulinum toxin injections and electrical stimulation for spastic paresis improve active hand function following stroke. *Toxins (Basel).* 2018;10(11):426. https://doi.org.10.3390/toxins10110426

53. Shaw LC, Price CI, van Wijck FM, et al. Botulinum toxin for the upper limb after stroke (BoTULS) trial: effect on impairment, activity limitation, and pain. Stroke 2011;42(5):1371–1379. https://doi.org.10.1161/STROKEAHA.110.582197

54. Andringa A, van de Port I, van Wegen E, Ket J, Meskers C, Kwakkel G. Effectiveness of botulinum toxin treatment for upper limb spasticity after stroke over different ICF domains: a systematic review and meta-analysis. *Arch Phys Med Rehabil.* 2019; 100(9):1703–1725. https://doi.org.10.1016/j.apmr.2019.01.016.

II Assessment and Evaluation

4 Measurements and Scales

Steven Escaldi and Laurie Dabaghian

INTRODUCTION

The development of a successful spasticity treatment plan requires a precise and thorough assessment and evaluation process. Measuring spasticity is important for monitoring the impact of a targeted treatment intervention. It establishes a baseline from which any future change can be noted which documents the efficacy of a treatment. Since there is no single unanimous definition of "spasticity," we are left with numerous and varied assessment tools and scales that have been developed to quantify it.

For the purpose of this chapter, the discussion will be geared toward the notion that spasticity is a clinical sign of the upper motor neuron syndrome (UMNS), and the primary objective of spasticity management is to minimize the physical impact and functional impairments resulting from the UMNS. In this context, spasticity assessment tools are clinically most useful when we focus on the evaluation of both the positive and negative signs of the UMNS, as well as the evaluation of the concurrent biomechanical changes (i.e., tissue stiffness, muscle shortening, and tendon contracture). The positive signs include those resulting in motor overactivity (i.e., spasticity, dystonia, co-contraction, and associated reactions) and the negative signs include those causing performance deficits (i.e., weakness, loss of dexterity, and fatigue). Selection of the assessment tool can then be tailored to focus on that clinical aspect of spasticity that is causing the most detrimental impact.

GETTING STARTED

It is important to start an initial assessment of spasticity with a thorough history from the patient, a caregiver, or from a member of the patient's therapy team.[1] Keeping true to team-based approach in rehabilitation medicine, it is beneficial to assess the patient with other team members in their care, including physical and occupational therapists. This communication between team members provides a more comprehensive understanding of how spasticity impacts a patient's function and mobility.

Important information to collect when obtaining history includes:

- Injury/illness type and date of onset
- Duration, onset, frequency, and severity of spasticity

- Impact of spasticity on patient's function, mobility, daily activities, sleep, pain, and skin
- Other relevant medical information including recent infections, deep venous thromboses, or wounds

Patients may use spasticity to their advantage, for example, helping them stand, transfer, or holding onto an object. It is necessary to gather this information because targeting/treating those muscles may negatively impact a patient's mobility and ability to complete their ADLs. Assessing the presence of medical information is important because treatment of underlying medical issues will improve spasticity.

A thorough history should be followed with a physical and functional exam which should include evaluation of:

- Motor strength, control, and quality of movement
- Reflexes
- Sensation
- Skin integrity
- Resting and dynamic limb positioning and postures
- Gait

MEASURING SPASTICITY

As mentioned earlier, there are many scales and measurements used to assess spasticity. For the purpose of this chapter, the scales will be broken down into broader categories including **clinical scales** and **quantitative measurements.**

I. Clinical Scales

Clinical scales are measures that the clinician can use at bedside. They have been created to measure the many different aspects of spasticity and therefore can be broken down into subcategories. The clinician should keep in mind that spasticity is not static and can change between evaluations, and results can be influenced by factors such as time of day, body position, environment, and illness.

Ia. Tone Intensity Scales

- **Name: Ashworth Scale**

Description: The Ashworth Scale (AS) (Table 4.1) is one of the most commonly used measures due to its ease and speed of use.[1,2] It was created by Ashworth as a simple way to assess the effects of carisoprodol in patients with multiple sclerosis.[3]

- 5-point scale ranging from 0 to 4
- Measures resistance to rapid passive range of motion
- Easy to complete at bedside

To test a flexor muscle group, the muscle is placed into maximum flexion and then ranged to maximum extension over 1 second. To test an extensor muscle group, the muscle group is placed into full extension and then moved to maximal flexion over 1 second.[4] This can be done across any muscle groups/joints that are involved.

Table 4.1 Ashworth Scale

Score	Definition
0	No increase in tone
1	Slight increase in tone (catch and release at the end of ROM)
2	Increase in tone through most of the ROM, but affected part is easily moved
3	Considerable increase in tone; affected part is difficult to move
4	Affected part is rigid

Table 4.2 Modified Ashworth Scale

Score	Definition
0	No increase in muscle tone
1	Slight increase in tone (catch and release or minimal resistance at the end of ROM) when affected part is moved in flexion or extension
1+	Slight increase in tone, with catch followed by minimal resistance throughout the remainder (less than half) of ROM
2	Increase in tone through most of the ROM, but affected part is easily moved
3	Considerable increase in tone; affected part is difficult to move
4	Affected part is rigid

Pandyan et al. concluded that the AS should be considered an ordinal level of measure of resistance to passive movement, not spasticity.[5]

- **Name: Modified Ashworth Scale**

Description: The Modified Ashworth Scale (MAS) (Table 4.2) is also very commonly used. Bohannon and Smith adjusted the AS by including an additional level (1+) to create the MAS and enhance the sensitivity of the scale.[2,6] The MAS should be considered a nominal measure of resistance to passive movement due to the ambiguity between the grades 1 and 1+.[5] When documenting the MAS score, it is recommended to document if pain or contracture are present as they may limit the assessment.

- Ranges from 0 to 4 but has additional level of 1+
- Moderate to high inter- and intra-rater reliability[7]
- Better when measuring upper limbs than lower limbs[7]

It should be noted that although used commonly, the MAS does not differentiate between mechanical and neural causes of resistance and does not distinguish spasticity across a range of velocities.[1] This scale and the AS measure the resistance to passive movement which is just one aspect of spasticity.

- **Name: Tone Assessment Scale**

Description: The Tone Assessment Scale (TAS) was created to address the shortcomings of the MAS. The TAS assigns a global spasticity score integrating resting postures, response to passive movement, and associated reactions. The section of the TAS that relates to passive movement was found to be reliable at multiple joints except the ankle. Measuring resting posture and associated reactions were not found to be reliable.[1,8]

- **Name: Tardieu Scale**

Description: Unlike the AS and MAS, the Tardieu Scale (Table 4.3) measures spasticity by incorporating velocity into its measure. This scale is based on comparing angles of muscle reaction to stretch at different velocities.

- Uses two parameters: X which is the spasticity angle and Y which is the spasticity grade
- Spasticity angle is calculated by measuring the angles at slow speed (V1) and fast speed (V3).
- The slow speed (V1) assesses passive range of motion.
- The high speed (V3) engages the stretch reflex and therefore measures spasticity.
- V2 is the velocity of the limb segment naturally falling with gravity and is used for knee extensors, wrist extensors, and elbow flexors in paretic patients.

The examiner moves the limb as slow as possible and determines at what angle the limb arrests, due to resistance or discomfort, and cannot be overcome without injuring the joint. The examiner then moves the limb as fast as possible and records the angle where the limb arrests. The spasticity angle is then determined as the difference between the angle at slow speed and the angle at fast speed (X_{V1}–X_{V3}) and demonstrates the extent of spasticity.[9] The reaction of the muscle being tested is then graded as follows:

All angles measured are relative to the muscle tested and 0° is defined as the position of minimal stretch for each muscle. Positioning to complete assessments includes maintaining the shoulder flexion angle at 0° for the upper arm, the knee at 45° when assessing the ankle, and the hip at 90° when assessing the knee flexors.[9]

The Tardieu Scale has good to excellent intra-rater and inter-rater reliability in both angle and grade parameters at the elbow and ankle plantar flexors as seen in a

Table 4.3 Tardieu Scale	
Y	**Spasticity Grade**
0	No resistance
1	Slight resistance throughout passive movement
2	Catch at a precise angle, interrupting passive movement, followed by release
3	Fatigable clonus (lasts <10 seconds) when maintaining pressure and appears at a precise angle, followed by release
4	Clonus that does not fatigue (lasts >10 seconds) when maintaining pressure at a precise angle

study in children with cerebral palsy, but only the spasticity grade is reliable at the knee flexors.[9]

- **Name: Modified Tardieu Scale**

Description: The Modified Tardieu Scale (MTS) (Table 4.4) standardized the testing speed and procedure of the Tardieu Scale.

- The MTS has four elements: R1, R2, R2–R1, and X.
- R1 is the angle of catch during fast passive stretch
- R2 is the angle of the tested muscle length at slow passive range of motion.
- R2-R1 helps differentiate spasticity from contracture (when the difference is big, it indicates spasticity and when it is small, it indicates contracture).
- X grades the muscle resistance when passive stretch is applied (rated 0–5) as in the Tardieu scale.[10]
- MTS has good to excellent reliability.[10]
- MTS has better inter-rater reliability relative to the MAS.[11]

Ib. Range of Motion Measurements
- The most fundamental tool for the assessment of joint motion.
- Range of motion can be used as a simple and objective measurement that can easily be done at bedside and is measured using a goniometer.
- Evaluates both passive and active motion to monitor treatment response.

Table 4.4 Modified Tardieu Scale

Y	Spasticity Grade
0	No resistance
1	Slight resistance throughout passive movement
2	Catch at a precise angle, followed by a release
3	Fatigable clonus (lasts <10 seconds) when maintaining pressure and appears at a precise angle, followed by release
4	Clonus that does not fatigue (lasts >10 seconds) when maintaining pressure at a precise angle
5	Fixed joint
V	**Velocity of stretch**
V1	As slow as possible
V2	Speed of limb falling due to gravity
V3	As fast as possible
X	**Angle of catch**

Ic. Spasm Frequency Scales
- **Name: Penn Spasm Frequency Scale[4,12] (Table 4.5)**

Description:

- Self-reported measure
- Describes the frequency and severity of spasms
- 5-point scale, 0 meaning no spasms and 4 meaning spontaneous spasms that occur more than 10 times per hour
- The second part of the scale rates severity of spasms on a three-point scale with 1 being mild and 3 being severe, and it is only used if a patient reports presence of spasms.
- **Name: Spasm Frequency Score (Table 4.6)**

Description:

- Alternate spasm frequency score
- Frequency of spasms rated per day

This scoring system was used as part of a composite spasticity score that also included the AS.[2,13]

Id. Disease-Specific Scales

- **Name: Spinal Cord Assessment Tool for Spastic Reflexes (SCATS)**

Description:

- Specific for patients with spinal cord injury
- Requires a trained physician
- Shown to have substantial inter-rater reliability
- Assesses clonus, flexor spasms, and extensor spasms

Table 4.5 Penn Spasm Frequency Scale

Spasm Score	Frequency of Spasms
0	No spasms
1	Mild spasms induced by stimulation
2	Infrequent full spasms occurring less than once per hour
3	Spasms occurring more than once per hour
4	Spasms occurring more than 10 times per hour

Table 4.6 Spasm Frequency Score

Spasm Score	Frequency of Spasms
0	No spasms
1	One or fewer spasms per day
2	Between 1 and 5 spasms per day
3	Five to less than 10 spasms per day
4	Ten or more spasms per day or continuous contraction

Clonus is examined with passive ankle dorsiflexion and is rated from 0, meaning no reaction to 3, meaning lasting greater than 10 seconds. Flexors spasms are triggered with pinprick to the medial arch with the knee and hip extended and are rated from 0, which is no reaction, to 3, which is 40° of hip and knee flexion. Extensor spasms are assessed by extending the hip and knee from the starting position of 90° hip flexion and 110° knee flexion and are rated on the same 4-point scale.[4] This tool is discussed in more details elsewhere.

Ie. Clinical Gait and Balance Measures

Gait should be evaluated in patients whose spasticity impacts the lower limbs. The Berg Balance Scale can be used to assess balance. It consists of 14 items, each rated 0–4. Scores <45 indicate a risk of falls.[14] Baseline gait speed should be compared to posttreatment gait speed to demonstrate treatment success.

Time walking tests that can be used include:

- 10-meter walk test
- 6-minute walk test
- Timed Up and Go Test

If. Functional Scales

Although functional scales do not directly measure spasticity, they may be used to indirectly measure how mobility and daily activities are limited due to spasticity. There is a correlation between spasticity and poor functional outcomes during the initial year after stroke,[15] but functional assessment is complex as multiple factors influence function including strength, balance, proprioception, sensation, and the environment.[4] There is no one functional scale that can be universally applicable.

In patients who have had a stroke, the Modified Rankin Scale (mRS), the Barthel Index (BI), the Functional Independence Measurement (FIM), and the Disability Assessment Scale (DAS) can be used.

- The mRS is rated from 0 to 6, with 0 rated as no disability, 2–5 ranging from slight to severe disability and 6 rated as dead.[16]
- The BI evaluates 10 aspects of activity including self-care and mobility.
- The FIM measures areas including self-care, mobility, locomotion, sphincter control, communication, and social expression, rating them from requiring total assistance to complete independence.[17]
- The DAS is specific for patients who have upper limb spasticity secondary to stroke[1] and assesses disability in four domains including hygiene, limb position, dressing, and pain with each area rated from 0–3, where 0 is no disability, 1 is mild disability, 2 is moderate disability, and 3 is severe disability.[18]

In patients with spinal cord injury, the Spinal Cord Independence Measure (SCIM) is used.[4] It is similar to the FIM, with three scales including self-care, respiration, and sphincter management and mobility.

In patients with multiple sclerosis, the Multiple Sclerosis Spasticity Scale is used, which is a patient-reported outcome that contains 88 items. It quantifies the impact of spasticity in eight areas including muscle stiffness, pain and discomfort, muscles spasms, ADLs, walking, body movements, emotional health, and social functioning.[19]

This scale has been proven to be valid and reliable in measuring the impact of spasticity in this patient population.[20]

I. Quantitative Measurements

Researchers and engineers have developed measurements to obtain objective data for quantitative measurement of spasticity. These methods quantify both the neural and nonneural (mechanical) components of spasticity.[21] There are different quantitative models including purely mechanical models, musculoskeletal models, neural dynamic models, and threshold control-based models. Unfortunately, some of these are not practical in the clinical setting and further investigation is needed prior to adapting these into practice.[22]

IIa. Electrophysiological Measures

- Electrophysiological measures are objective measurements that assess the electrical manifestation of abnormal motor movement and control.
- **Electromyography (EMG)**

EMG through surface electrodes can be used to monitor the electrical current generated in muscles during contraction.[22] EMG data can be used to monitor agonist and antagonist muscle groups, giving information on muscle co-contraction.

- **Hoffman Reflex (H-reflex)**

The H-reflex is a low-threshold spinal reflex that is elicited through stimulation of a peripheral nerve. Ia sensory fibers are stimulated which then stimulate motor neurons. This reflex was first recorded in the soleus but can also be recorded at the quadriceps muscle and the flexor carpi radialis.[23]

The H-reflex provides information about changes in inhibition and excitability of the motor neuron pool due to supraspinal influences. In patients with spasticity, there is a decrease in H-reflex latency and increase in H-reflex amplitude demonstrating increased excitability of the motor neurons.[24] The latency and amplitudes have not been shown to be correlated with the MAS.[24]

- **H_{max}/M_{max} Ratio**

The M wave is a direct activation of motor neurons. The ratio of the maximal H-reflex amplitude and maximal M-response amplitude reflects the numbers of motor units activated by a reflex, influenced by excitatory and inhibitory inputs, compared to the total number of motor units, thereby indicating the level of excitability of the motor neuron pool. Increased H/M ratio is associated with increased excitability.

The H-reflex has been used while studying the impacts of intrathecal baclofen (ITB) for spasticity treatment. Studies have shown that the H-reflex is suppressed with intrathecal baclofen.[25] The H/M ratio significantly decreases with increase in the intrathecal baclofen dose.[26] Measurement of this reflex and ratio allows for dosing adjustments of ITB, as it has been seen that decrease in the H-reflex is dependent on time, concentration, and programming of ITB administration.[27]

- **Vibratory Inhibition Index**

The Vibratory Inhibition Index (VII) of the H-reflex is used to calculate presynaptic inhibition. It represents the percentage of the H-reflex amplitude that is reduced by vibration of the muscle tendon ($H_{vibration}/H_{control}$). The H-reflex is optimally inhibited with vibration of the Achilles tendon applied 20 to 60 ms before the H-reflex is tested. In healthy young subjects, the H-reflex is reduced by 40% to 50% after vibration. In spastic patients, vibratory inhibition is reduced, and the H-reflex is only reduced by 20%, indicating reduced presynaptic inhibition and increased motor neuron excitability.[24]

- **Tendon Reflex**

The tendon reflex is the mechanical counterpart of the H-reflex and is the muscle's response to tendon percussion. Tapping of a tendon activates a reflex through Ia afferents that synapse with alpha motor neurons, ultimately causing muscle contraction which is recorded with surface electromyography. In spastic muscles, less intensity is required to trigger the reflex due to decreased threshold, and the latency of the T-reflex is decreased while the amplitude increased as the excitability of alpha motor neurons is increased.

- T_{max}/M_{max}

The maximum amplitude of the T-reflex as a proportion of the maximum amplitude of the M wave is a ratio that increases with spasticity and gives more information regarding alpha motor neuron excitability. This ratio is a better indicator of motor neuron excitability than just the T-reflex amplitude.[24]

IIb. Biomechanical Measurements

Biomechanical measurement methods use apparatuses with manual or motorized movement that measure torque and kinematic information including joint angle. Biomechanical measurements require equipment and therefore are often done in research or lab settings and have limited use in the clinical setting.

- **Isokinetic Dynamometers**

Isokinetic dynamometers standardize stretch velocity and amplitude and then quantify the velocity-dependent resistance in the muscle being tested to passive movement.[2,28] Isokinetic dynamometers offer objective and reproducible measures. These are highly reliable measures but are limited for research use.[22,28]

- **Pendulum Testing**

The pendulum test, also known as Wartenberg test, measures spasticity during passive swing of the lower limb.[29] It is used to evaluate knee spasticity, but there have been modified versions used to test the upper limbs.[30] The leg is released from an extended position and drops due to gravity. The pendular movement of the knee is measured using electrogoniomety, videography, magnetic tracking, or wearable systems. Pendulum testing has excellent reliability and validity.[31]

IIc. New Methods of Measurement

- **Ultrasound elastography** is a newer modality used to measure the elastic properties (flexibility) of tissues. Studies have used this technique to measure muscle properties in patients with spasticity due to multiple sclerosis.[20,32]
- **Myotonometry** quantifies tissue displacement response to a perpendicular compression force and has also been used to assess spasticity.[28,33]

KEY POINTS

- Spasticity is a multifactor entity, with neural and nonneural contributions.
- There is no single scale or measurement that is able to evaluate spasticity and all its components.
- There remains a need to develop a system that objectively, accurately, and reliably assesses spasticity, to be able to evaluate the impact of treatment and rehabilitation.
- Clinicians should use a combination of the above scales as it pertains to their unique patient presentation and may be guided and correlated with specific treatment goal setting.

REFERENCES

1. Sunnerhagen KS, Olver J, Francisco GE. Assessing and treating functional impairment in poststroke spasticity. *Neurology.* 2013;80(3 Suppl 2):S35–44. https://doi.org/10.1212/WNL.0b013e3182764aa2

2. Biering-Sørensen F, Nielsen JB, Klinge K. Spasticity-assessment: a review. *Spinal Cord.* 2006;44(12):708–722. https://doi.org/10.1038/sj.sc.3101928

3. Ashworth B. Preliminary trial of carisoprodol in multiple sclerosis. *The Practitioner.* 1964;192:540–542.

4. Nene AV, Rainha Campos A, Grabljevec K, et al. Clinical assessment of spasticity in people with spinal cord damage: recommendations from the ability network, an international initiative. *Arch Phys Med Rehabil.* 2018;99(9):1917–1926. https://doi.org/10.1016/j.apmr.2018.01.018

5. Pandyan AD, Johnson GR, Price CI, et al. A review of the properties and limitations of the ashworth and modified ashworth scales as measures of spasticity. *Clin Rehabil.* 1999;13(5):373–383. https://doi.org/10.1191/026921599677595404

6. Bohannon RW, Smith MB. Interrater reliability of a modified ashworth scale of muscle spasticity. *Physical Therapy.* 1987;67(2):206–207. https://doi.org/10.1093/ptj/67.2.206

7. Meseguer-Henarejos AB, Sánchez-Meca J, López-Pina JA, Carles-Hernández R. Inter- and intra-rater reliability of the modified ashworthsScale: a systematic review and meta-analysis. *Eur J Phys Rehabil Med.* 2018;54(4):576–590. https://doi.org/10.23736/s1973-9087.17.04796-7

8. Gregson JM, Leathley M, Moore AP, Sharma AK, Smith TL, Watkins CL. Reliability of the tone assessment scale and the modified ashworth scale as clinical tools for assessing poststroke spasticity. *Arch Phys Med Rehabil.* 1999;80(9):1013–1016. https://doi.org/10.1016/s0003-9993(99)90053-9

9. Gracies JM, Burke K, Clegg NJ, et al. Reliability of the tardieu ccale for assessing spasticity in children with cerebral palsy. *Arch Phys Med Rehabil.* 2010;91(3):421–428. https://doi.org/10.1016/j.apmr.2009.11.017

10. Shu X, McConaghy C, Knight A. Validity and reliability of the modified tardieu scale as a spasticity outcome measure of the upper limbs in adults with neurological conditions: a systematic review and narrative analysis. *BMJ Open.* 2021;11(12):e050711. https://doi.org/10.1136/bmjopen-2021-050711

11. Synnot A, Chau M, Pitt V, et al. Interventions for managing skeletal muscle spasticity following traumatic brain injury. *Cochrane Database Syst Rev.* 2017;11(11):Cd008929. https://doi.org/10.1002/14651858.CD008929.pub2

12. Penn RD, Savoy SM, Corcos D, et al. Intrathecal baclofen for severe spinal spasticity. *N Engl J Med.* 1989;320(23):1517–1521. https://doi.org/10.1056/nejm198906083202303

13. Snow BJ, Tsui JK, Bhatt MH, Varelas M, Hashimoto SA, Calne DB. Treatment of spasticity with botulinum toxin: a double-blind study. *Ann Neurol.* 1990;28(4):512–515. https://doi.org/10.1002/ana.410280407

14. Berg KO, Wood-Dauphinee S L, Williams JI, Maki B. (1992). Measuring balance in the elderly: validation of an instrument. *Can J Public Health.* 1992;83 Suppl 2:S7–S11

15. Shin YI, Kim SY, Lee HI, et al. Association between spasticity and functional impairments during the first year after stroke in korea: the KOSCO study. *Am J Phys Med Rehabil.* 2018;97(8):557–564. https://doi.org/10.1097/phm.0000000000000916

16. Broderick JP, Adeoye O, Elm J. Evolution of the modified rankin scale and its use in future stroke trials. *Stroke.* 2017;48(7):2007–2012. https://doi.org/10.1161/strokeaha.117.017866

17. Dodds TA, Martin DP, Stolov WC, Deyo RA. A validation of the functional independence measurement and its performance among rehabilitation inpatients. *Arch Phys Med Rehabil.* 1993;74(5):531–536. https://doi.org/10.1016/0003-9993(93)90119-u

18. Brashear A, Zafonte R, Corcoran M, et al. Inter- and intrarater reliability of the ashworth scale and the disability assessment scale in patients with upper-limb poststroke spasticity. *Arch Phys Med Rehabil.* 2002;83(10):1349–1354. https://doi.org/10.1053/apmr.2002.35474

19. Hobart JC, Riazi A, Thompson AJ, et al. Getting the measure of spasticity in multiple sclerosis: the Multiple Sclerosis Spasticity Scale (MSSS-88). *Brain: A J Neurol.* 2006;129(1):224–234. https://doi.org/10.1093/brain/awh675

20. Hugos CL, Cameron MH. Assessment and measurement of spasticity in MS: state of the evidence. *Curr Neurol Neurosci Rep.* 2019;19(10):79. https://doi.org/10.1007/s11910-019-0991-2

21. Luo Z, Lo WLA, Bian R, Wong S, Li L. Advanced quantitative estimation methods for spasticity: a literature review. *J Intmed Res.* 2020;48(3):300060519888425. https://doi.org/10.1177/0300060519888425

22. Cha Y, Arami A. Quantitative modeling of spasticity for clinical assessment, treatment and rehabilitation. *Sensors (Basel, Switzerland).* 2020;20(18). https://doi.org/10.3390/s20185046

23. Decq P, Filipetti P, Lefaucheur JP. Evaluation of spasticity in adults. *Oper Tech Neuro.* 2004;7(3):100–108.

24. Voerman GE, Gregoric M, Hermens HJ. Neurophysiological methods for the assessment of spasticity: the Hoffmann reflex, the tendon reflex, and the stretch reflex. *Disabil Rehabil.* 2005;27(1–2):33–68. https://doi.org/10.1080/09638280400014600

25. Azouvi P, Roby-Brami A, Biraben A, Thiebaut JB, Thurel C, Bussel B. Effect of intrathecal baclofen on the monosynaptic reflex in humans: evidence for a postsynaptic action. *J Neurol Neurosurg Psychiatry.* 1993;56(5):515–519. https://doi.org/10.1136/jnnp.56.5.515

26. Bowden M, Stokic DS. Clinical and neurophysiologic assessment of strength and spasticity during intrathecal baclofen titration in incomplete spinal cord injury: single-subject design. *J Spinal Cord Med.* 2009;32(2):183–190. https://doi.org/10.1080/10790268.2009.11760770

27. Stokic DS, Yablon SA. Effect of concentration and mode of intrathecal baclofen administration on soleus H-reflex in patients with muscle hypertonia. *Clin Neurophysiol.* 2012;123(11):2200–2204. https://doi.org/10.1016/j.clinph.2012.04.007

28. Balci BP. Spasticity measurement. *Arch Clin Neuropsychol.* 2018;55(1):S49–s53. https://doi.org/10.29399/npa.23339

29. Joghtaei M, Arab AM, Hashemi-Nasl H, Joghataei MT, Tokhi MO. Assessment of passive knee stiffness and viscosity in individuals with spinal cord injury using pendulum test. *J Spinal Cord Med.* 2015;38(2):170–177. https://doi.org/10.1179/2045772314y.0000000265

30. Rahimi F, Eyvazpour R, Salahshour N, Azghani MR. Objective assessment of spasticity by pendulum test: a systematic review on methods of implementation and outcome measures. *Biomed Eng Online.* 2020;19(1):82. https://doi.org/10.1186/s12938-020-00826-8

31. Huang YD, Li W, Chou YL, Hung ES, Kang JH. Pendulum test in chronic hemiplegic stroke population: additional ambulatory information beyond spasticity. *Sci Rep.* 2021;11(1):14769. https://doi.org/10.1038/s41598-021-94108-5

32. Illomei G. Muscle elastography in multiple sclerosis spasticity. *Neurodegener Dis Manag.* 2016;6(6s):13–16. https://doi.org/10.2217/nmt-2016-0048

33. Li X, Shin H, Li S, Zhou P. Assessing muscle spasticity with myotonometric and passive stretch measurements: validity of the myotonometer. *Sci Rep.* 2017;7:44022. https://doi.org/10.1038/srep44022.s

5 Evaluation and Treatment of Spastic Gait

Alberto Esquenazi

INTRODUCTION

Ambulation is the end result of a well-choreographed pattern of phasic muscle activation and deactivation that is modulated by complex interactions within and between the central and peripheral nervous system and the gravitational forces. Given the multiple and complex neural pathways involved in producing ambulation, it is not surprising that disorders of the neurologic system result in gait disturbances. The various hemiparetic gait patterns are the result of an upper motor neuron syndrome (UMNS) (frequently associated with stroke, tumor, and traumatic brain injuries) which can impair movement through muscle paresis, problems with muscle overactivity (e.g., spasticity, co-contraction, clonus), and increased muscle stiffness. UMNS is an umbrella term encompassing any dysfunction disrupting the sensorimotor pathways of the central nervous system. Normally, a relationship exists between muscle activation and development of muscle tension; however, in UMNS, this relationship is altered and contributes to the presenting movement disorder.[1]

Many supraspinal structures are involved in the control of ambulation, including the brainstem reticular formation; basal ganglia; motor, premotor, and supplementary motor area of the motor cortex; and the cerebellum.[2,3]

Peripheral nerves located in tendons, muscles, ligaments, and joints relay information regarding limb position and kinesthesia. Proprioceptive information transmitted to the cortex assists with controlling volitional movements planned by the motor cortex. Proprioceptive information transferred to the cerebellum assists with involuntary modulation of motor control.[4] Load information sensed by mechanical receptors in the sole of the feet and from proprioceptive inputs in the extensor muscles of the foot,[5] as well as afferents that signal hip-joint position,[6] play a role in muscle activation patterns and stance-swing phase transitions during ambulation.

The objective evaluation of walking and its underlying muscle activation patterns can be performed by the collection of joint kinematics, kinetics, and dynamic electromyography (EMG) data simultaneously as an extension of the physical examination and visual assessment to better discern primary gait deviations from compensatory gait deviations as well as underlying muscle forces than need to be differentiated from contracture.

Despite the available literature supporting instrumented three-dimensional (3D) gait analysis for adults with neurologic injuries, its specific use in clinical and surgical decision-making has been limited because of its associated cost, the incorrect view by some insurance companies of gait analysis as mostly a research tool, the limited number of qualified clinical gait and motion analysis laboratories for adult patients, and limited access to physicians and surgeons who have experience in the treatment of neurologic-related gait disfunction.[7]

The objective of this chapter is to review the use of instrumented gait analysis in the management of adults with spastic gait dysfunction and describe an organized approach to the multiple deviations that can be observed in this population.

Neurologic recovery can be arbitrarily divided into an early period during which motor recovery may be expected and a late period during which, for all practical purposes, motor recovery has ended. During the period of motor recovery, temporizing interventions such as targeted chemodenervation with botulinum toxin A or neurolysis with phenol or ethanol can be used to address muscle overactivity. When these agents wear off in approximately 3 to 6 months, reevaluation is performed to determine whether additional motor recovery has taken place and whether there is further indication for treatment.[8]

Functional recovery is different from neurologic recovery and can occur many years after the initial neurologic injury. For instance, a patient who is unable to walk because of an equinovarus ankle foot deformity may regain the ability to walk through medical or surgical interventions to correct the problem.

The treatment of focal problems compared to diffuse problems will also guide the approach. When restricted motion can be attributed to a small number of muscles, chemodenervation or tendon lengthening or surgical releases or transfers of these muscles is feasible. If the problem is diffuse or generalized, oral or intrathecal antispasticity agents may be best.[9]

Traumatic brain injuries and stroke produce highly variable presentations of coexisting residual voluntary function and patterns of muscle overactivity and must be carefully assessed using an individualized objective and functional approach for surgical planning. Observational gait analysis is commonly used but has been identified as an inadequate diagnostic method in the evaluation of gait abnormalities. Therefore, these treatment selections should not be based on physical examination and observation alone but should include instrumented gait analysis to provide a sound basis for implementing conservative and surgical interventions.[10]

For patients with walking dysfunction after a neurologic injury, clinical examination and 3D instrumented gait analysis should attempt to answer the following questions:

- Which muscles can be voluntarily activated?
- Is the muscle spastic?
- Is the muscle co-contracting as an antagonist during active movement?
- Does the joint have limitations in motion due to contracture?[11,12]

Gait Analysis

Normal human locomotion consists of complex movement sequence of the legs, arms, head, and trunk with the goal of moving the center of mass from one point to another

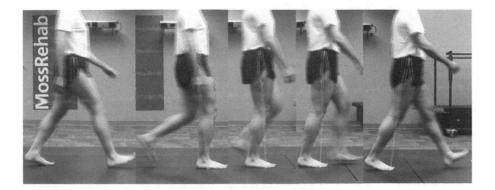

Figure 5.1 Right leg depiction of the stance phase components of the normal gait cycle (from initial contact to toe off) and for the swing phase on the left leg (from toe off to initial contact).

in a safe and efficient manner. Gait is a cyclic event and can be characterized by the timing of foot contact with the ground. An entire sequence of walking that includes two steps is identified as a gait cycle (Figure 5.1).

Instrumented gait analysis is a useful and validated clinical tool used for the assessment of gait. The evaluation of a single patient may take approximately 1 hour because of the need of a thorough clinical examination, application of instrumentation, and multiple trials of walking. For instrumented gait analysis evaluation to be clinically useful, the measured parameters should supply additional and more pertinent information than that of the clinical examination; should be accurate, repeatable, and functionally correlated; and should not alter the patient natural performance. Instrumented gait analysis is not indicated for every patient with UMN syndrome-related gait dysfunction. Clinicians should be trained and experienced in the instrumentation and equipment limitations and the data interpretation and should be able to relate these features to the observed deviations during walking to effectively diagnose and address the problems presented by pathologic gait.[9,7]

Kinematics

The analysis of motion, regardless of what external or internal forces are producing it, is referred to as kinematics. Temporal spatial parameters are simple to obtain, are useful for evaluating gait, and can be recorded with instrumented walkways (Figure 5.2) and wearable inertial sensors.[9]

Step length is the distance covered from one foot to the other. The stride period is defined from an event in one foot until repeated on the same foot (e.g., right initial contact to next right initial contact).

Cadence refers to the number of steps in a period of time and is commonly reported as steps per minute.

PABLO GAIT ASSESSMENT

MossRehab EINSTEIN HEALTHCARE NETWORK *tyromotion*

Personal data

| Name: | Birthdate: | Date: | 24.04 | Time: | 14:53 |

| Sex: | | Number of evaluated Steps: 90 | | Distance: | 93.1 m |

Gait parameters:

Velocity: 2.96 ± 0.07 km/h   Cadence: 95.36 steps/minute   Stride length: 103.45 ± 3.41 cm

Gait cycle

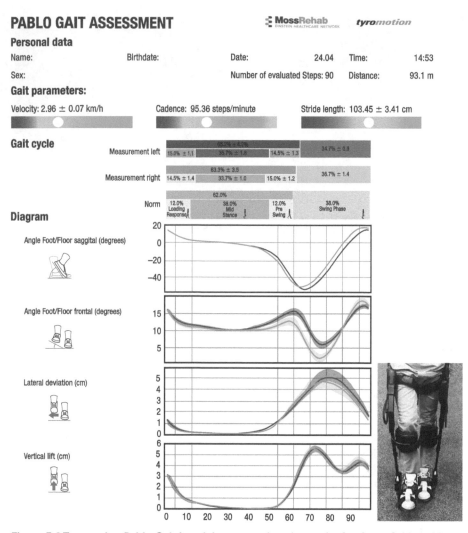

Measurement left	15.0% ± 1.1	35.7% ± 1.8	14.5% ± 1.3	34.7% ± 0.9
		65.2% ± 4.3%		
Measurement right	14.5% ± 1.4	33.7% ± 1.0	15.0% ± 1.2	36.7% ± 1.4
		83.3% ± 3.5		
Norm	12.0% Loading Response	38.0% Mid Stance	12.0% Pre Swing	38.0% Swing Phase
		62.0%		

Diagram

Angle Foot/Floor saggital (degrees)

Angle Foot/Floor frontal (degrees)

Lateral deviation (cm)

Vertical lift (cm)

Figure 5.2 Tyromotion Pablo Gait inertial sensors placed over the forefoot of this subject (white boxes), used to measure temporal spatial gait parameters and foot angles on a person using an Ekso exoskeleton device.

A 3D motion analysis is used to quantitatively describe the movement of body segments. Modern gait laboratories use specialized optoelectronic tracking systems to determine marker positions in space and time measuring joint angles (Figure 5.3), while linear and angular velocities and accelerations are some of the available calculated measures.

Kinetics

Joint kinetics are calculated when kinematic data are combined with ground reaction forces. The ground reaction force is a reflection of the body's mass and acceleration

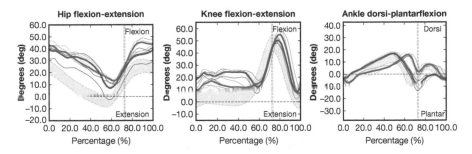

Figure 5.3 A 3D kinematic normalized data recorded with CODA CX1 active marker system from a patient with right hemiparesis. Red represents the right leg and blue is the left leg. Darker lines are the mean with ± 1 standard deviation. Grey envelope represents velocity matched normative data.

as it contacts the ground. Moment is the rotatory force on a joint that is affected by the distance from the center of rotation. Internal forces, generated primarily by muscles, ligaments, joint capsule, and the geometry of the articulating joint surfaces, counteract external rotational forces. In normal subjects, muscles will activate to counter this moment.[9]

Electromyography

The EMG signal is a recording of the electrical activity that reflects skeletal muscle activation. These recordings can be analyzed to determine the timing and relative intensity of the muscular activity during walking. Abnormalities in activation patterns can be classified as absence of activity, abnormal onset of activation (early or delayed), abnormal duration of activation (abbreviated or prolonged), and abnormal activation pattern timing (out-of-phase activity).[13] EMG can also assist in identifying spasticity as evidenced by inappropriate activity associated with motion or stretch. Clonus can be seen as short-duration bursts of repetitive electrical activity that occur in response to stretch.[13] To better identify problems with muscle activation timing and coordination that may be responsible for the gait dysfunction, studies should include all muscles capable of producing the target movement, not just the muscles that cross the affected joint.[14]

Pathological Gait

Gait dysfunction resulting from muscle overactivity, contracture, and impaired motor control after UMN injury is complex because of the involvement of multiple muscles and the difficulty discerning primary from compensatory gait deviations. Weakness of the hip flexor, knee extensor, and ankle plantar flexor muscles are the primary factors impairing walking in patients with hemiparesis due to acquired brain injury.[15,16]

Initial contact with the forefoot and decreased ankle dorsiflexion are typically observed. The plantar-flexed attitude of the ankle can result from muscle overactivity of plantar flexors and/or ankle contracture. Excessive knee extension or knee flexion may also be present. These deviations result primarily in stance phase limb instability that are correlated with a decrease in stance time on the affected limb, shortening of step length for the unaffected limb and increased duration of double support. During the swing phase, decreased hip and knee flexion and ankle equinovarus can lead to impairment in limb clearance on the affected side with compensatory hip hiking or in some cases circumduction. Swing phase may be delayed and more effortful, consistent with the findings of increased swing time on the affected side.[17–20]

The knee can be flexed or hyperextended along with the ankle in equinus, further impairing swing phase limb clearance and stance phase stability.

The goal of gait dysfunction management and treatment following an acquired brain injury should target improving lower limb stability in stance and during swing addressing limb clearance and advancement.

Instrumented gait analysis can help better identify the presence of muscle overactivity and differentiate joint contracture in gait dysfunction.

In the following paragraphs, we review common abnormal postures that impair gait in the UMNS and their underlying biomechanics, muscle overactivity patterns, and treatment.

Equinovarus Deformity

Equinovarus foot deformity is the most frequently observed lower limb deformity resulting from an acquired brain injury. The foot and ankle is plantar flexed (equinus) and frequently is also inverted (varus). Initial contact occurs with the forefoot, with weight applied primarily on the anterior and lateral border of the foot with or without coexisting toe flexion. Limited ankle dorsiflexion in midstance restricts the forward progression of the tibia over the stationary foot, potentially producing knee hyperextension and increasing pressure under the metatarsal.

During the swing phase, plantar flexion of the foot may result in impaired limb clearance.

Overactivation of ankle plantar flexors during the swing phase, or reduction of activation of the ankle dorsiflexors during the swing phase, can result in this deformity. The muscles capable of contributing to the deformity and those that should be studied include the gastrocnemius, soleus, tibialis anterior, tibialis posterior, extensor hallucis longus, flexor digitorum longus, and flexor hallucis longus.[38,39]

At times, it is difficult to differentiate the force contribution of the tibialis anterior and tibialis posterior to a varus deformity, and the use of a diagnostic tibial nerve block with lidocaine can be of help. In some cases, lengthening of the Achilles tendon, a split transfer of the tibialis anterior tendon, and myotendinous lengthening of the extensor hallucis longus may be considered.[21–24]

To supplement the force generation of weak ankle plantar flexors and reduce uncomfortable toe curling, a release and transfer of the long toe flexors to the calcaneus can be performed.[25]

Stiff Knee Gait Pattern

Stiff knee gait frequently is the result of a dynamic deformity caused by abnormal timing of muscle activation and external moments rather than a structural deformity of the knee joint. This gait deviation is characterized by sustained knee extension throughout the swing phase resulting in an increase in the lower limb moment of inertia which may interfere with hip flexion as well. The reduction in hip and knee flexion range can produce impairment of limb clearance caused by foot drag, even if the ankle has adequate dorsiflexion posture.

Compensatory mechanisms at the trunk (pelvic hike), ipsilateral hip (e.g., circumduction), and contralateral limb (e.g., early heel rise) may be called upon. A 3D gait analysis typically demonstrates peak swing phase knee flexion to be diminished and/or delayed. Out-of-phase muscle activation of the rectus femoris as recorded by EMG in the swing phase can be a major contributor to this pattern. The rectus femoris crosses both the hip and knee joints and can restrict knee flexion. Out-of-phase activation of the vasti muscles of the knee in the swing phase can further contribute to the gait deviation. At the hip, overactivity of the gluteus maximus and hamstrings during the swing phase may restrain flexion of the hip which in turn reduces the force transmission for adequate knee flexion generation. Iliopsoas weakness can also result in reduced hip flexion in the swing phase, impairing knee flexion. In the stance phase, ankle equinus can result in knee hyperextension by restricting forward progression of the tibia and delaying timely start of knee flexion.

When a concomitant ankle deformity is observed with a stiff knee, in general, the ankle should be addressed first, as addressing the ankle alone may help address the stiff knee gait pattern.

A stiff knee gait can be further evaluated by performing a diagnostic lidocaine block of the motor branch of the femoral nerve to the rectus femoris to reduce the force contribution of knee extensor muscles and permit evaluation of the hip extensor muscles contribution to the gait deviation. This can then be followed by using longer-acting agents such as phenol neurolysis or intramuscular botulinum toxin A injections.[26,27]

Selective surgical release of the rectus femoris alone or in combination with vastus intermedius can be considered,[28] and a transfer of the rectus femoris to the hamstrings can, in some patients, increase knee flexion.[8,29]

Hyperextended Great Toe (Hitchhiker's Toe)

Observation of barefoot walking can reveal extension of the great toe during the swing and stance phases. A frequent accompanying deformity is ankle equinovarus. The patient may report pain at the tip of the great toe and under the first metatarsal head when wearing shoes. Dynamic poly-EMG will demonstrate increased activity of the extensor hallucis longus. Weakness of the flexor hallucis longus may contribute to the deformity. Equinovarus may also be present. If so, contribution from muscles that can invert and plantar flex the foot should be evaluated. These include the tibialis posterior, tibialis anterior, gastrocnemius, soleus, and long toe flexors.[30] Treatment with botulinum toxin A intramuscular injection to the extensor hallucis longus is an effective intervention in reducing this deformity and addressing the patient's complaints. In selected cases, surgery may be performed to lengthen the extensor hallucis longus tendon.[31]

Flexed Knee Deformity

The flexed knee deformity presents as a stance phase problem of the knee that may also be observed during swing phases. This deformity impairs limb stability and negatively affects contralateral limb clearance, while the lack of knee extension in terminal swing results in a shortening of the step length. This gait pattern is often associated with medial and lateral hamstring muscle overactivity or contracture. Other factors that can contribute to this dysfunction include weakness of knee extensors or plantar flexors resulting in knee flexion in early stance phase.

When the hamstring muscles are the primary contributors, a temporary sciatic nerve block can differentiate between muscle overactivity and contracture. Intramuscular injection of botulinum toxin A to the hamstrings or phenol injections to the motor points of hamstrings may be performed to reduce knee flexor overactivity. If knee flexion deformity is persistent or is due to contracture, tendon lengthening of the involved muscles may need to be considered.[32,33]

Adducted Hip Deformity

Also referred to as a scissoring gait pattern results from severe hip adduction during the swing phase that can interfere with limb advancement and promotes a narrow base of support during the stance phase which can produce instability and increase risk for falls. In addition, this deformity may interfere with perineal hygiene, sitting, dressing, sexual intimacy, and, in some cases, transfers. In children and young adults with severe adductor overactivity, hip subluxation or dislocation can occur.

The 3D kinematic studies demonstrate increase in hip adduction in the swing phase. Overactive adductor longus, adductor brevis, and adductor magnus are most frequently involved. Gracilis and/or pectineus overactivity or weakness of iliopsoas, sartorius, and/or gluteus medius muscles evident in the swing phase can also contribute to this deformity. A diagnostic lidocaine block of the obturator nerve can help differentiate hip adductor muscle overactivity of the adductors from contracture. Phenol neurolysis of the obturator nerve or botulinum toxin A injections can reduce dynamic hip adduction deformity and are possible longer-term intervention strategies. Surgical release of the adductor muscles can be performed.[33] Obturator neurectomy can also be performed if the hip range of motion is adequate and increased tone is the principal problem.[30]

Flexed Hip Deformity

Hip extension limitations are a common physical examination finding and may be due to contracture from prolonged sitting or overactivity of the hip flexor muscles (e.g., iliacus, psoas, pectineus, and rectus femoris). Hip flexion deformity may also contribute to knee flexion posturing and can restrain hip extension during the late stance phase resulting in shortening of step length. The 3D kinematic studies may reveal excessive anterior pelvic tilt, forward trunk flexion, and reduced hip extension in mid and terminal stance.[32]

Intramuscular botulinum toxin A injections or phenol motor point injections to the offending muscles may be able to address the problem. Surgical release of persistent overactive or contracted flexor muscles can be considered and a postoperative rehabilitation program implemented to promote correction of the residual deformity.[33]

KEY POINTS

- Ambulation is the result of a well-choreographed pattern muscle activation and interactions within and between the central and peripheral nervous system and gravity.
- Instrumented gait analysis involves assessing kinematics, kinetics, and EMG.
- Gait analysis may be helpful for diagnosis, treatment, and outcomes.
- Common abnormal gait patterns assessed include equinovarus, hyperextended great toe, stiff knee gait, flexed knee, adducted hip, and flexed hip.

REFERENCES

1. O'Dwyer NJ, Ada L, Nielson PD. "Spasticity and muscle contracture following stroke." *Brain.* 1996;119(Pt 5):1737–49. https://doi.org.10.1093/brain/119.5.1737

2. Dietz V. "Neurophysiology of gait disorders: present and future applications." *Electroencephalogr Clin Neurophysiol.* 1997;103(3):333 55. https://doi.org.10.1016/s0013-4694(97)00047-7

3. Duysens J, Van De Crommert HW. "Neural control of locomotion; part 1: the central pattern generator from cats to humans." *Gait Posture* 1998;7(2):131–41. https://doi.org/10.1016/S0966-6362(97)00042-8

4. Schneider RJ, Kulics AT, Ducker TB. "Proprioceptive pathways of the spinal cord." *J Neurol Neurosurg Psychiatry.* 1977;40(5):417–33. https://doi.org.10.1136/jnnp.40.5.417

5. Dietz V, Duysens J. "Significance of load receptor input during locomotion: A review." *Gait Posture.* 2000;11(2):102–10. https://doi.org.10.1016/s0966-6362(99)00052-1

6. Pang MY, Yang JF. "The nitiation of the swing phase in human infant stepping: importance of hip position and leg loading." *J Physiol (Lond).* 2000;15(Pt 2):389–404. https://doi.org.10.1111/j.1469-7793.2000.00389.x

7. Baker R, Esquenazi A, Benedetti MG, Desloovere K. Gait analysis: clinical facts. *Eur J Phys Rehabil Med.* 2016;52(4):560–574.

8. Esquenazi A, Mayer NH. Laboratory analysis and dynamic polyEMG for assessment and treatment of gait and upper limb dysfunction in upper motoneuron syndrome. *Eura Medicophys.* 2004;40(2):111–22.

9. Moon D, Esquenazi A. Instrumented gait analysis. A tool in the treatment of spastic gait dysfunction. *JBJS Rev.* 2016;4(6):1–11. http://doi.org/10.2106/JBJS.RVW.15.00076

10. Vachranukunkiet T, Esquenazi A. Pathophysiology of gait disturbance in neurologic disorders and clinical presentations. *Phys Med Rehabil Clin N Am.*2013;24(2):233–246. https://doi.org.10.1038/nrneurol.2017.128

11. Keenan MA, Fuller DA, Whyte J, Mayer N, Esquenazi A, Fidler-Sheppard R. The influence of dynamic polyelectromyography in formulating a surgical plan in treatment of spastic elbow flexion deformity. *Arch Phys Med Rehabil.* 2003;84(2):291–6. https://doi.org.10.1053/apmr.2003.50099

12. Roche N, Bonnyaud C, Reynaud V, Bensmail D, Pradon D, Esquenazi A. Motion analysis for the evaluation of muscle overactivity: a point of view. *Ann Phys Rehabil Med.* 2019;62(6):442–452. https://doi.org.10.1016/j.rehab.2019.06.004

13. Mayer NH, Esquenazi A, Keenan MAE. Patterns of upper motoneuron dysfunction in the lower limb. In: Ruzicka E, Hallet M, Jankovic J, eds. *Gait Disorders, Advances in Neurology.* Philadelphia: Lippincot; 2001;87:311–319. https://doi.org.10.1093/brain/awaa052

14. Esquenazi A, Cionni M, Mayer NH. Assessment of muscle overactivity and spasticity with dynamic polyelectromyography and motion analysis. *Am J Phys Med Rehabil.* 2010;3:143–8. https://doi.org.10.1097/01.phm.0000141127.63160.3e

15. Hsu AL, Tang PF, Jan MH. Analysis of impairments influencing gait velocity and asymmetry of hemiplegic patients after mild to moderate stroke. *Arch Phys Med Rehabil.* 2003;84(8):1185–93. https://doi.org.10.1016/s0003-9993(03)00030-3

16. Ochi F, Esquenazi A, Hirai B, Talaty M. Temporal-spatial feature of gait after traumatic brain injury. *J Head Trauma Rehabil.* 1999;14(2):105–15. https://doi.org.10.1097/00001199-199904000-00002

17. Jonkers I, Delp S, Patten C. Capacity to increase walking speed is limited by impaired hip and ankle power generation in lower functioning persons post-stroke. *Gait Posture*. 2009;29(1):129–37. Epub 2008 Sep 11. https://doi.org.10.1016/j.gaitpost.2008.07.010

18. Brandstater ME, de Bruin H, Gowland C, Clark BM. Hemiplegic gait: analysis of temporal variables. *Arch Phys Med Rehabil*. 1983;64(12):583–7. https://doi.org. 10.3390/ijerph18020720

19. Mayer NH, Esquenazi A, Childers MK. Common patterns of clinical motor dysfunction. *Muscle Nerve Suppl*. 1997;6:S21–35.

20. Keenan MA, Creighton J, Garland DE, Moore T. Surgical correction of spastic equinovarus deformity in the adult head trauma patient. *Foot Ankle*. 1984;5(1):35–41. https://doi.org.10.1177/107110078400500105

21. Fulford GE. Surgical management of ankle and foot deformities in cerebral palsy. *Clin Orthop Relat Res*. 1990;253:55–61. https://doi.org.10.1016/j.cpm.2021.09.001

22. Vogt JC. Split anterior tibial transfer for spastic equinovarus foot deformity: retrospective study of 73 operated feet. *J Foot Ankle Surg*. 1998;37(1):2–7. htttps://doi.org.10.1016/s1067-2516(98)80003-3

23. Keenan MA, Lee GA, Tuckman AS, Esquenazi A. Improving calf muscle strength in patients with spastic equinovarus deformity by transfer of the long toe flexors to the os calcis. *J Head Trauma Rehabil*. 1999;14(2):163–75. https://doi.org.10.1097/00001199-199904000-00006

24. Robertson JV, Pradon D, Bensmail D, Fermanian C, Bussel B, Roche N. Relevance of botulinum toxin injection and nerve block of rectus femoris to kinematic and functional parameters of stiff knee gait in hemiplegic adults. *Gait Posture*. 2009;29(1):108–12. Epub 2008 3. https://doi.org.10.1016/j.gaitpost.2008.07.005

25. Tenniglo MJ, Nederhand MJ, Prinsen EC, Nene AV, Rietman JS, Buurke JH. Effect of chemodenervation of the rectus femoris muscle in adults with a stiff knee gait due to spastic paresis: a systematic review with a meta-analysis in patients with stroke. *Arch Phys Med Rehabil*. 2014;95(3):576–87. Epub 2013. https://doi.org.10.1016/j.apmr.2013.11.008

26. Waters RL, Garland DE, Perry J, Habig T, Slabaugh P. Stiff-legged gait in hemiplegia: surgical correction. *J Bone Joint Surg Am*. 1979;61(6A):927–33

27. Ounpuu S, Muik E, Davis RB 3rd, Gage JR, DeLuca PA. Rectus femoris surgery in children with cerebral palsy. Part I: the effect of rectus femoris transfer location on knee motion. *J Pediatr Orthop*. 1993;13(3):325–30. https://doi.org.10.1097/01241398-199305000-00010

28. Scully WF, McMulkin ML, Baird GO, Gordon AB, Tompkins BJ, Caskey PM. Outcomes of rectus femoris transfers in children with cerebral palsy: effect of transfer site. *J Pediatr Orthop*. 2013;33(3):303–8. https://doi.org.10.1097/BPO.0b013e3182784b0c

29. Mayer N, Esquenazi A. Managing upper motoneuron muscle overactivity. In: Zasler N, Katz D, Zafonte R, eds. *Brain Injury Medicine*. New York, NY: DEMOS, Chapter 50; 2012:821–849.

30. Keenan MA, Ure K, Smith CW, Jordan C. Hamstring release for knee flexion contracture in spastic adults. *Clin Orthop Relat Res*. 1988;236:221–6.

31. Vachranukunkiet T, Esquenazi A. Pathophysiology of gait disturbance in neurologic disorders and clinical presentations. *Phys Med Rehabil Clin N Am*. 2013;24(2):233–246. https://doi.org.10.1038/nrneurol.2017.128

32. Wheeler ME, Weinstein SL. Adductor tenotomy-obturator neurectomy. *J Pediatr Orthop*. 1984;4(1):48–51. https://doi.org.10.1097/01241398-198401000-00011

33. Haftek I. Clinical and electromyographic evaluation of obturator neurectomy in severe spasticity. *Paraplegia*. 1987;25(5):394–6. https://doi.org.10.1038/sc.1987.69

6 Management of Poststroke Spasticity With Botulinum Toxin Type A Based on Patient-Centered Treatment Goals

Jorge Jacinto

INTRODUCTION

Why Should Spasticity Treatment Be Patient-Centered and Goal-Oriented?

Even if the underlying pathology is similar across a population of patients, each patient is unique and the way spasticity manifests and impacts their lives is diverse between individuals, as well as in the same individual, according to the influence of many personal and environmental factors, that eventually enters into play during the course of their lives.[1]

Spasticity management, as stated by the most recognized international guidelines and expert consensuses, should be multimodal, and it should involve the input of knowledge and know-how of a specialized multi-professional team,[2] who respects the values, needs, and expectations of each patient, while providing to their best ability the highest standard of clinical/treatment practices.[3]

The patient and/or their caregivers must also have an active participation in the completion of any treatment plan, which implies a change in behavior. Schedules, routines, habits, postures, and exercises must change, according to a global plan to enhance the effects of the pharmacologic and rehabilitation modalities of the treatment. Scientific evidence shows that all human behavior is driven by goals, even if the individual is not always aware of it. So it is fundamental that patients, caregivers, and healthcare professionals (HCP), who are to be involved in pursuing a certain number of treatment goals, actually know exactly what those are so that they are motivated and coordinated during the process of developing the efforts needed to succeed.

Scientific publications have reported that HCPs, patients, and informal caregivers often have different perspectives when analyzing needs, impacts, and treatment outcomes related to spasticity assessment and management. Studies have also shown that the degree of motivation during the implementation of the treatment strategies and the degree of satisfaction with the achievements in the end are significantly greater when the patient/caregivers have been actively involved in the process of defining the goals.[4,5]

At present, all recognized international guidelines and expert consensus statements, in their most recent versions, recommend that spasticity management programs should be based on patient-centered, goal-oriented treatment plans. And that

57

treatment plans should be defined and implemented in interactive collaboration between the specialized multi-professional rehabilitation teams and the patients and/or caregivers.[2,3,6]

GOAL-SETTING AND USE OF THE GOAL-ATTAINMENT SCALING METHODOLOGY

What Are Patient-Centered SMART Treatment Goals?

Patient-centered goals are those that arise from the problems that the patient feels and manifests, which relate to the fact that the patient has developed spasticity in one or more body segments, in the context of some disease or lesion of the central nervous system that affects the pyramidal tract. The HCPs must acknowledge them and evaluate if, in fact, they are related to the presence of spasticity and, on the other hand, if the problems are susceptible to be changed by the different types of therapeutic interventions available. If so, then these become patient-centered treatment goals (PCTG), for that particular patient at that particular time.[3,7]

PCTGs must be clearly stated and recorded so that the HCP team and the patient and caregivers are well aware of them at baseline (before the intervention begins) and remain so through the whole time it will last and also at the moment of assessing the outcomes achieved. To make this possible and to ensure that all players involved are on the same page all the time and have the same interpretation of expected results and of when they are expected to be achieved, it's crucial that PCTGs are stated in a SMART way.

A SMART goal is[7]:

- Specific – It states exactly what we want to change with the treatment and if it focuses on one problem and not in multiple problems (symptom/functional limitation).
- Measurable – It can be associated to some parameter, through which the expected change can be measured before and after the treatment is implemented (known as the rule 1 goal = 1 parameter).
- Attainable – It must be estimated to be achievable with the multimodal intervention planned.
- Realistic – The change expected must be compatible with the underlying global pathophysiological condition of the patient as well as with the resources available and the intensity planned for the intervention.
- Timed – The goal statement must include the time when the expected results should be obtained and if the treatment plan is implemented as predicted.

According to the above explanation, a SMART goal statement must be formulated as follows (Figure 6.1):

"We will change the symptom/limitation (X), by so much, as measured by the goal parameter (Y), in so many weeks."

Here are some more concrete examples:

1. "We will improve the difficulty in performing hygiene of the right axilla, from very difficult to easy on a Likert-like scale (**very difficult** – difficult – fairly easy – **easy** – very easy), in 4 to 6 weeks."
2. "We will reduce the associated reaction of left elbow flexion during gait, from 80°–90° to 30°–45°, in 4 to 6 weeks."

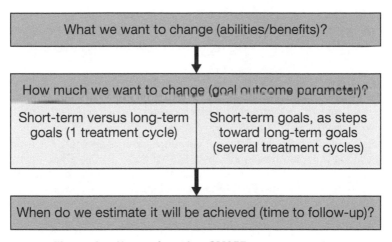

Figure 6.1 How to formulate SMART treatment goals.

3. "We will improve the velocity of gait on even grounds, by 10% to 20%, as measured by the 10-m walk test, in 6 to 8 weeks."
4. "We will reduce the pain on passive mobilization of the fingers of the right hand, from 8/10 to 2/10–3/10 on an NRS (0 = no pain; 10 = unbearable pain), in 2 to 4 weeks."

In the context of spasticity management, including botulinum toxin A (BoNTA) as part of the multimodal treatment plan, HCPs and patients usually talk about treatment cycles. This relates to the fact that the therapeutic effects of BoNTA typically have a profile of improvement to a peak effect at 4 to 6 weeks than sustaining effects until 10 to 12 weeks, followed by progressive wane of the benefits until another BoNTA treatment is administered.[6,8,9]

At each new BoNTA treatment session, goals should be assessed and new or the same goals should be established, according to which the new treatment will be designed and implemented. Some goals are achievable within the time of one treatment cycle; those are usually called short-term goals. Others must be worked on for longer periods of time, in view of the magnitude of change desired or of the complexity of the change that requires different stages of learning/reeducation. These are called long-term goals and they are usually achieved in 3 to 4 treatment cycles.

When treating for long-term goals, it is recommended that they should be broken into smaller "steps," to be reached in each treatment cycle. In this way, one long-term goal develops as a sequence of several short-term goals that allow the assessment of the achievement after each cycle while keeping patient, caregivers, and HCP team focused on the bigger purpose of the long-term goal.

One of the most difficult aspects of implementing this methodology in routine clinical practice seems to be the choice of one parameter per PCTG to measure the change. It is common knowledge that despite the great variety of clinical measurement tools available, HCPs do not use them frequently in routine clinical practice to record baseline and outcome findings. This is even more so when trying to capture changes in real-life situations, which are not reproduced in the standardized outcome measures described in scientific literature as measures of functionality in neurologic patients.

The lack of data hence existing and the heterogeneity of measures used by different authors are the reasons behind the massive lack of information regarding functional benefits of spasticity management with BoNTA. Let us propose possible solutions for both problems:

1. *Lack of data due to the fact that existing functional outcome measures are too cumbersome to use in routine clinical practice (with limited time slots for assessment and treatment of each patient) and do not reflect most of the concrete real-life situations that patients refer to when establishing their PCTGs:*

   To try and overcome this hurdle, we must adopt parameters that arise from simple and practical outcome measurement tools like the ones described on the "Goal Attainment Scaling–Evaluation of Outcome for Upper Limb Spasticity Tool" (http://www.csi.kcl.ac.uk/files/GASeoustool3pdf), for example, numeric or analogic rating scales for symptoms or difficulty in performing activities/tasks; Likert-like scales to describe improvement as perceived by patient/caregiver; 10-m walk test, TUG test, or FAC for gait; and ArmA/LegA for active/passive function of upper and lower limbs respectively.[10,11]

   By adhering to such practice, HCPs will create a virtuous compromise between the practical/logistics concerns of spasticity centers and the need to generate real-world data about the benefits accomplished by the treatment of spasticity with BoNTA. The fact that heterogeneity of measures used would hence be reduced might allow for larger pools of data to be analyzed and for the sub-analysis of outcomes achieved by different types of patients, for different types of goals, with different types of multimodal approaches. This would in turn lead to a better understanding of "who needs what," "for which goals" to be successfully achieved, when treated with BoNTA for spasticity.

2. *Trying to compare success obtained in the treatment of different patients or in the same patient in two different moments in time:*

   Because the success in spasticity management depends on an array of factors as mentioned before in this chapter, we need to have a methodology that allows these comparisons by scoring the success in a common "numeric scale." The scores allow us to know if the goals of a certain patient, for each treatment cycle, were achieved as expected, underachieved, or overachieved. That is to say to use the GAS methodology applied to spasticity management with BoNTA.[12]

What Is Goal Attainment Scaling and How to Use It in Routine Clinical Practice?

GAS is a methodology to measure attainment of success in achieving pre-set goals and scoring it according to a 5-point scale. The original scale described and validated in the 1960s[11] includes the possibility of weighting the goals (importance x difficulty), but for routine clinical purposes, the GAS-light version is the most commonly used: (−2) "achieved much less than expected"; (−1) "achieved a little less than expected" or "no change from baseline"; (0) "achieved as expected"; (+1) "achieved a little more than expected"; (+2) "achieved much more than expected." To assess global success for the number of PCTGs in a certain cycle, the score of each goal is entered into a calculation formula to determine the so-called GAS T-score. If that score is 50±10, it means that goals were quite well achieved (and the nearest to 50 the better). If the T-score is <40, it usually means goals were unrealistic, treatment was insufficient, or outcomes were underestimated. When T-score is >60, often it is related to underestimation of patients' ability to change, underestimation of treatment efficacy, or overestimation of outcomes. The change of GAS T-score from baseline to outcome evaluation moment (GAS change) should be 10 or more to be considered clinically relevant.

Ideally, during the goal-setting process, expected outcomes should be defined (according to the selected parameter for each goal) in collaboration with patient/ caregiver and the time for the assessment of outcomes should be fixed. At baseline, all goals should be scored (−1), unless the limitation/symptom cannot get any worse, in which case it should be scored (−2)*. GAS baseline T-score can then be calculated, using the GAS formula. Outcome GAS T-score is calculated once the results are assessed, as well as GAS change.[12]

Timing of reevaluation can be key to determine success or failure, when measuring goal achievement. For example, goals that depend mostly on the pharmacologic effect of BoNTA can be evaluated at 4 to 6 weeks, according to the efficacy profile of the product. Differently, goals that depend on the pharmacologic effect as well as on rehabilitation interventions (physiotherapy, occupational therapy, exercise/ stretching programs) that will then allow for learning of new movements/functional strategies should be reevaluated no earlier than 6 to 10 weeks (depending on intensity of rehabilitation program, patient motivation and cognition/behavior, difficulty of goal, etc.).

Evaluating goal achievement should take into consideration more than just the magnitude of change produced in each goal parameter defined *ab initium*. The therapeutic profile of BoNTA tells us that at approved doses, the benefits felt usually start to wane after 10 to 12 weeks. On the other hand, manufacturers do not recommend reinjection intervals of less than 12 weeks.[13-15] So in order to avoid that patients live their "spasticity journey" as if they were riding in a roller coaster, benefits (at least partial benefit) should last until the next injection date. This means that apart from the magnitude of change in each goal parameter, we must take into consideration if that change lasts as much as expected.[7] This methodology allows us to learn from each injection cycle and eventually introduce adjustments to the treatment protocol: doses, muscles, guidance technique, adjuvant therapy type or intensity, patient/caregiver education, and time to reevaluation. Under this perspective, I propose that all GAS outcomes can be considered positive:

a. GAS scores (+1) and (+2): We are happy and we raise the bar for next treatment cycle considering them the expected outcomes.

b. GAS score (0): We are happy and must decide with the patient/caregiver whether it is as good as they wish/can or if we may try to raise the bar for the next treatment cycle (never forgetting the SMART goal A and R principles).

c. GAS scores (−1) and (−2): In these cases, we are not happy and we must analyze several possibilities and act accordingly, to try and obtain better results for our patient in the next treatment cycle: poor patient selection, poor muscle selection, poor injection technique (dilution, guidance, etc.), insufficient dosing of BoNTA, insufficient or poor adjuvant therapies combination, and unrealistic goals. So in the end, it is a learning opportunity.

(*) when baseline score for a certain PCTG is (−2), at outcome evaluation, the scores should be (−2) "no change from baseline"; (−1) "achieved a little less than expected"; (0), (+1), and (+2), same as when baseline is (−1).

Goal-Based Treatment Design and Action Plan

The different components of the treatment, in each treatment cycle, must be determined according to the goals pursued for that cycle.

a. Concerning BoNTA: The muscles to target should be the ones limiting the functions/activities or generating the symptoms that we want to treat and not necessarily all those that are spastic in a certain limb or body segment. This allows the clinicians to use effective dosing per muscle while keeping within clinical reasonability for total doses.
b. Regarding adjuvant therapies: The modalities used and their intensities and durations should be decided on the basis of whether the goals at hand are symptomatic, associated reactions/involuntary movements, of passive function, of active function, etc. More functional and more complex goals, or even more ambitious expected outcomes, in general, may require more modalities, more intensity, and more duration of treatment.

Any set of goals for a treatment cycle must be associated to a "plan of action."[4] Typically, it may involve BoNTA injections, multimodal rehabilitation adjuvant treatment, concomitant systemic medication, and medical devices such as orthosis, positioning systems, walking aids, etc..

Success may rely on planning and implementing the optimal combination, in a customized way for each patient, set of goals, and treatment cycle. Patients and/or caregivers should be aware that compliance with any of the parts of the plan of action will contribute, as much as the BoNTA treatment, for the overall success in goal attainment.[3,7]

KEY POINTS

- Spasticity management should be multimodal and involve a specialized multi-professional team, who respects patients' values, needs, and expectations and provides the highest standard of clinical/treatment practices and resources available.
- The patient and/or their caregivers must also have an active participation in the design and implementation of any treatment plan.
- Patients, caregivers, and HCPs must be clearly aware of what the treatment goals are so that they are motivated and act synergistically toward goal attainment.
- Treatment goals should be defined at the baseline of each new BoNTA treatment cycle and should be stated in a SMART manner and patient-centered (PCTG).
- For each SMART goal, there must be a goal parameter to measure the change. Upon scoring the success in goal attainment, we should value the magnitude, as well as the duration of the benefits felt/achieved.
- We propose the GAS methodology applied to spasticity management with BoNTA. Assessment and clinical interpretation of goal attainment, using GAS and the principle of one goal–one parameter, should inform the decisions for the fine-tuning of the next treatment cycle: target muscles; BoNTA doses; injection technique; modality combination; intensity and duration of adjuvant therapies; and outcome assessment timing.

REFERENCES

1. Barnes M, Kocer S, Fernandez MM, Balcaitiene J, Fheodoroff K. An international survey of patients living with spasticity. *Disabil Rehabil.* 2017;39(14):1428–1434. https://doi.org/10.1080/09638288.2016.1198432

2. Royal College of Physicians. *Spasticity in Adults: Management Using Botulinum Toxin.* NationalGuidelines2018.https://www.rcplondon.ac.uk/guidelines-policy/spasticity -adults-management-using-botulinum-toxin (Accessed: January 2021); 2018.

3. Turner-Stokes L, Ashford L, Esquenazi A, et al. A comprehensive person-centered approach to adult spastic paresis: a consensus-based framework. *Eur J Phys Rehabil Med.* 2018;54(4):605–617. https://doi.org/10.23736/S1973-9087.17.04808-0. Epub 2017 Dec 21.

4. Scobbie L, Dixon D, Wyke S. Goal setting and action planning in the rehabilitation setting: development of a theoretically informed practice framework. *Clin Rehabil.* 2011;25(5):468–82. https://doi.org/10.1177/0269215510389198. Epub 2010 Dec 3.

5. Holliday RC, Cano S, Freeman FA, Playford ED. Should patients participate in clinical decision making? An optimised balance block design controlled study of goal setting in a rehabilitation unit. *J Neurol Neurosurg Psychiatry.* 2007;78(6):576–80. https://doi.org/10.1136/jnnp.2006.102509. Epub 2006 Dec 18.

6. Bensmail D, Hanschmann A, Wissel. Satisfaction with botulinum toxin treatment in post-stroke spasticity: results from two cross-sectional surveys (patients and physicians). *J Med Econ.* 2014;17(9):618–25.https://doi.org/10.3111/13696998.2014.925462. Epub 2014 Jun 12.PMID: 24841450

7. Francisco GE, Balbert A, Bavikatte G, et al. A practical guide to optimizing the benefits of post-stroke spasticity interventions with botulinum toxin A: an international group consensus. *J Rehabil Med.* 2021;53(1):jrm00134. https://doi.org/ 10.2340/16501977-2753

8. Patel AT, Wein T, Bahroo LB, Wilczynski O, Rios CD, Murie-Fernández M. Perspective of an international online patient and caregiver community on the burden of spasticity and impact of botulinum neurotoxin therapy: survey study. *JMIR Public Health Surveill.* 2020;6(4):e17928. http://doi.org/10.2196/17928.PMID: 33284124

9. Jacinto J, Varriale P, Pain E, Lysandropoulos A, Esquenazi A. Patient perspectives on the therapeutic profile of botulinum neurotoxin type a in spasticity. *Front Neurol.* 2020;11:388. https://doi.org/10.3389/fneur.2020.00388. eCollection 2020.PMID: 32477251

10. Turner-Stokes L, Jacinto J, Fheodoroff K, et al. Longitudinal goal attainment with integrated upper limb spasticity management including repeat injections of botulinum toxin A: findings from the prospective, observational Upper Limb International Spasticity (ULIS-III) cohort study. *J Rehabil Med.* 2021;53(2):jrm00157. https://doi.org/10.2340/16501977-2801.PMID: 33616192

11. Kiresuk T, Sherman R. Goal attainment scaling: a general method of evaluating comprehensive mental health programmes. *Community Ment Health J.* 1968;4(6):443–453. https://doi.org/10.1007/BF01530764

12. Turner-Stokes L. Goal Attainment Scaling (GAS) in rehabilitation: a practical guide. *Clin Rehabil.* 2009;23(4):362–70. http://doi.org/10.1177/0269215508101742. Epub 2009 Jan 29.PMID: 19179355

13. Botox® (onabotulinumtoxinA) [Prescribing Information]. Irvine, CA: Allergan, Inc.

14. Xeomin® (incobotulinumtoxinA) [Prescribing Information]. Raleigh, NC: Merz Pharmaceuticals, LLC.

15. Dysport® (abobotulinumtoxinA) [Prescribing Information]. Basking Ridge, NJ: Ipsen Biopharmaceuticals, Inc.

III Principles of Treatment

7 Physical Therapy and Management of Spasticity

Sandeep K. Subramanian, Anjali Sivaramakrishnan, and
Selina M. Morgan

INTRODUCTION

Spasticity is a frequent disabling consequence of neurologic disorders that can impact function and results in decreased quality of life (QOL). Physical therapists play an important role in the rehabilitation of individuals with spasticity. Different interventions are performed to enhance function by decreasing spasticity if it is an impediment to independent functioning or working with spasticity if it enables functioning.

The aim of physical therapy (PT) interventions is to regain motor control in hypertonic and spastic musculature regardless of the diagnosis and severity of the injury. PT interventions are considered as a conservative, yet highly functional approach to managing spasticity. The aim of PT with neuro-recovery is to elicit even traces of volitional muscle activation through adapted manual muscle testing and surface electromyography (EMG). Physical therapists are obligated to search for and treat both remaining active motor control as well as facilitating new function. More often, a patient with spasticity demonstrates reduced motor control and limited functional mobility. Depending on the pathology, the limbs are held in fixed and abnormal postures with a predominant involvement of the anti-gravity muscles. In patients with stroke, the upper extremity typically adopts a posture with abnormal flexion while the lower extremity adopts a posture with abnormal extension. While considering the management of a patient with spasticity, the therapist must weigh the patient's goals, benefits versus deleterious effects of spasticity, etiology of spasticity, administration and timing of medical and surgical interventions, and muscle groups affected.

Hypertonicity and spasticity do not always require intervention. There are obvious benefits of hypertonicity and spasticity including reduction in the extent of disuse atrophy. Some patients use spastic responses to empty their bladder, perform activities of daily living (ADLs), transfer, stand, and walk. To suppress spasticity in this scenario can be counterproductive for functional task performance. Spasticity can also adversely affect function and interfere with transfers, bed mobility, and ADLs such as walking, eating, and dressing. Moreover, spasticity can cause disabling pain, affect sleep, and reduce QOL.[1] Spasticity has also been reported to occur more frequently in individuals with spinal cord injury (SCI), particularly in those with neuropathic pain.[2]

Considering the abovementioned factors, important goals that need to be considered for managing spasticity include improving functional mobility, restoring postural alignment, improving sensorimotor control, preventing the development of contractures, and improving independence. Although there are several approaches for managing spasticity, a multimodal approach for managing spasticity would produce optimal results.

EDUCATION

Prior to starting any rehabilitation program, it is important that physical therapists explain spasticity in simpler terms to the patient and caregiver in terms of the basic anatomy of the muscle and how the length of the muscle changes with exercise. A good understanding of these concepts can improve patient compliance and increase self-management of spasticity. Moreover, patients must be informed about internal and external spasticity triggers such as noxious stimuli, pressure sores, bowel and bladder retention or infection, environmental heat or cold, and other factors.[3]

PHYSICAL THERAPY TECHNIQUES

Stretching and Passive Techniques

Stretching refers to the application of either manual or mechanical forces to lengthen muscle and other connective tissue structures that have shortened over time. Spasticity is characterized by changes in muscle length and tone as a function of the biomechanical, viscoelastic, and excitability properties of the muscle. The shortened state of a spastic muscle causes a loss of sarcomeres, which alters the muscle length–tension relationship. Increasing the muscle length via interventions such as positioning or stretching has shown to increase the number of sarcomeres in the muscle.[4] Stretching applies tension to different soft tissue structures that can normalize muscle tone and improve the length–tension relationship thus improving function.

Static Stretching

Static stretching refers to slowly lengthening of the muscle based on patient's tolerance, and the end position (maximal lengthened state) is held for 30 seconds or so. It is either passive, that is, where the stretch is performed by another person, or active, that is, where the patient initiates and/or maintains the stretch. A sustained stretch reduces the activation of the muscle spindle and increased firing of the Golgi tendon organ that results in inhibition of the muscle and increased length via autogenic inhibition. *Mechanical stretching* using devices such as a feedback-controlled device, mechanical weights, pulleys, orthotic devices, or the dynamometer can be applied for several hours. Recent research has reported that positioning or weightbearing on a tilt table resulted in significant improvements in muscle tone in patients with stroke.[5] Moreover, standing on a tilt table or standing frame can activate the anti-gravity muscles in the trunk and lower extremities, increase the flexibility of the soft tissues, and improve postural alignment.[6] *Prolonged positioning* refers to positioning the limb out spastic pattern to achieve a longer duration stretch of a particular muscle or muscle group. Positioning can be performed either in recumbent postures (supine, side lying, or prone) or on a wheelchair for improving proximal stability and management of a deformity or in standing. While positioning, the physical therapist needs to ensure that pressure is uniformly distributed to prevent the formation of pressure areas.

Stretching can vary in *intensity* (amount of tension that is applied to the muscle), *velocity* (speed at which the muscle is being elongated), *repetitions* (number of stretches), *dosage* (total duration of muscle elongation), and frequency (number of sessions).[7] Although stretching can be beneficial from a physical therapist's standpoint, a systematic review reported that the clinical benefits on outcomes such as range of motion (ROM) are inconclusive.[7] Stretching can be expected to produce temporary improvements in muscle tone and length and should be considered as preparatory techniques to improve muscle range of ROM and functional mobility. There is evidence to support that stretching for 30 minutes can prevent soft tissue shortening. Combining stretching with other interventions such as strengthening can be optimal for improving function.[8]

Casting and Splinting

A variety of splints are used in order to reduce spasticity or maintain the gain in range obtained using stretching techniques. A systematic review on use of splints for stroke found a low level of evidence to support the utility of splints in reducing spasticity.[9] The same review found that dynamic splints were more useful than static splints for individuals sustaining strokes. In individuals sustaining traumatic brain injuries, a recent systematic review reported large effect sizes for static stretching (improved elbow extension range) and moderate effect sizes for soft splints in decreasing finger spasticity.[10]

Range of Motion Exercises

ROM exercises can be performed passively by the physical therapist or using devices such as robots for providing continuous passive motion. Continuous passive motion can improve functional mobility across a joint, lengthen soft tissue, reduce tone, and cause cortical activation in the sensorimotor cortex similar to while performing an active movement.[11] Previous research has shown that devices using robots (EMG robots/electromechanical robots) can reduce spasticity in the upper limb and improve muscle coordination via upper limb motor training,[12,13] which suggests that such therapies although expensive can be used for managing spasticity.

Active Exercises

Strengthening Exercises

Spasticity may often coexist with muscle weakness. For instance, a patient with stroke may not be able to perform overhead activities due to weakness in the upper arm and shoulder muscles. In such a scenario, the physical therapist can focus on strengthening the weaker muscles for achieving a balance between the agonist and antagonist to improve the movement. Previous research has suggested that progressive resistance training can improve upper limb strength, activity, motor function, and ADLs without increasing spasticity in individuals with stroke.[14] In another recent study, resistance training was proposed as a possible intervention for reducing spasticity after stroke; however, only limited studies directly assessed the effectiveness of strength training on spasticity.[15] Overall, strength training is recommended in stroke rehabilitation, and these findings also extend to other populations such as cerebral palsy (CP). A recent meta-analysis found that strength training can improve function, muscle strength, balance, and gait without adversely affecting spasticity in CP.[16] Although spasticity does not directly reduce with strength training, the physical therapist should incorporate strength training and weigh its beneficial effects in a rehabilitation program.

Aerobic Exercise
Aerobic exercise (i.e., walking, cycling, swimming, etc.) is an integral part of a rehabilitation program for individuals with disorders such as stroke, SCI, CP, and multiple sclerosis (MS). Several studies have shown that aerobic exercise can improve aerobic capacity and cardiorespiratory fitness,[17] walking endurance,[18] and spasticity[19] in individuals with neurologic disorders.

Gait Training
Gait training performed with or without body support can reduce spasticity by retraining postural and stepping reactions that are important during walking. Gait training allows for early training of postural and stepping reactions and improves gait symmetry. Thus, it can be utilized for facilitating motor learning of physiological gait patterns. The evidence in this domain is not very clear, and there is a paucity of studies showing direct effects of gait training on reducing spasticity. However, given that gait training integrates repetitive task-oriented practice and is generally safe, it can be integrated into a treatment plan depending on the patient's level of impairment.

MODALITIES

Thermal Modalities
Prolonged icing can be used to reduce spasticity and is typically applied with ice packs, cold baths, or crushed ice. Cooling is usually performed for approximately 20 minutes,[20] and the effects on reducing spasticity may last for 15 to 20 minutes. Heating modalities are less used compared to cooling but could include hot packs, therapy with ultrasound and infrared, and warm baths. Overall, the evidence supporting the evidence of thermotherapy for reducing spasticity is not definitive and future studies are required to prove their effects.[21]

Electrical Stimulation
Electrical stimulation has been recommended for reducing spasticity and the pain that is associated with spasticity. There are several types of electrical stimulation and the commonly used modalities include transcutaneous electrical stimulation (TENS) and functional electrical stimulation (FES). It is thought that TENS can reduce spasticity by stimulating the large-diameter mechanoceptive afferents and/or modulating spinal inhibition. A recent study reported that TENS in combination with other PT techniques was more effective in reducing spasticity compared to PT alone.[22] FES has been frequently used for neuromuscular reeducation and functional movement training by stimulating the muscles to produce a movement. The putative mechanisms for reducing spasticity include recurrent inhibition and/or Renshaw cell inhibition or reciprocal inhibition depending on the muscle being stimulated (spastic muscle/antagonist). Although FES cycling is a common mode of treatment that is administered to individuals with SCI, the evidence about its effectiveness remains inconclusive.[23] Guidelines with respect to dosage remain inconsistent; however, a single session of electrical stimulation for 30 to 60 minutes appears to reduce spasticity in individuals with stroke.[22]

OTHER TECHNIQUES

Neurodevelopmental Treatment

Neurodevelopmental treatment (NDT) is a common approach that is used in rehabilitation of CP and stroke. This approach aims on encouraging normal movement patterns and postural reactions while attempting to reduce abnormal movement and reflexes. Specifically, NDT also integrates functional movement training with an emphasis on postural control. Only few studies have assessed the effects of NDT on spasticity and motor function. One study incorporated 1 year of NDT for children with CP and found significant improvements in spasticity but not muscle strength and gross motor function.[24] From a neurophysiological perspective, this approach can be integrated into a treatment plan depending on how the patient presents in the clinic and whether he/she will benefit from performance of more normalized movement patterns.

Neurofacilitatory Techniques

Proprioceptive neuromuscular facilitation (PNF) is a neurophysiological approach that integrates motor learning and uses different movement patterns with superimposed facilitatory or inhibitory techniques that can help with muscle contraction and relaxation, ROM, and tone reduction. One such technique is *rhythmic rotation* where the limb is slowly rotated out of the spastic pattern (with repetitions as tolerated) up to a point where the therapist notes a limitation. Once the muscles relax, the limb is slowly moved into the new range and the process is repeated. For instance, rhythmic rotation can be used to move the paretic limb from flexed and adducted posture into a weight-bearing position with a focus on elbow extension and wrist and finger extension. A recent systematic review indicated beneficial effects of PNF on poststroke spasticity.[25]

In addition to these traditionally used treatments, several newer interventions can cause a change in spasticity levels. These interventions include the use of noninvasive brain stimulation, virtual reality (VR), constraint-induced movement therapy (CIMT), and robotic rehabilitation.

Virtual Reality

VR technology can help design personalized training environments (virtual environments [VEs]) in which events and objects appear, sound, and feel similar to real-world environments.[26] The use of VEs has been increasing substantially to deliver rehabilitation interventions, with the availability of a variety of options.[27] Intensive and repetitive training delivered using VR technology has been useful to decrease spasticity with large effect sizes in the upper[28] and lower[29] limbs in individuals with stroke. Use of VR should be encouraged if available, given its benefits in increasing motivation and incorporating high-intensity practice.

Constraint-Induced Movement Therapy

CIMT is based on the principle of shaping and involves task performance using the more-affected upper limb. The less-affected side is encased in a mitt, which prevents it from helping in task completion. A recent randomized controlled trial (RCT) reported beneficial effects of CIMT in reducing biceps brachii[30] and knee extensor[31] spasticity. CIMT should be used when possible and has been recommended with highest levels of evidence in available practice guidelines.[32]

Robotics

The use of robotics is also correspondingly increasing in rehabilitation after neurologic injuries. These robots are useful in assisting movements in those with inadequate strength and provide resistance once improvements are noted in muscle strength.[33] There are a variety of robotic devices available for upper and lower limb rehabilitation. Use of robotic devices to help enhance hand functioning led to decreased spasticity in finger flexor muscles (small effect size[34]; in individuals with stroke). Similarly, robotic devices led to decreased plantar flexor spasticity and increase in strength of ankle muscles in children with CP[35] and decreased lower limb spasticity in individuals with MS.[36] Although robotic devices are useful and should be used when available, the high cost does raise questions on feasibility.

Combination Treatments

Given the effects of individual interventions, many studies have tried various combinations of interventions to assess the synergistic effects of these interventions. No significant change in spasticity levels were obtained, when CIMT was combined with action observation therapy in children with CP.[37] Similarly, a recent meta-analysis of two good quality RCTs reported that a combination of CIMT and botulinum toxin injections does not lead to a decrease in upper limb spasticity levels in individuals with stroke.[38] However, provision of 0.7 mA anodal transcranial direct current stimulation (tDCS) followed by CIMT resulted in a significant decrease in poststroke upper limb spasticity.[39] A combination of 2 mA anodal tDCS and VR-based training resulted in more individuals having minimal clinically important difference (MCID) level changes in spasticity for poststroke wrist flexors compared to sham stimulation.[40] Pilot results also support the efficacy of combining focal vibration along with robotic-assisted therapy in decreasing upper limb spasticity in individuals with incomplete SCIs.[41] Although preliminary evidence is encouraging, no definitive suggestions can be made about the use of combination therapies without additional well-designed and adequately powered RCTs.

KEY POINTS

- Spasticity can influence motor functioning and motor learning after a stroke.
- Physical therapists have a wide repertoire of treatments available including traditionally used techniques and emerging innovative combinations of interventions. These treatment techniques can help potentially to manage spasticity and improve functioning.
- Recent advances in research including the use of innovative combinations of interventions have provided interesting results on the effects of these combinations.
- Answers to emergent questions will help more information on the best techniques to manage spasticity and improve the QOL of those afflicted by it.

REFERENCES

1. Finnerup NB. Neuropathic pain and spasticity: intricate consequences of spinal cord injury. *Spinal Cord*. 2017;55(12):1046–1050. https://doi.org.10.1038/sc.2017.70

2. Andresen SR, Biering-Sorensen F, Hagen EM, Nielsen JF, Bach FW, Finnerup NB. Pain, spasticity and quality of life in individuals with traumatic spinal cord injury in Denmark. *Spinal Cord*. 2016;54(11):973–979. https://doi.org.10.1038/sc.2016.46

3. Cheung J, Rancourt A, Di Poce S, et al. Patient-identified factors that influence spasticity in people with stroke and multiple sclerosis receiving botulinum toxin injection treatments. *Physiother Can*. Spring 2015;67(2):157–66 https://doi.org.10.3138/ptc.2014-07

4. Williams PE, Goldspink G. Longitudinal growth of striated muscle fibres. *J Cell Sci*. 1971;9(3):751–67. https://doi.org.10.1242/jcs.9.3.751

5. Kumar S, Yadav R, Aafreen. Comparison between Erigo tilt-table exercise and conventional physiotherapy exercises in acute stroke patients: a randomized trial. *Arch Physiother*. 2020;10:3. https://doi.org.10.1186/s40945-020-0075-2

6. Stevenson V. Rehabilitation in practice: spasticity management. *Clin Rehabil*. 2010;24(4):293–304. https://doi.org.10.1177/0269215509353254

7. Bovend'Eerdt TJ, Newman M, Barker K, Dawes H, Minelli C, Wade DT. The effects of stretching in spasticity: a systematic review. *Arch Phys Med Rehabil*.2008;89(7):1395–406. https://doi.org.10.1016/j.apmr.2008.02.015

8. You YY, Her JG, Woo JH, Ko T, Chung SH. The effects of stretching and stabilization exercise on the improvement of spastic shoulder function in hemiplegic patients. *J Phys Ther Sci*. 2014;26(4):491–5. https://doi.org.10.1589/jpts.26.491

9. Kerr L, Jewell VD, Jensen L. Stretching and splinting interventions for post-stroke spasticity, hand function, and functional tasks: a systematic review. *Am J Occup Ther*. 2020;74(5):7405205050p1–7405205050p15. https://doi.org.10.5014/ajot.2020.029454

10. Subramanian SK, Fountain MK, Hood AF, Verduzco-Gutierrez M. Upper limb motor improvement after traumatic brain injury: systematic review of interventions. *Neurorehabil Neural Repair*. 2022;36(1):17–37. https://doi.org.10.1177/15459683211056662

11. Weiller C, Jüptner M, Fellows S, et al. Brain representation of active and passive movements. *Neuroimage*.1996;4(2):105–10. https://doi.org.10.1006/nimg.1996.0034

12. Mayr A, Kofler M, Saltuari L. ARMOR: an electromechanical robot for upper limb training following stroke. A prospective randomised controlled pilot study. *Handchir Mikrochir Plast Chir*. 2008;40(1):66–73. https://doi.org.10.1055/s-2007-989425

13. Hu XL, Tong KY, Song R, Zheng XJ, Leung WW. A comparison between electromyography-driven robot and passive motion device on wrist rehabilitation for chronic stroke. *Neurorehabil Neural Repair*. 2009;23(8):837–46. https://doi.org.10.1177/1545968309338191

14. Harris JE, Eng JJ. Strength training improves upper-limb function in individuals with stroke: a meta-analysis. *Stroke*. 2010;41(1):136–40. https://doi.org.10.1161/STROKEAHA.109.567438

15. Veldema J, Jansen P. Resistance training in stroke rehabilitation: systematic review and meta-analysis. *Clin Rehabil*. 2020;34(9):1173–1197. https://doi.org.10.1177/0269215520932964

16. Merino-Andres J, Garcia de Mateos-Lopez A, Damiano DL, Sanchez-Sierra A. Effect of muscle strength training in children and adolescents with spastic cerebral palsy: a systematic review and meta-analysis. *Clin Rehabil*. 2022;36(1):4–14. https://doi.org.10.1177/02692155211040199

17. Ginis KA, Hicks AL, Latimer AE, et al. The development of evidence-informed physical activity guidelines for adults with spinal cord injury. *Spinal Cord*. 2011;49(11):1088–96. https://doi.org.10.1038/sc.2011.63

18. Luft AR, Macko RF, Forrester LW, et al. Treadmill exercise activates subcortical neural networks and improves walking after stroke: a randomized controlled trial. *Stroke*. 2008;39(12):3341–50. https://doi.org.10.1161/STROKEAHA.108.527531

19. Adar S, Dündar Ü, Demirdal Ü S, Ulaşlı AM, Toktaş H, Solak Ö. The effect of aquatic exercise on spasticity, quality of life, and motor function in cerebral palsy. *Turk J Phys Med Rehabil*. 2017;63(3):239–248. https://doi.org.10.5606/tftrd.2017.280

20. Ko H-Y, Huh S. Spasticity. *Handbook of Spinal Cord Injuries and Related Disorders: A Guide to Evaluation and Management*. Springer Singapore; 2021:467–482.

21. Kumaran B. Superficial heating. In: Watson T, Nussbaum T, eds. *Electrophysical Agents Evidence-based Practice*. 7th ed. Elsevier; 2020:118–131.

22. Mahmood A, Veluswamy SK, Hombali A, Mullick A, Natarajan M, Solomon JM. Effect of transcutaneous electrical nerve stimulation on spasticity in adults with stroke: a systematic review and meta-analysis. *Arch Phys Med Rehabil*. 2019;100(4):751–768. https://doi.org.10.1016/j.apmr.2018.10.016

23. Barbosa P, Glinsky JV, Fachin-Martins E, Harvey LA. Physiotherapy interventions for the treatment of spasticity in people with spinal cord injury: a systematic review. *Spinal Cord*. 2021;59(3):236–247. https://doi.org.10.1038/s41393-020-00610-4

24. Park EY, Kim WH. Effect of neurodevelopmental treatment-based physical therapy on the change of muscle strength, spasticity, and gross motor function in children with spastic cerebral palsy. *J Phys Ther Sci*. 2017;29(6):966–969. https://doi.org.10.1589/jpts.29.966

25. Alashram AR, Alghwiri AA, Padua E, Annino G. Efficacy of proprioceptive neuromuscular facilitation on spasticity in patients with stroke: a systematic review. *Phys Ther Rev*. 2021;26(3):168–76. htps://doi,org,10.1136/bmjopen-2017-016739

26. Weiss PL, Kizony R, Feintuch U, Katz N. Virtual reality in neurorehabilitation. In: Selzer M, Clarke S, Cohen L, Duncan P, Gage F, eds. *Textbook of Neural Repair and Rehabilitation*. Cambridge University Press; 2006:182–97.

27. Subramanian SK, Cross MK, Hirschhauser CS. Virtual reality interventions to enhance upper limb motor improvement after a stroke: commonly used types of platform and outcomes. *Disabil Rehabil Assist Technol*. 2022;17(1):107–115. https://doi.org.10.1080/17483107.2020.1765422

28. Abd El-Kafy EM, Alshehri MA, El-Fiky AA-R, Guermazi MA, Mahmoud HM. The effect of robot-mediated virtual reality gaming on upper limb spasticity poststroke: a randomized-controlled trial. *Games Health J*. 2022;11(2):93–103. https://doi.org.10.1089/g4h. 2021.0197

29. Luque-Moreno C, Cano-Bravo F, Kiper P, et al. Reinforced feedback in virtual environment for plantar flexor poststroke spasticity reduction and gait function improvement. *BioMed Res Int*. 2019;2019:6295263. https://doi.org. 10.1155/2019/6295263.

30. Rocha LSO, Gama GCB, Rocha RSB, et al. Constraint induced movement therapy increases functionality and quality of life after stroke. *J Stroke Cerebrovasc Dis*. 2021; 30(6):105774. https://doi.org. 10.1016/j.jstrokecerebrovasdis.2021.105774.

31. Abdullahi A, Aliyu NU, Useh U, et al. Comparing two different modes of task practice during lower limb constraint-induced movement therapy in people with stroke: A randomized clinical trial. *Neural Plast*. 2021;2021:6664058. https://doi.org.10.1155/2021/6664058

32. Hebert D, Lindsay MP, McIntyre A, et al. Canadian stroke best practice recommendations: stroke rehabilitation practice guidelines, update 2015. *Int J Stroke*. 2016;11(4): 459–484. https://doi.org.10.1177/1747493016643553.

33. Gassert R, Dietz V. Rehabilitation robots for the treatment of sensorimotor deficits: a neurophysiological perspective. *J Neuroeng Rehabil*. 2018;15(1):46. https://doi.org.10.1186/s12984-018-0383-x

34. Zhao M, Wang G, Wang A, Cheng LJ, Lau Y. Robot-assisted distal training improves upper limb dexterity and function after stroke: a systematic review and meta-regression. *Neurol Sci*. 2022;43(3):1641–1657. https://doi.org.10.1007/s10072-022-05913-3

35. Coley C, Kovelman S, Belschner J, et al. PedBotHome: A video game-based robotic ankle device created for home exercise in children with neurological impairments. *Pediatr Phys Ther*. 2022;34(2):212–219. https://doi.org.10.1097/pep.0000000000000881

36. Calabrò RS, Cassio A, Mazzoli D, et al. What does evidence tell us about the use of gait robotic devices in patients with multiple sclerosis? a comprehensive systematic review on functional outcomes and clinical recommendations. *Eur J Phys Rehabil Med*. 2021;57(5):841–849. https://doi.org.10.23736/s1973-9087.21.06915-x

37. Simon-Martinez C, Mailleux L, Jaspers E, et al. Effects of combining constraint-induced movement therapy and action-observation training on upper limb kinematics in children with unilateral cerebral palsy: a randomized controlled trial. *Sci Rep*. 2020;10(1):1–15. https://doi.org.10.1038/s41598-020-67427-2.

38. Nasb M, Shah SZA, Chen H, et al. Constraint-Induced Movement Therapy combined with botulinum toxin for post-stroke spasticity: a systematic review and meta-analysis. *Cureus*. 2021;13(9):e17645. https://doi.org.10.7759/cureus.17645

39. Andrade SM, Batista LM, Nogueira LLRF, et al. Constraint-induced movement therapy combined with transcranial direct current stimulation over premotor cortex improves motor function in severe stroke: a pilot randomized controlled trial. *Rehab Res Pract*. 2017;2017:6842549.https://doi.org.10.1155/2017/6842549

40. Viana RT, Laurentino GE, Souza RJ, et al. Effects of the addition of transcranial direct current stimulation to virtual reality therapy after stroke: a pilot randomized controlled trial. *NeuroRehabilitation*. 2014;34(3):437–46. https://doi.org.10.3233/NRE-141065

41. Vojinovic TJ, Linley E, Zivanovic A, Loureiro CR. Effects of focal vibration and robotic assistive therapy on upper limb spasticity in incomplete spinal cord injury. *Proc Int Conf on Rehab Robotics*, IEEE; 2019:542–547. https://doi.org. 10.1109/ICORR.2019.8779566

8 Pharmacologic Treatments

Sindhoori Nalla and Thomas Watanabe

INTRODUCTION

The treatment of spasticity as a result of upper motor neuron syndrome (UMNS) requires a multifaceted thought process and approach. While there are a variety of different oral pharmacologic treatment options available for the management of spasticity, it is imperative to consider the indications, risk versus benefit profile, and adjunctive treatment options to use in conjunction with oral medications.

As detailed in prior chapters, one must appropriately assess spasticity (and more broadly, the UMNS) in a patient and how it affects an individual's function, range of motion (ROM), hygiene, pain, and caregiver burden. Spasticity can be beneficial in maintaining muscle mass, assisting with transfers and function, increasing venous blood flow, and assisting with bowel and bladder functioning.[1]

Oral medications are commonly initiated prior to trialing more invasive spasticity management. Traditionally, oral pharmacologic medications are thought to be more useful in treating spasticity of spinal origin compared to cerebral origin, although they are widely used in a variety of clinical spasticity presentations.[2,3] Systemic pharmacologic management is also usually considered when spasticity is more generalized.

This chapter highlights the various oral pharmacologic medications used to treat spasticity and the different factors, including indications to treat, side effect profile, and evidence of efficacy, to consider when deciding on the most appropriate medication for each patient's clinical presentation and treatment goals. Common medications are outlined in Table 8.1. Selected less common oral medications used to treat spasticity are highlighted in Table 8.2.

PHARMACOLOGIC TREATMENTS

Baclofen

Mechanism of Action

- It is a GABA-B agonist that crosses the blood–brain barrier and acts on both presynaptic and postsynaptic GABA-B receptors in the central nervous system (CNS), including at the levels of the dorsal horn of the spinal cord and brainstem.[14–18]
- Its activity on GABA-B receptors causes membrane hyperpolarization and restriction of calcium influx, resulting in inhibition of monosynaptic and polysynaptic

Table 8.1 Common Oral Pharmacologic Agents

Medication	Mechanism of Action	Dosing Recommendations[4-7]	Common Side Effects	Additional Comments
Baclofen	• GABA-B agonist • Acts on presynaptic and postsynaptic GABA-B receptors to inhibit excitatory neurotransmitter release	Initial: 5 mg TID Max: 80 mg/day	Sedation, confusion, fatigue, dizziness, hepatotoxicity, muscle weakness	Avoid abrupt withdrawal due to risk of withdrawal-related seizures
Tizanidine	• Centrally acting selective alpha-2 adrenergic agonist and imidazole agonist • Inhibits presynaptic excitatory neurotransmitter release	Initial: 2 mg TID Max: 36 mg/day	Sedation, dizziness, hepatotoxicity, hypotension, xerostomia	Recommended to monitor LFTs due to potential for transaminitis
Dantrolene	• Peripherally acting, direct skeletal muscle relaxant • Inhibits calcium release from the sarcoplasmic reticulum, resulting in uncoupling of electrical excitation and inhibition of skeletal muscle contraction	Initial: 25 mg 1–3 times/day Max: 400 mg/day	Hepatotoxicity, generalized weakness	Less concern for cognitive impairment or sedation due to peripherally acting mechanism Can be particularly useful in treating clonus
Diazepam	• CNS depressant with postsynaptic GABA-A receptor effects • Promotes GABA release, which inhibits activity in descending lateral and ascending reticular system	Initial: 2 mg BID or 5 mg qHS Max: 40–60 mg/day	Fatigue, sedation, impaired coordination, confusion, memory impairment, paradoxical agitation, potential for dependence/abuse	Abrupt withdrawal may result in tremors, nausea, irritability, and seizures
Clonidine	• Centrally acting alpha-2 agonist and imidazole agonist • Inhibits presynaptic sensory afferent transmission	Initial: 0.1 mg BID Max: 2.4 mg/day	Hypotension, bradycardia, drowsiness, dry mouth, edema, and depression	Has alpha-1 agonist properties that can result in hypotension

Table 8.2 Less Commonly Used Oral Pharmacologic Agents

Medication	Mechanism of Action	Dosing Recommendations[8–13]	Common Side Effects	Additional Comments
Cyclobenzaprine	• Centrally acting muscle relaxant • Reduces somatic motor activity through influence on the serotonin system	Initial: 5 mg prn (1–3 times daily) Max: 10 mg TID	Somnolence	Risk of serotonin syndrome has been documented in literature
Cyproheptadine	• Anticholinergic and antihistamine agent • Acts as a serotonin receptor blocker	Initial: 2–4 mg TID Max: 8 mg TID	Sedation, weight gain	May help improve clonus
Gabapentin	• Structurally similar to GABA • Acts as a calcium channel blocker	Initial: 100–300 mg 1–3 times daily Max: 1.2–2.4 g/day in divided doses	Sedation, dizziness, ataxia, headache, nystagmus, tremor, and nausea/vomiting	Adjunct to first-line treatment; useful for patients with neuropathic pain
Cannabinoids	• Act on the CB-1 and CB-2 cannabinoid receptors • Effect on CB-1 receptors results in inhibition of neurotransmitter release and reduction in spasticity	Variable dosing depending on formulation	Heightened psychiatric symptoms, euphoria, dizziness, diarrhea, difficulty concentrating, xerostomia	Most studied in the multiple sclerosis population
Riluzole	• Glutaminergic modulating medication, thought to block sodium channels and reduce glutamate release	Varies based on drug interactions and comorbidities	Nausea, headache, dizziness, decreased lung function, drowsiness, abdominal pain	Neuroprotective in spinal cord injury

(continued)

Table 8.2 Less Commonly Used Oral Pharmacologic Agents (*continued*)

Medication	Mechanism of Action	Dosing Recommendations[8-13]	Common Side Effects	Additional Comments
Modafinil	• Centrally acting stimulant that acts on the brainstem and works as a dopamine reuptake inhibitor	Initial: 100 mg/daily Max: 400 mg/day divided into two doses	Headache, nausea, decreased appetite, anxiety, insomnia, diarrhea, dizziness	Studied primarily in pediatric population; may help improve Modified Ashworth Scale scores and gait speed in patients with cerebral palsy
Glycine	• Amino acid that crosses blood–brain barrier and has inhibitory effects on neurons in the central nervous system	3–4 g/day	Typically well tolerated as a supplement	Limited human studies; may be more beneficial in spasticity of spinal origin

spinal reflexes that facilitate spasticity and inhibition of endogenous excitatory neurotransmitter release.[14,18–20]

- The summative effect of the above is reduction in the overactive reflex response to muscle stretch.
- Note: Efficacy may be limited at lower doses due to inadequate penetration of the blood–brain barrier and may require titration of dose until intended effects are seen.[21]

Indications

- It is commonly used as an initial pharmacologic treatment option for spasticity. It is most heavily studied in spinal cord injury (SCI) and multiple sclerosis (MS) populations, and it is considered a first-line treatment in these population groups.[4]
- Although it may still be commonly used as an initial treatment option in the brain injury and stroke populations, it has been less formally studied in these groups.
- It can also be administered intrathecally.

Common Adverse Effects

- Sedation, confusion, fatigue, dizziness, hepatotoxicity, and muscle weakness.[22–25]
- Use with caution in patients with brain injury due to its potential cognitive effects in brain recovery.[14]
- Avoid abrupt medication withdrawal as this may result in withdrawal-related seizures.[26,27]

Tizanidine

Mechanism of Action

- It is a selective alpha-2 adrenergic agonist and imidazole agonist with centrally acting properties similar to clonidine.[28]
- Its activity on alpha-2 receptors causes presynaptic inhibition of excitatory neurotransmitter (glutamate and aspartate) release from spinal interneurons.[14,4]
- It also has effects at the supraspinal level, inhibiting activity in the locus coeruleus and resulting in inhibition of facilitation of the descending cerebrospinal tract.[29]
- It does not have effects at the levels of the neuromuscular junction, monosynaptic reflexes, or skeletal muscle fibers and, as such, does not result in muscle weakness to the same degree as other oral antispasticity agents.[29–35]
- Some studies have shown increases in strength as a result of central relaxation within opposing musculature.[32]
- The half-life of tizanidine is about 2 to 4 hours, thus requiring frequent dosing (every 6–8 hours) to maintain effectiveness.[36,37]

Indications

- It is typically used for spasticity in the SCI, traumatic brain injury (TBI), MS, stroke, and cerebral palsy (CP) populations. Several randomized controlled trials have highlighted its efficacy in decreasing Modified Ashworth scores in these populations.[32–34,38]
- It can be used in conjunction with medications such as baclofen, for additive antispasticity benefits.[39]

Common Adverse Effects

- Sedation, dizziness, hepatotoxicity, hypotension, xerostomia, and, to a lesser extent, hallucinations, nightmares, QT prolongation, and constipation.[4,32–34,36,39,40]
- It is imperative to check liver enzymes at medication initiation and at periodic time intervals afterward, especially when titrating the dose.[28]
- Given its receptor selectivity, it has a relatively lower effect in decreasing blood pressure and heart rate when compared to clonidine.[30]

Dantrolene

Mechanism of Action

- It is a peripherally acting, direct skeletal muscle relaxant that inhibits calcium release from the sarcoplasmic reticulum by acting on the ryanodine receptors.[41]
- Inhibition of calcium results in uncoupling of electrical excitation and inhibition of skeletal muscle contraction.[42]

Indications

- Because dantrolene is peripherally acting, it has a significant benefit of not contributing to cognitive impairment or sedation. It can be considered a first-line oral pharmacologic agent for the treatment of spasticity in the TBI population for this reason.[43]
- Conversely, given its direct effect at the muscle level resulting in general weakness, it should be used judiciously in populations of patients with spinal spasticity and it should be avoided in patients with MS, particularly in those with bulbar and respiratory symptoms.[43–47]
- It can be a useful medication to aid in the treatment of clonus.[47–50]
- It can also be utilized as an adjunctive treatment to other oral pharmacologic agents.[4]

Common Adverse Effects

- The most significant and concerning side effect of dantrolene is hepatotoxicity. It is imperative to monitor liver function tests (LFTs) every week for the first month after initiating treatment and then periodically afterward.[21]
- As stated above, another important side effect to be aware of is generalized weakness due to its direct effect on the muscles.[22]

Benzodiazepines

Mechanism of Action

- It is a CNS depressant that hase postsynaptic effects on the GABA-A receptors, promoting GABA release through facilitation of sodium.[21,51–54]
- The release of GABA, in turn, presynaptically inhibits activity in the descending lateral and ascending reticular system.[1]

Indications

- While all benzodiazepines can in theory be effective in targeting spasticity, diazepam and clonazepam are most commonly used in the management of spasticity.[51,55]

- Diazepam is more commonly utilized in the adult spasticity population and clonazepam in the pediatric spasticity population, but they can both be used across the span of age groups.[1]
- Many clinical trials highlight the benefit of diazepam in the MS population as well as the CP population, especially in the context of pain-related spasticity.[48,56–61] Data are available to a lesser extent in the SCI population, although it is still used frequently.
- Diazepam may have a greater primary effect on flexor hypertonia compared to extensor tone, and with spinal spasticity commonly affecting flexor reflexes, this medication may serve more useful in spasticity of spinal origin compared to cerebral origin.[62]
- There are only a handful of studies with small sample sizes in the stroke population, but it has been found to be effective for this diagnosis.[58,63–66]
- It shows less evidence for clonazepam use and is primarily focused on the MS and pediatric CP populations.[67,68]

Common Adverse Effects

- Fatigue, sedation, impaired coordination, confusion, memory impairment, paradoxical agitation, and potential for physical and psychological dependence/abuse.[24,27,51,52,55,66,69,70]
- Use with caution in the geriatric and brain injury/stroke populations.[53]
- Sedative effects may prove to be useful when dosing the medication at night, particularly in cases where spasticity results in pain and difficulty sleeping.[21]
- Caution should be taken to avoid abrupt withdrawal as this may result in tremors, nausea, irritability, and seizures.[51,55]

Clonidine
Mechanism of Action

- It is a centrally acting alpha-2 agonist and imidazole agonist that acts in the CNS at both the spinal cord level and the locus coeruleus.[4,28] It inhibits presynaptic sensory afferent transmission, reducing spasticity.[71,72]
- Also, it acts as an alpha-1 agonist, which is an important detail to consider when weighing its side effect profile.[28,73]

Indications

- Because of its effects at the spinal cord level, as well as the centrally acting nature of its mechanism of action, its use is typically seen more in the SCI population.[28,72,74–76]
- This can be particularly useful in people with SCI with hypertension, especially those with incomplete injuries, as it has additional effects in reducing blood pressure through its alpha-1 agonist activity.[71]

Common Adverse Effects

- Hypotension, bradycardia, drowsiness, dry mouth, edema, and depression.[28,77]
- Hypotensive effects are less likely to impact patients with complete SCI.[78,79]
- It may adversely affect motor recovery in the brain injury population due to centrally acting properties and should thus be used with caution.[80]

Cyclobenzaprine

Mechanism of Action

- It is a centrally acting muscle relaxant with a primary mechanism of action targeting the brainstem rather than the spinal cord.[81]
- It reduces somatic motor activity through influence on the serotonin system.[81]

Indications

- While there are not specific studies highlighting its use on spasticity itself, it can be used as an adjunctive treatment for pain and muscle spasms as a result of spasticity.[81]

Common Adverse Effects

- The most limiting side effect is somnolence.[81]
- Given its effects on the serotonin system, it is important to be aware of its possible interactions with serotonin agonists, and there are some case reports in literature documenting its association with serotonin syndrome.[81]

Cyproheptadine

Mechanism of Action

- It is an anticholinergic and antihistamine agent that acts as a serotonin receptor blocker.
- It was traditionally utilized for treatment of serotonin syndrome, vascular headaches, anorexia, and hives.[82] Studies, though limited, later showed its effect on spasticity.[83–86]

Indications

- It has been found in some studies to improve ankle clonus in MS and SCI, as well as walking speed in people with SCI.[84–85]
- A study comparing cyproheptadine, clonidine, and baclofen showed that cyproheptadine was superior to clonidine and equal to baclofen when evaluating spasticity in patients based on pendulum test and Ashworth Scale.[85]

Common Adverse Effects

- Sedation and weight gain.[28]

Gabapentin

Mechanism of Action

- It is an anticonvulsant medication structurally similar to GABA but does not bind to GABA receptors or convert into GABA itself.[62,87,88]
- While the specific mechanism of action is not clearly known, it is thought to act similarly to a calcium channel blocker.[21,89]

Indications

- It is typically used as an adjunct to first-line oral pharmacologic spasticity treatments.[77] It is more specifically utilized when a patient has complaints of neuropathic pain in addition to spasticity.[24]

- There are some studies documenting effectiveness in treating spasticity particularly of spinal origin when assessing reduction in Ashworth score; however, results appear to be marginal in the said studies.[90–93]

Common Adverse Effects

- Sedation, dizziness, ataxia, headache, nystagmus, tremor, and nausea/vomiting.[51,62,94,95]
- Because it is renally excreted, caution must be taken for patients with renal impairment.[89,94,96]

Cannabinoids

Mechanism of Action

- While its mechanism of action is not completely understood, it is thought to act on the CB-1 (found in the CNS) and CB-2 (more widely distributed through the body) cannabinoid receptors.
- Its effects on the CB-1 receptors result in inhibition of neurotransmitter release and thus reduction in spasticity.[97]

Indications

- The use of cannabinoids in spasticity has been a topic of growing interest in the recent years, with most research studies focused on the MS population.[98]
- Various forms can be utilized for the treatment of spasticity, including dronabinol, delta-9-tetrahydrocannabinol (THC), cannabidiol (CBD), and nabilone, among other synthetic derivatives.[82, 98]
- Studies have shown that it may aid in slowing the progression of MS through its anti-inflammatory effects and in some cases can improve spastic neurogenic bladder-related symptoms in this population.[99,100]
- Its use can be considered as an adjunctive treatment for patients with severe spasticity that is uncontrolled on medications such as baclofen and tizanidine.[101]

Common Adverse Effects

- It is generally well tolerated in its use for spasticity, but effects of THC on the more widespread CB-2 receptors can result in heightened psychiatric symptoms such as anxiety and psychosis in some patients.[102] This adverse effect can be reduced by combining THC treatment with CBD.[103]
- Other adverse effects include dizziness, euphoria, diarrhea, difficulty concentrating, and xerostomia.[104]

Other Pharmacologic Options

Other systemic medication options to consider in the treatment of spasticity include riluzole, modafinil, and glycine.

Riluzole

- It is a glutaminergic modulating medication that can be used particularly in the SCI population. While its mechanism of action is not completely understood, it is known to block sodium channels that play a role in emergence of spastic reflexes, and is also thought to reduce glutamate release, which can further reduce spasticity and serve as neuroprotection in SCI.[105–107]

- Studies have shown decrease in spastic reflexes, improvement in motor function, and decreased nociception in patients with SCI.[105]
- Adverse effects include nausea, headache, dizziness, decreased lung function, drowsiness, and abdominal pain.[108]

Modafinil

- It is a centrally acting stimulant that works as a dopamine reuptake inhibitor.[8,109,110]
- While it is traditionally used in the treatment of narcolepsy, shift work sleep disorder, obstructive sleep apnea, and other arousal-related conditions, some studies have shown improvement in Modified Ashworth Scale (MAS) scores and gait speed in patients with CP.[109,110]
- Mechanism of action related to its spasticity effects are not clear, but it is thought that its centrally acting effects on the brainstem play a role.[8]
- Adverse effects include headache, nausea, decreased appetite, anxiety, insomnia, diarrhea, and dizziness.[8]

Glycine

- It is an amino acid that crosses the blood–brain barrier and has inhibitory effects on neurons in the CNS.[23]
- It is thought that reduced levels of glycine results in decreased neuronal inhibition, which in turns contributes to the clinical presentation of spasticity.[111]
- There are a few animal and limited human case studies in literature showing that administration of glycine may help improve measures of spasticity of spinal origin.[111,112]
- Its use as a supplement is typically well tolerated at doses of 3 g to 5 g daily.[9]

Treatment Considerations

As highlighted, there are numerous oral pharmacologic agents that can be used in the treatment of spasticity. A multitude of factors, including origin of neurologic injury, patient comorbidities, goals for treatment, and clinical presentation of spasticity, must be taken into consideration when determining the appropriate medication to initiate.

The majority of the oral medications listed above were initially designated to treat spasticity of spinal origin, but over time, treatment approaches with these medications have been adapted to account for patient profile as well as side effect implications. The centrally acting nature and associated cognitive impairments of many of these pharmacologic agents should be taken into consideration when deciding on a medication for spasticity management, particularly in the brain injury and stroke populations. This is particularly important in the initial few months of recovery, as certain medications and their associated side effects may contribute to inhibiting neurologic recovery.[80,113–115]

In patients with cerebral origins of spasticity, particularly after TBI, it is reasonable to start with dantrolene as a first-line agent given its peripherally acting mechanism of action directly at the muscle level, thus limiting the concern for cognitive effects. As previously mentioned, its potential for hepatoxicity requires cautious monitoring, especially if patients are already on other hepatically metabolized medications including antiepileptics such as valproic acid or phenytoin, which may increase the hepatic load systemically.[116] Other medications to consider in brain injury and stroke patients include baclofen and tizanidine. Some research indicates that baclofen may

Table 8.3 Common Oral Pharmacologic Medications by Diagnosis

Diagnosis	Medications (Studies)
Traumatic Brain Injury	Dantrolene (*Zafonte et al.*[43]) Baclofen (*Maythaler et al.*[119]) Tizanidine (*Meythaler et al.*[32])
Stroke	Baclofen (*Medaer et al.*[120]) Tizanidine (*Maupas et al.*[121]; *Gelber et al.*[122])
Spinal Cord Injury	Baclofen (*Duncan et al.*[123]) Tizanidine (*Nance*[86]; *Taricco et al.*[124]) Benzodiazepines (*Corbett et al.*[125]) Clonidine (*Maynard*[76]; *Nance et al.*[71]; *Donovan et al.*[75]) Gabapentin (*Gruenthal et al.*[92]) Cannabinoids (*Hagenbach et al.*[126])
Multiple Sclerosis	Baclofen (*Brar et al.*[127]; *Duncan et al.*[123]; *Sawa and Paty*[59]) Tizanidine (*UK Tizanidine Trial Group*[128]) Benzodiazepines (*Cendrowski and Sobczyk*[67]; *Wilson and McKechnie*[57]) Cannabinoids (*Wade et al.*[129]; *Collin et al.*[100]; *Ungerleider et al.*[130]) Gabapentin (*Mueller et al.*[90]; *Cutter et al.*[91]) Cyproheptadine (*Barbeau et al.*[84])
Cerebral Palsy	Baclofen (*Milla and Jackson*[131]; *Scheinberg et al.*[102]) Tizanidine (*Vasquez-Briceno et al.*[132]) Benzodiazepines (*Dahlin et al.*[68]; *Matthew et al.*[133]) Dantrolene (*Denhoff et al.*[46])
Spastic Hemiplegia	Gabapentin (*Scheuer et al.*[134])

be particularly useful in predominantly lower limb spasticity, whereas tizanidine may be more useful in predominantly upper limb spasticity.[117,118]

In patients with spinal origins of spasticity, it is reasonable to consider baclofen or benzodiazepines as first-line agents for treatment.[1] Table 8.3 highlights various oral pharmacologic options that may be used for a given diagnosis related to spasticity.

KEY POINTS

- Oral medications are commonly initiated prior to trialing more invasive spasticity management.
- Oral pharmacologic medications are thought to be more useful in treating spasticity of spinal origin compared to cerebral origin but are commonly used across all etiologies of spasticity.
- Consideration must be made for origin of neurologic injury, patient comorbidities, goals for treatment, and clinical presentation of spasticity when selecting oral medications.

REFERENCES

1. Meythaler J, Smith R. Pharmacologic management of spasticity: oral medications. In: Brashear A, ed. *Spasticity Diagnosis and Management*. 2nd ed. Demos Medical Publishing, LLC; 2016:251–285.

2. Katz RT, Rymer WZ. Spastic hypertonia: mechanisms and measurement. *Arch Phys Med Rehabil.* 1989;70(2):144–155.

3. Katz RT. Management of spasticity. *Am J Phys Med Rehabil.* 1988;67(3):108–116. https://doi.org/10.1097/00002060-198806000-00004

4. Ripley DL, Driver S, Stork R, Maneyapanda M. Pharmacologic management of the patient with traumatic brain injury. In: *Rehabilitation After Traumatic Brain Injury.* Elsevier; 2019:133–163. https://doi.org/10.1016/B978-0-323-54456-6.00011-6

5. Lexicomp. *Dantrolene: Drug Information.* UpToDate.

6. Lexicomp. *Diazepam: Drug information.* UpToDate.

7. Lexicomp. *Clonidine: Drug Information.* UpToDate.

8. Greenblatt K, Adams N. *Modafinil*; 2022.

9. Hall P V., Smith JE, Lane J, Mote T, Campbell R. Glycine and experimental spinal spasticity. *Neurology.* 1979;29(2):262–262. https://doi.org/10.1212/WNL.29.2.262

10. Lexicomp. *Cyclobenzaprine: Drug Information.* UpToDate.

11. Lexicomp. *Cyproheptadine: Drug Information.* UpToDate.

12. Lexicomp. *Gabapentin.* UpToDate.

13. Lexicomp. *Riluzole: Drug Information.* UpToDate.

14. Simon O, Yelnik AP. Managing spasticity with drugs. *Eur J Phys Rehabil Med.* 2010;46(3):401–410.

15. Terrence CF, Fromm GH. Complications of baclofen withdrawal. *Arch Neurol.* 1981;38(9):588–589. https://doi.org/10.1001/archneur.1981.00510090082011

16. Wilson PR, Yaksh TL. Baclofen is antinociceptive in the spinal intrathecal space of animals. *Eur J Pharmacol.* 1978;51(4):323–330. https://doi.org/10.1016/0014-2999(78)90423-5

17. Yaksh TL, Reddy SV. Studies in the primate on the analgetic effects associated with intrathecal actions of opiates, alpha-adrenergic agonists and baclofen. *Anesthesiology.* 1981;54(6):451–467. https://doi.org/10.1097/00000542-198106000-00004

18. Awaad Y, Rizk T, Siddiqui I, Roosen N, McIntosh K, Waines GM. Complications of intrathecal baclofen pump: prevention and cure. *ISRN Neurol.* 2012;2012:575168. https://doi.org/10.5402/2012/575168

19. Kheder A, Nair KPS. Spasticity: pathophysiology, evaluation and management. *Pract Neurol.* 2012;12(5):289–298. https://doi.org/10.1136/practneurol-2011-000155

20. Eisenberg M, Jasey N. Spasticity and muscle overactivity as components of the upper motor neuron syndrome. In: Frontera W, ed. *Delisa's Physical Medicine & Rehabilitation.* Vol 5. Lippincott Williams & Wilkins; 2010.

21. Chang E, Ghosh N, Yanni D, Lee S, Alexandru D, Mozaffar T. A review of spasticity treatments: pharmacological and interventional approaches. *Crit Rev Phys Rehabil Med.* 25(1-2):11–22. https://doi.org/10.1615/CritRevPhysRehabilMed.2013007945

22. Chou R, Peterson K, Helfand M. Comparative efficacy and safety of skeletal muscle relaxants for spasticity and musculoskeletal conditions: a systematic review. *J Pain Symptom Manage.* 2004;28(2):140–175. https://doi.org/10.1016/j.jpainsymman.2004.05.002

23. Abbruzzese G. The medical management of spasticity. *Eur J Neurol.* 2002;9 Suppl 1:30–34; discussion 53–61. https://doi.org/10.1046/j.1468-1331.2002.0090s1030.x

24. Keenan E. Spasticity management, part 2: choosing the right medication to suit the individual. *Br J Neurosci Nurs.* 2009;5(9):419–424. https://doi.org/10.12968/bjnn.2009.5.9.44099

25. Dario A, Tomei G. A benefit-risk assessment of baclofen in severe spinal spasticity. *Drug Saf.* 2004;27(11):799–818. https://doi.org/10.2165/00002018-200427110-00004

26. Kofter M, Leis AA. Prolonged seizure activity after baclofen withdrawal. *Neurology.* 1992;42(3):697. https://doi.org/10.1212/WNL.42.3.697

27. Verrotti A, Greco R, Spalice A, Chiarelli F, Iannetti P. Pharmacotherapy of spasticity in children with cerebral palsy. *Pediatr Neurol.* 2006;31(1).1–6. https://doi.org/10.1016/j.pediatrneurol.2005.05.001

28. Nance PW. Alpha adrenergic and serotonergic agents in the treatment of spastic hypertonia. *Phys Med Rehabil Clin N Am.* 2001;12(4):889–905.

29. Honda M, Sekiguchi Y, Sato N, Ono H. Involvement of imidazoline receptors in the centrally acting muscle-relaxant effects of tizanidine. *Eur J Pharmacol.* 2002;445(3):187–193. https://doi.org/10.1016/s0014-2999(02)01664-3

30. Coward DM. Tizanidine: neuropharmacology and mechanism of action. *Neurology.* 1994;44(11 Suppl 9):S6–10; discussion S10-1.

31. Wallace JD. Summary of combined clinical analysis of controlled clinical trials with tizanidine. *Neurology.* 1994;44(11 Suppl 9):S60–8; discussion S68-9.

32. Meythaler JM, Guin-Renfroe S, Johnson A, Brunner RM. Prospective assessment of tizanidine for spasticity due to acquired brain injury. *Arch Phys Med Rehabil.* 2001;82(9):1155–1163. https://doi.org/10.1053/apmr.2001.25141

33. Nance PW, Bugaresti J, Shellenberger K, Sheremata W, Martinez-Arizala A. Efficacy and safety of tizanidine in the treatment of spasticity in patients with spinal cord injury. North American Tizanidine Study Group. *Neurology.* 1994;44(11 Suppl 9):S44–51; discussion S51–2.

34. Smith C, Birnbaum G, Carter JL, Greenstein J, Lublin FD. Tizanidine treatment of spasticity caused by multiple sclerosis: results of a double-blind, placebo-controlled trial. US Tizanidine Study Group. *Neurology.* 1994;44(11 Suppl 9):S34–42; discussion S42–3.

35. Kamen L, Henney HR, Runyan JD. A practical overview of tizanidine use for spasticity secondary to multiple sclerosis, stroke, and spinal cord injury. *Curr Med Res Opin.* 2008;24(2):425–439. https://doi.org/10.1185/030079908x261113

36. Wagstaff AJ, Bryson HM. Tizanidine. A review of its pharmacology, clinical efficacy and tolerability in the management of spasticity associated with cerebral and spinal disorders. *Drugs.* 1997;53(3):435–452. https://doi.org/10.2165/00003495-199753030-00007

37. Stevenson V, Playford D. Neurological rehabilitation and the management of spasticity. *Medicine (Baltimore).* 2012;40(9):513–517. https://doi.org/10.1016/j.mpmed.2012.06.008

38. Medici M, Pebet M, Ciblis D. A double-blind, long-term study of tizanidine ('Sirdalud') in spasticity due to cerebrovascular lesions. *Curr Med Res Opin.* 1989;11(6):398–407. https://doi.org/10.1185/03007998909110141

39. Lance JW. What is spasticity? *Lancet (London, England).* 1990;335(8689):606. https://doi.org/10.1016/0140-6736(90)90389-m

40. Halpern R, Gillard P, Graham GD, Varon SF, Zorowitz RD. Adherence associated with oral medications in the treatment of spasticity. *PM R.* 2013;5(9):747–756. https://doi.org/10.1016/j.pmrj.2013.04.022

41. Krause T, Gerbershagen MU, Fiege M, Weisshorn R, Wappler F. Dantrolene—a review of its pharmacology, therapeutic use and new developments. *Anaesthesia.* 2004;59(4):364–373. https://doi.org/10.1111/j.1365-2044.2004.03658.x

42. Tilton A, Vargus-Adams J, Delgado MR. Pharmacologic treatment of spasticity in children. *Semin Pediatr Neurol.* 2010;17(4):261–267. https://doi.org/10.1016/j.spen.2010.10.009

43. Zafonte R, Elovic EP, Lombard L. Acute care management of post-TBI spasticity. *J Head Trauma Rehabil.* 19(2):89–100. https://doi.org/10.1097/00001199-200403000-00002

44. Ketel WB, Kolb ME. Long-term treatment with dantrolene sodium of stroke patients with spasticity limiting the return of function. *Curr Med Res Opin.* 1984;9(3):161–169. https://doi.org/10.1185/03007998409109576

45. Weiser R, Terenty T, Hudgson P, Weightman D. Dantrolene sodium in the treatment of spasticity in chronic spinal cord disease. *Practitioner.* 1978;221(1321):123–127.

46. Denhoff E, Feldman S, Smith MG, Litchman H, Holden W. Treatment of spastic cerebral-palsied children with sodium dantrolene. *Dev Med Child Neurol.* 1975;17(6):736–742. https://doi.org/10.1111/j.1469-8749.1975.tb04697.x

47. Pinder RM, Brogden RN, Speight TM, Avery GS. Dantrolene sodium: a review of its pharmacological properties and therapeutic efficacy in spasticity. *Drugs.* 1977;13(1):3–23. https://doi.org/10.2165/00003495-197713010-00002

48. Schmidt RT, Lee RH, Spehlmann R. Comparison of dantrolene sodium and diazepam in the treatment of spasticity. *J Neurol Neurosurg Psychiatry.* 1976;39(4):350–356. https://doi.org/10.1136/jnnp.39.4.350

49. Steinberg FU, Ferguson KL. Effect of dantrolene sodium on spasticity associated with hemiplegiat. *J Am Geriatr Soc.* 1975;23(2):70–73. https://doi.org/10.1111/j.1532-5415.1975.tb00386.x

50. Joynt RL. Dantrolene sodium: long-term effects in patients with muscle spasticity. *Arch Phys Med Rehabil.* 1976;57(5):212–217.

51. Francisco GE, Kothari S, Huls C. GABA agonists and gabapentin for spastic hypertonia. *Phys Med Rehabil Clin N Am.* 2001;12(4):875–888, viii.

52. Barbee JG. Memory, benzodiazepines, and anxiety: integration of theoretical and clinical perspectives. *J Clin Psychiatry.* 1993;54 Suppl:86–97; discussion 98–101.

53. Hesse S, Werner C. Poststroke motor dysfunction and spasticity: novel pharmacological and physical treatment strategies. *CNS Drugs.* 2003;17(15):1093–1107. https://doi.org/10.2165/00023210-200317150-00004

54. Olsen RW. GABA-benzodiazepine-barbiturate receptor interactions. *J Neurochem.* 1981;37(1):1–13. https://doi.org/10.1111/j.1471-4159.1981.tb05284.x

55. Meythaler JM, Yablon SA. Antiepileptic drugs. *Phys Med Rehabil Clin N Am.* 1999;10(2):275–300. https://doi.org/10.1016/S1047-9651(18)30197-9

56. Roussan M, Terrence C, Fromm G. Baclofen versus diazepam for the treatment of spasticity and long-term follow-up of baclofen therapy. *Pharmatherapeutica.* 1985;4(5):278–284.

57. Wilson LA, McKechnie AA. Oral diazepam in the treatment of spasticity in paraplegia a double-blind trial and subsequent impressions. *Scott Med J.* 1966;11(2):46–51. https://doi.org/10.1177/003693306601100202

58. Basmajian J V, Shankardass K, Russell D, Yucel V. Ketazolam treatment for spasticity: double-blind study of a new drug. *Arch Phys Med Rehabil.* 1984;65(11):698–701.

59. Sawa GM, Paty DW. The use of baclofen in treatment of spasticity in multiple sclerosis. *Can J Neurol Sci.* 1979;6(3):351–354. https://doi.org/10.1017/s0317167100023994

60. Smolenski C, Muff S, Smolenski-Kautz S. A double-blind comparative trial of new muscle relaxant, tizanidine (DS 103-282), and baclofen in the treatment of chronic spasticity in multiple sclerosis. *Curr Med Res Opin.* 1981;7(6):374–383.

61. Mugglestone MA, Eunson P, Murphy MS, Guideline development group. Spasticity in children and young people with non-progressive brain disorders: summary of NICE guidance. *BMJ*. 2012;345:e4845. https://doi.org/10.1136/bmj.e4845

62. Lapeyre E, Kuks JBM, Meijler WJ. Spasticity: revisiting the role and the individual value of several pharmacological treatments. *NeuroRehabilitation*. 2010;27(2):193–200. https://doi.org/10.3233/NRE-2010-0596

63. Glass A, Hannah A. A comparison of dantrolene sodium and diazepam in the treatment of spasticity. *Paraplegia*. 1974;12(3):170–174. doi:10.1038/sc.1974.27

64. KendallPH. News drugs—I: the use of diazepam in hemiplegia. *Rheumatology*. 1964;7(6):225–228. https://doi.org/10.1093/rheumatology/7.6.225

65. Cocchiarella A, Downey JA, Darling RC. Evaluation of the effect of diazepam on spasticity. *Arch Phys Med Rehabil*. 1967;48(8):393–396.

66. Rowland T, Depalma L. Current neuropharmacologic interventions for the management of brain injury agitation. *Neuro Rehabil*. 1995;5(3):219–232. https://doi.org/10.3233/NRE-1995-5305

67. Cendrowski W, Sobczyk W. Clonazepam, baclofen and placebo in the treatment of spasticity. *Eur Neurol*. 1977;16(1–6):257–262. https://doi.org/10.1159/000114906

68. Dahlin M, Knutsson E, Nergårdh A. Treatment of spasticity in children with low dose benzodiazepine. *J Neurol Sci*. 1993;117(1–2):54–60. https://doi.org/10.1016/0022-510x(93)90154-q

69. Henriksen O. An overview of benzodiazepines in seizure management. *Epilepsia*. 1998;39(s1):S2–S6. https://doi.org/10.1111/j.1528-1157.1998.tb05110.x

70. Kischka U. Neurological rehabilitation and management of spasticity. *Medicine (Baltimore)*. 2008;36(11):616–619. https://doi.org/10.1016/j.mpmed.2008.08.007

71. Nance PW, Shears AH, Nance DM. Clonidine in spinal cord injury. *Can Med Assoc J*. 1985;133(1):41–42.

72. Nance PW, Shears AH, Nance DM. Reflex changes induced by clonidine in spinal cord injured patients. *Paraplegia*. 1989;27(4):296–301. https://doi.org/10.1038/sc.1989.44

73. Kobinger W, Walland A. Investigations into the mechanism of the hypotensive effect of 2-(2,6-dichlorphenylamino)-2-imidazoline-HCl. *Eur J Pharmacol*. 1967;2(3):155–162. https://doi.org/10.1016/0014-2999(67)90080-5

74. Yablon SA, Sipski ML. Effect of transdermal clonidine on spinal spasticity. A case series. *Am J Phys Med Rehabil*. 1993;72(3):154–157. https://doi.org/10.1097/00002060-199306000-00009

75. Donovan WH, Carter RE, Rossi CD, Wilkerson MA. Clonidine effect on spasticity: a clinical trial. *Arch Phys Med Rehabil*. 1988;69(3 Pt 1):193–194.

76. Maynard FM. Early clinical experience with clonidine in spinal spasticity. *Spinal Cord*. 1986;24(3):175–182. https://doi.org/10.1038/sc.1986.24

77. Rabchevsky AG, Kitzman PH. Latest approaches for the treatment of spasticity and autonomic dysreflexia in chronic spinal cord injury. *Neurotherapeutics*. 2011;8(2):274–282. https://doi.org/10.1007/s13311-011-0025-5

78. Kooner JS, Birch R, Frankel HL, Peart WS, Mathias CJ. Hemodynamic and neurohormonal effects of clonidine in patients with preganglionic and postganglionic sympathetic lesions. Evidence for a central sympatholytic action. *Circulation*. 1991;84(1):75–83. https://doi.org/10.1161/01.cir.84.1.75

79. Kooner JS, Edge W, Frankel HL, Peart WS, Mathias CJ. Haemodynamic actions of clonidine in tetraplegia - effects at rest and during urinary bladder stimulation. *Spinal Cord*. 1988;26(3):200–203. https://doi.org/10.1038/sc.1988.31

80. Goldstein LB. Common drugs may influence motor recovery after stroke. The Sygen In Acute Stroke Study Investigators. *Neurology*. 1995;45(5):865–871. https://doi.org/10.1212/wnl.45.5.865

81. Shprecher D, Sloan CT, Sederholm B. Neuropsychiatric side effects of cyclobenzaprine. *BMJ Case Rep*. 2013;2013. https://doi.org/10.1136/bcr-2013-008997

82. Nance P, Meythaler J. Spasticity management. In: Braddom R, ed. *Physical Medicine and Rehabilitation*. Saunders; 2006:651–662.

83. D'Amico JM, Murray KC, Li Y, et al. Constitutively active 5-HT2/α1 receptors facilitate muscle spasms after human spinal cord injury. *J Neurophysiol*. 2013;109(6):1473–1484. https://doi.org/10.1152/jn.00821.2012

84. Barbeau H, Richards CL, Bédard PJ. Action of cyproheptadine in spastic paraparetic patients. *J Neurol Neurosurg Psychiatry*. 1982;45(10):923–926. https://doi.org/10.1136/jnnp.45.10.923

85. Wainberg M, Barbeau H. Modulatory action of cyproheptadine on the locomotor pattern of spastic paretic patients. *Soc Neurosci*. 1986;308(5).

86. Nance PW. A comparison of clonidine, cyproheptadine and baclofen in spastic spinal cord injured patients. *J Am Paraplegia Soc*. 1994;17(3):150–156. https://doi.org/10.1080/01952307.1994.11735927

87. Ramsay RE. Clinical efficacy and safety of gabapentin. *Neurology*. 1994;44(6 Suppl 5):S23–30; discussion S31–2.

88. Rose MA, Kam PCA. Gabapentin: pharmacology and its use in pain management. *Anaesthesia*. 2002;57(5):451–462. https://doi.org/10.1046/j.0003-2409.2001.02399.x

89. Hendrich J, Van Minh AT, Heblich F, et al. Pharmacological disruption of calcium channel trafficking by the alpha2delta ligand gabapentin. *Proc Natl Acad Sci USA*. 2008;105(9):3628–3633. https://doi.org/10.1073/pnas.0708930105

90. Mueller ME, Gruenthal M, Olson WL, Olson WH. Gabapentin for relief of upper motor neuron symptoms in multiple sclerosis. *Arch Phys Med Rehabil*. 1997;78(5):521–524. https://doi.org/10.1016/s0003-9993(97)90168-4

91. Cutter NC, Scott DD, Johnson JC, Whiteneck G. Gabapentin effect on spasticity in multiple sclerosis: a placebo-controlled, randomized trial. *Arch Phys Med Rehabil*. 2000;81(2):164–169. https://doi.org/10.1016/s0003-9993(00)90135-7

92. Gruenthal M, Mueller M, Olson WL, Priebe MM, Sherwood AM, Olson WH. Gabapentin for the treatment of spasticity in patients with spinal cord injury. *Spinal Cord*. 1997;35(10):686–689. https://doi.org/10.1038/sj.sc.3100481

93. Priebe MM, Sherwood AM, Graves DE, Mueller M, Olson WH. Effectiveness of gabapentin in controlling spasticity: a quantitative study. *Spinal Cord*. 1997;35(3):171–175. https://doi.org/10.1038/sj.sc.3100366

94. Shorvon S, Stefan H. Overview of the safety of newer antiepileptic drugs. *Epilepsia*. 1997;38 Suppl 1:S45– S51. https://doi.org/10.1111/j.1528-1157.1997.tb04519.x

95. McLean MJ. Gabapentin. *Epilepsia*. 1995;36 Suppl 2:S73–S86. https://doi.org/10.1111/j.1528-1157.1995.tb06001.x

96. Leppik IE. Antiepileptic drugs in development: prospects for the near future. *Epilepsia*. 1994;35 Suppl 4:S29–S40. https://doi.org/10.1111/j.1528-1157.1994.tb05953.x

97. Baker D, Pryce G. The endocannabinoid system and multiple sclerosis. *Curr Pharm Des*. 2008;14(23):2326–2336. https://doi.org/10.2174/138161208785740036

98. Baker D, Pryce G, Giovannoni G, Thompson AJ. The therapeutic potential of cannabis. *Lancet Neurol*. 2003;2(5):291–298. https://doi.org/10.1016/s1474-4422(03)00381-8

99. de Lago E, Moreno-Martet M, Cabranes A, Ramos JA, Fernández-Ruiz J. Cannabinoids ameliorate disease progression in a model of multiple sclerosis in mice, acting preferentially through CB1 receptor-mediated anti-inflammatory effects. *Neuropharmacology*. 2012;62(7):2299–2308. https://doi.org/10.1016/j.neuropharm.2012.01.030

100. Collin C, Davies P, Mutiboko IK, Ratcliffe S, Sativex Spasticity in MS Study Group. Randomized controlled trial of cannabis-based medicine in spasticity caused by multiple sclerosis. *Eur J Neurol*. 2007;14(3):290–296. https://doi.org/10.1111/j.1468-1331.2006.01639.x

101. Oreja-Guevara C, Montalban X, de Andrés C, et al. [Consensus document on spasticity in patients with multiple sclerosis. Grupo de Enfermedades Desmielinizantes de la Sociedad Española de Neurología]. *Rev Neurol*. 2013;57(8):359–373.

102. Koppel BS, Brust JCM, Fife T, et al. Systematic review: efficacy and safety of medical marijuana in selected neurologic disorders: report of the guideline development subcommittee of the american academy of neurology. *Neurology*. 2014;82(17):1556–1563. https://doi.org/10.1212/WNL.0000000000000363

103. Zuardi AW, Crippa JAS, Hallak JEC, Moreira FA, Guimarães FS. Cannabidiol, a Cannabis sativa constituent, as an antipsychotic drug. *Brazilian J Med Biol Res = Rev Bras Pesqui medicas e Biol*. 2006;39(4):421–429. https://doi.org/10.1590/s0100-879x2006000400001

104. Nielsen S, Germanos R, Weier M, et al. The use of cannabis and cannabinoids in treating symptoms of multiple sclerosis: a systematic review of reviews. *Curr Neurol Neurosci Rep*. 2018;18(2):8. https://doi.org/10.1007/s11910-018-0814-x

105. Kitzman PH. Effectiveness of riluzole in suppressing spasticity in the spinal cord injured rat. *Neurosci Lett*. 2009;455(2):150–153. https://doi.org/10.1016/j.neulet.2009.03.016

106. Theiss RD, Hornby TG, Rymer WZ, Schmit BD. Riluzole decreases flexion withdrawal reflex but not voluntary ankle torque in human chronic spinal cord injury. *J Neurophysiol*. 2011;105(6):2781–2790. https://doi.org/10.1152/jn.00570.2010

107. Srinivas S, Wali AR, Pham MH. Efficacy of riluzole in the treatment of spinal cord injury: a systematic review of the literature. *Neurosurg Focus*. 2019;46(3):E6. https://doi.org/10.3171/2019.1.FOCUS18596

108. Rossi S ed. *Australian Medicines Handbook (2013 Ed.)*. Adelaide: The Australian Medicines Handbook Unit Trust; 2013.

109. Murphy AM, Milo-Manson G, Best A, Campbell KA, Fehlings D. Impact of modafinil on spasticity reduction and quality of life in children with CP. *Dev Med Child Neurol*. 2008;50(7):510–514. https://doi.org/10.1111/j.1469-8749.2008.03019.x

110. Hurst DL, Lajara-Nanson W. Use of modafinil in spastic cerebral palsy. *J Child Neurol*. 2002;17(3):169–172. https://doi.org/10.1177/088307380201700303

111. Smith JE, Hall P V., Galvin MR, Jones AR, Campbell RL. Effects of glycine administration on canine experimental spinal spasticity and the levels of glycine, glutamate, and aspartate in the lumbar spinal cord. *Neurosurgery*. 1979;4(2):152–156. https://doi.org/10.1227/00006123-197902000-00008

112. Stern P, Bokonjic R. Glycine therapy in 7 cases of spasticity. *Pharmacology*. 1974;12(2):117–119. https://doi.org/10.1159/000136529

113. Goldstein LB. Prescribing of potentially harmful drugs to patients admitted to hospital after head injury. *J Neurol Neurosurg Psychiatry*. 1995;58(6):753–755. https://doi.org/10.1136/jnnp.58.6.753

114. Goldstein LB. Neuropharmacology of TBI-induced plasticity. *Brain Inj*. 2003;17(8):685–694. https://doi.org/10.1080/0269905031000107179

115. Schallert T, Hernandez TD, Barth TM. Recovery of function after brain damage: severe and chronic disruption by diazepam. *Brain Res.* 1986;379(1):104–111. https://doi.org/10.1016/0006-8993(86)90261-1

116. Vidaurre J, Gedela S, Yarosz S. Antiepileptic drugs and liver disease. *Pediatr Neurol.* 2017;77:23–36. https://doi.org/10.1016/j.pediatrneurol.2017.09.013

117. Olvey EL, Armstrong EP, Grizzle AJ. Contemporary pharmacologic treatments for spasticity of the upper limb after stroke: a systematic review. *Clin Ther.* 2010;32(14):2282–2303. https://doi.org/10.1016/j.clinthera.2011.01.005

118. Ertzgaard P, Campo C, Calabrese A. Efficacy and safety of oral baclofen in the management of spasticity: a rationale for intrathecal baclofen. *J Rehabil Med.* 2017;49(3):193–203. https://doi.org/10.2340/16501977-2211

119. Meythaler JM, Clayton W, Davis LK, Guin-Renfroe S, Brunner RC. Orally delivered baclofen to control spastic hypertonia in acquired brain injury. *J Head Trauma Rehabil.* 2004;19(2):101–108. https://doi.org/10.1097/00001199-200403000-00003

120. Medaer R HHVD et al. Treatment of spasticity due to stroke. A double-blind, cross-over trial comparing baclofen to placebo. *Acta Ther.* 1991;17(4):323–331.

121. Maupas E, Marque P, Roques CF, Simonetta-Moreau M. Modulation of the transmission in group II heteronymous pathways by tizanidine in spastic hemiplegic patients. *J Neurol Neurosurg Psychiatry.* 2004;75(1):130–135.

122. Gelber DA, Good DC, Dromerick A, Sergay S, Richardson M. Open-label dose-titration safety and efficacy study of tizanidine hydrochloride in the treatment of spasticity associated with chronic stroke. *Stroke.* 2001;32(8):1841–1846. https://doi.org/10.1161/01.STR.32.8.1841

123. Duncan GW, Shahani BT, Young RR. An evaluation of baclofen treatment for certain symptoms in patients with spinal cord lesions: a double-blind, cross-over study. *Neurology.* 1976;26(5):441–441. https://doi.org/10.1212/WNL.26.5.441

124. Taricco M, Pagliacci MC, Telaro E, Adone R. Pharmacological interventions for spasticity following spinal cord injury: results of a Cochrane systematic review. *Eura Medicophys.* 2006;42(1):5–15.

125. Corbett M, Frankel HL, Michaelis L. A double blind, cross-over trial of valium in the treatment of spasticity. *Spinal Cord.* 1972;10(1):19–22. https://doi.org/10.1038/sc.1972.4

126. Hagenbach U, Luz S, Ghafoor N, et al. The treatment of spasticity with Δ9-tetrahydrocannabinol in persons with spinal cord injury. *Spinal Cord.* 2007;45(8):551–562. https://doi.org/10.1038/sj.sc.3101982

127. Brar SP, Smith MB, Nelson LM, Franklin GM, Cobble ND. Evaluation of treatment protocols on minimal to moderate spasticity in multiple sclerosis. *Arch Phys Med Rehabil.* 1991;72(3):186–189.

128. Barnes MP, Bates D, Corston RN, et al. A double-blind, placebo-controlled trial of tizanidine in the treatment of spasticity caused by multiple sclerosis. United Kingdom Tizanidine Trial Group. *Neurology.* 1994;44(11 Suppl 9):S70–8.

129. Wade DT, Robson P, House H, Makela P, Aram J. A preliminary controlled study to determine whether whole-plant cannabis extracts can improve intractable neurogenic symptoms. *Clin Rehabil.* 2003;17(1):21–29. https://doi.org/10.1191/0269215503cr581oa

130. Ungerleider JT, Andyrsiak T, Fairbanks L, Ellison GW, Myers LW. Delta-9-THC in the Treatment of spasticity associated with multiple sclerosis. *Adv Alcohol Subst Abuse.* 1988;7(1):39–50. https://doi.org/10.1300/J251v07n01_04

131. Milla PJ, Jackson ADM. A controlled trial of baclofen in children with cerebral palsy. *J Int Med Res*. 1973;1(2):398–404. https://doi.org/10.1177/030006057300100203

132. Vásquez-Briceño A, Arellano-Saldaña ME, León-Hernández SR, Morales-Osorio MG. The usefulness of tizanidine. A one-year follow-up of the treatment of spasticity in infantile cerebral palsy. *Rev Neurol*. 43(3):132–136.

133. Mathew A, Mathew MC. Bedtime diazepam enhances well being in children with spastic cerebral palsy. *Pediatr Rehabil*. 8(1):63–66. https://doi.org/10.1080/13638490410001731180

134. Scheuer KH, Svenstrup K, Jennum P, et al. Double-blind crossover trial of gabapentin in SPG4-linked hereditary spastic paraplegia. *Eur J Neurol*. 2007;14(6):663–666. https://doi.org/10.1111/j.1468-1331.2007.01812.x

9 Toxins

Natasha L. Romanoski and Shivani Patel

INTRODUCTION

Botulinum toxin (BoNT) is an agent used in the focal management of spasticity as well as various other clinical and cosmetic applications. Its use as a therapeutic treatment option for spasticity management has been supported by various patient-specific goals, which include but are not limited to decreasing spasms, improving active and passive range of motion (ROM), improving ability to perform activities of daily living (ADLs), improving functional mobility, improving gait mechanics, improving positioning and posturing, preventing contractures, preventing skin breakdown, decreasing caregiver burden, improving hygiene, and managing pain. The first therapeutic use of botulinum toxin A (BoNTA) for muscle overactivity was reported in 1973 by an ophthalmologist to treat strabismus.[1] It was later approved by the Food and Drug Administration (FDA) in 1989 for the treatment of blepharospasm, strabismus, and hemifacial spasm. Its use for spasticity in the extremities was not widely known until 1989 when Das and Park revealed selective weakening of spastic muscles when injected for post-stroke spasticity.[2] The use of BoNT across various indications in adult and pediatric populations continues to expand as our understanding of its safety and efficacy continues to grow.

MECHANISM OF ACTION

BoNT is a neurotoxin that is derived from the anaerobic, rod-shaped, gram-positive, and spore-forming bacterium *Clostridium botulinum*. BoNTs consist of a group of seven well-established serotypes (A–G) with recent discoveries of serotypes H and X that are still being investigated regarding their safety and clinical use. Serotypes A and B were first identified in 1919 and each of the subsequent serotypes were discovered through 1969 when serotype G was discovered. It was not until 2013 when serotype H was discovered and more recently serotype X in 2017. Only two serotypes, A and B, are currently used in clinical practice for therapeutic treatment due to a longer-lasting effect than other serotypes.[3] Serotype H has been determined to be a mosaic toxin, which is a designation that identifies substantial similarities to other previously discovered serotypes, notably Type A1 and Type F toxin. Type

X, the most recent discovery, has been found to have a different site for protein cleavage and is still being investigated regarding the safety and efficacy of its use.[4]

All serotypes consist of a 150-kilodalton (kDa) protein that is organized into heavy chains and light chains linked by a disulfide bond.[5] At the cellular level, the neurotoxin binds presynaptically to the cholinergic nerve endings and undergoes endocytosis into the vesicle. Once inside the presynaptic cell, the toxin cleaves a soluble N-ethylmaleimide-sensitive attachment protein receptor (SNARE) protein complex that then inhibits acetylcholine (Ach) from binding to the intracellular membrane that ultimately leads to the inhibition of its release. A specific component of the SNARE protein, SNAP-25, is the site of attachment of type A toxin's light chain, whereas for type B toxin, the SNARE protein is attached directly to the proteins on the surface of the vesicle, otherwise known as vesicle-associated membrane proteins (VAMP). The reduction in Ach release is also thought to occur within the autonomic system, thereby producing clinical effects of dry mouth and sweat reduction. This is why BoNT also has clinical indications within these areas. In animal models, it is also known to inhibit Substance P release that can be analgesic. As the toxin wears off, collateral nerve sprouting occurs and allows for regeneration of the nerve.[6]

Despite many similarities between serotypes, there are some notable differences in regard to the complexing proteins within each formulation. The proteins are not directly involved within the known mechanism of action of neurotoxins, and the effect on immunogenicity and potency at the cellular level is still being investigated.[7] All neurotoxins used in clinical practice contain human serum albumin (HSA), which is used as a protein stabilizer. HSA has theoretical risk of transmitting viral disease, although this has never been reported. In 2020, a new formulation by the name of MT10107 was studied. MT10107 is a substance containing a 150-kDa neurotoxin that is free from both complexing proteins and HSA contents. Instead, it utilizes methionine, polysorbate 20, and sucrose to stabilize the toxin. A clinical trial comparing MT10107 and onabotulinumtoxinA (ona-BoNTA) shows similar efficacy and safety for poststroke spasticity; however, it is not approved in the United States for clinical use.[8]

Clinical Indications

Toxin Formulations

There are four commercially available BoNT formulations in the United States approved for therapeutic use. Serotype A exists in three formulations: onaBoNTA, abobotulinumtoxinA (aboBoNTA), and incobotulinumtoxinA (incoBoNTA), whereas serotype B exists in one formulation: rimabotulinumtoxinB (rimaBoNTB).

All four of these BoNT formulations are approved by the FDA for cervical dystonia; however, their approved indications for spasticity remain variable and are constantly evolving. FDA indications across the different toxin formulations are represented in Table 9.1.[9-12] The available vial sizes listed in units per vial can be found in Figure 9.1.

As of this writing, there are two other BoNT formulations available in the United States: daxibotulinumtoxinA-lanm (daxiBoNT) and prabotulinumtoxinA-xvfs (pra-BoNT).[13,14] However, these are currently only approved for dermatologic use.

Table 9.1 FDA-Approved Indications for Clinical Use

		FDA Indications			
OnaBoNTA (Botox)	**AboBoNTA (Dysport)**	**IncoBoNTA (Xeomin)**	**RimaBoNTB (Myobloc)**	**DaxiBoNTA (Daxxify)**	**PraBoNTA (Jeuveau)**
Cervical Dystonia	Cervical Dystonia	Cervical Dystonia	Cervical Dystonia	Glabellar Lines	Glabellar Lines
Overactive Bladder**	Glabellar Lines	Chronic Sialorrhea***	Chronic Sialorrhea		
Detrusor Overactivity associated with a Neurologic Condition**	Spasticity*	Upper Limb Spasticity***			
Chronic Migraine		Glabellar Lines			
Spasticity*		Blepharospasm			
Primary Axillary Hyperhidrosis					
Blepharospasm and Strabismus**					
Glabellar Lines					

*Spasticity in patients 2 years of age and older.
**OnaBoNTA is FDA approved for pediatric patients 12 years of age or older in the following conditions: strabismus, blepharospasm associated with dystonia, and overactive bladder. It is also approved for neurogenic detrusor overactivity for patients 5 years and old who have had a poor response to anticholinergics.
***IncoBoNTA is FDA approved for sialorrhea for those 2 years and older as well as upper limb spasticity in patients 2 years and older, excluding those with spasticity due to cerebral palsy.

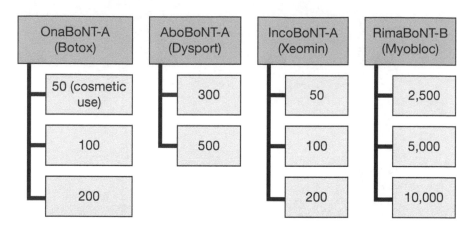

Figure 9.1 Available vial sizes (units/vial) for each FDA-approved BoNT.

Off-Label Uses

While the only forms of dystonia that have FDA approval for BoNT injections are cervical dystonia and blepharospasm, BoNT has been routinely applied off-label to treat other forms of dystonia but is beyond the scope of this text. These uses have included but are not limited to limb dystonia, oromandibular dystonia or bruxism, spasmodic dysphonia, and tardive and truncal dystonia.[15]

Procedural Considerations

When considering BoNT therapy for patients with spasticity, clinicians should have an understanding of the unique reconstitution required, as well as all safety considerations. In addition, optimal use of BoNT for spasticity relies on an in-depth understanding of neuroanatomy in order to effectively perform the procedure and optimize outcomes. Suggested equipment needed for the procedure is listed in Figure 9.2.

Reconstitution

Reconstitution of the lyophilic form of BoNTA in physiological saline varies from provider to provider based on clinical experience, product label recommendations, and provider preference. The desired amount of sterile preservative-free 0.9% normal saline should be drawn into a sterile syringe. As an example, 1 mL of 0.9% normal saline is drawn up and inserted into the vacuum-sealed onaBoNTA vial. The vacuum seal should pull the saline into the vial, and without this, the vial should be considered defective and not used. The vial should be gently swirled to mix the contents without inverting the vial. The reconstituted solution, which should be clear, colorless, and free of particulate matter, is then drawn into the preferred injectable syringe. AboBoNTA and incoBoNTA have individual recommendations for reconstitution and dilution options, while rimaBoNTB does not require reconstitution with normal saline and is generally drawn up directly from the manufactured vial.

The dilution used for reconstitution varies per manufacturer product label and clinicians may adjust the amount of saline used for dilution in order to achieve various clinical effects.

Equipment needed	Botulinum toxin
	Preservative-free 0.9% sodium chloride (for BoNT-A formulations)
	Needle to draw up medication (i.e., 21 gauge 1.5 inch)
	Syringe to draw up medication (i.e., 1 mL)
	Antiseptic (i.e., alcohol prep pads or ChloraPrep)
	Sterile gauze (i.e., 4×4 inch gauze)
	Band-aid
	(Optional) topical anesthetic (i.e., ethyl chloride spray or lidocaine cream)
	Preferred guidance method (i.e., EMG, stimulation or ultrasound)

Figure 9.2 **Equipment needed.**

STORAGE OF TOXIN

BoNTs must be stored at specific temperatures prior to use. BoNTA is stored in powder form and botulinum toxin B (BoNTB) is stored in liquid form.

- OnaBoNTA must be refrigerated between temperatures of 2°C to 8°C for up to 36 months before reconstitution.[9]
- AboBoNTA must be refrigerated between temperatures of 2°C to 8°C for up to 24 months before reconstitution.[10]
- IncoBoNTA should be stored at or below 25°C for up to 36 months before reconstitution.[11]
- RimaBoNTB must be kept refrigerated between temperatures of 2°C to 8°C for up to 36 months before use.[12]

Once reconstituted, all BoNTA formulations should either be used immediately or refrigerated and used within 24 hours of reconstitution.[9–12] BoNTB does not require reconstitution; however, it may be diluted with 0.9% normal saline, per provider preference, and if this occurs, it should be used within 4 hours.[12]

Safety
Informed consent should occur prior to treatment with BoNT and should include a thorough discussion of potential adverse reactions, contraindications, and precautions.

Adverse Events
Adverse events, usually transient and mild, have been reported with the use of BoNT injections. These include localized bruising, bleeding, edema, focal weakness, and

most commonly, pain at the site of injection. Flu-like symptoms may also occur.[9–12] Other reported adverse effects include muscular weakness or falls,[10] seizure, nasopharyngitis, dry mouth, and upper respiratory tract infection.[11]

Contraindications and Precautions

- Contraindications to BoNT injections include hypersensitivity to BoNT or any of its components, allergic reaction to other BoNT products, and active infection at the site of injection.[9–12]
- Precaution should be taken in patients with neuromuscular disorders as the clinical effects of toxin may be exacerbated.[9–12]
- Use of aminoglycoside antibiotics may potentiate the effects of toxin by interfering with neuromuscular transmission.[9–12]
- Systemic anticholinergic effects may be potentiated with the use of anticholinergic drugs.[10–12]
- Caution should be taken in patients with compromised respiratory function.[9–12]
- All BoNT labels contain a black box warning regarding the risk of distant spread. The warning states: "The effects of [BoNT formulation] and all botulinum toxin products may spread from the area of injection to produce symptoms consistent with botulinum toxin effects. These symptoms have been reported hours to weeks after injection. Swallowing and breathing difficulties can be life threatening and there have been reports of death. The risk of symptoms is probably greatest in children treated for spasticity but symptoms can also occur in adults, particularly in those patients who have an underlying condition that would predispose them to these symptoms."[9–12]

Concomitant Anticoagulation Use

Localized bleeding at the site of injection is a common risk of any intramuscular injection. If there is concern for increased risk of bleeding based on a history and physical exam, provider-dependent practices, such as the utilization of ultrasound (US) guidance, aspiration prior to injecting, and direct localized pressure upon needle removal, can be implemented. Several studies have shown that BoNT injections are safe with concomitant use of anticoagulation,[16,17] and thus there is no need to hold antiplatelets or anticoagulants prior to procedure.

Dosing

Each FDA-approved BoNT has recommended dosages per muscle and total dose per injection visit as listed in Figure 9.3.[9–11] Due to the rapidly changing approval of new on-label muscles, each product label should be referenced for specific dosage recommendations for both adult and pediatric populations. There is no recommended dose conversion between toxins as the potency of each toxin is dependent on the specific preparation and assay method used for each toxin.

Dosing should always be individualized after considering the patient's intended goals and outcomes. When choosing dosage for treatment, the clinician should consider product label dose recommendations, dilution options, the number of muscles involved, passive and active goals, other concomitant treatments, and past response to BoNT products. A dose-dependent response is anticipated[18] and there should be continuous reassessment of goals at each visit.

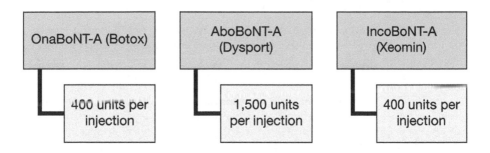

Figure 9.3 Current FDA recommendations for total injectable dose per visit, when used for adult spasticity management.

High Dosing

Despite approved recommendations, off-label use of higher dosages of various BoNTA products have been increasingly utilized in recent years.

In 2009, a European Consensus recommended maximum doses of 600 units for onaBoNTA and 1500 units for aboBoNTA, respectively. These recommendations were either at or above FDA approved recommendations with suggestions for maximum dosage per injection site of 50 units onaBoNTA toxin and 125 units for aboBoNTA.[19] Since this report, there have been various studies looking at the safety and efficacy of high dose BoNTA use, however, safety concerns remain variable.

A 2020 study by Kirshblum reported no difference in reported adverse effects for those injected with 401 to 600 units of onaBoNTA. In those treated with greater than 600 units, there was an increase in reported adverse effects, including dysphagia at 1.6%, compared to 0.4% in the lower group. Weakness, a common and expected outcome, was reported at 1.7% across all groups.[20] In 2015, a study looked at onaBoNTA dosage of 600 to 800 units that resulted in a positive Modified Ashworth Scale (MAS) reduction, a positive functional improvement, and no change in adverse events.[21] A similar more recent report in 2020 by Intiso reviewed onaBoNT dosages of 600 to 840 units, and again, no significant changes in adverse effects were reported; however, this study did not report functional changes.[22] For incoBoNT, the TOWER study in 2017 revealed no increase in adverse effects when doses of incoBoNT 800 units were used over three series of injections.[23]

With several studies confirming either little or no increase in adverse effects with high dosages, a 2017 registry revealed that more experienced physicians tend to use dosages higher than manufacturer label recommendations. Experienced clinicians who utilize higher dosages have shown larger gains in MAS reduction at the knee and ankle while often utilizing larger dilutions and fewer injection sites per visit.[24]

Special Populations

Pregnancy

There have been limited reports of BoNT use in pregnant women; however, the safety remains unknown as there are no known human studies. Clinicians should consider the potential for fetal harm, based on the use of the neurotoxin in animal studies.[9]

Lactation
There have been no documented reports of the transfer of BoNT from a lactating woman to an infant; however, the risks of botulism from the neurotoxin should be considered.

Pediatrics
Various BoNTA preparations have FDA approval for spasticity in pediatric populations and dose recommendations are generally weight based per product label. BoNTA is often utilized in attempts to prevent or delay definitive surgical intervention during periods of rapid bone growth.

Concomitant Botulinum Toxin Use With Other Clinical Indications
Due to the rapidly evolving indications for BoNT use, it is not uncommon that patients may seek treatment for various medical conditions (i.e., detrusor overactivity). When this occurs, the total BoNT dosage between all treatments should be considered when assessing dosage recommendations as well as risks for adverse effects related to high dosage. Evidence regarding the timing of each treatment is lacking; however, it is commonly recommended to arrange the timing of treatments in close proximity to one another to prevent the potential formation of neutralizing antibodies.

Suspected Treatment Failure

Treatment failure can be defined as those who do not achieve a satisfactory response to BoNT therapy; however, adjustments to the treatment plan should first be considered to optimize therapy. Patient care plans should be approached in a patient-centered and goal-oriented way to determine if the treatment plan has been optimized.

The following should be considered prior to consideration for treatment failure:

Injection protocol

- Consider if the dose to each muscle needs to be adjusted.
- Consider if new muscles need to be injected and/or determine muscles that no longer need to be injected.
- Recognize variations in different dilution options and consider adjustment to dilution technique.
- Evaluate localization method and consider alternatives (i.e., add US or electrical stimulation [e-stim]).
- Determine if expectations were realistic and goal-oriented and modify accordingly.

Concomitant treatments

- Consider if adjunct treatments are needed (i.e., intrathecal baclofen [ITB] pump).
- Determine if adequate therapeutic modalities were utilized (i.e., orthoses or physical therapy).

Associated or secondary diagnoses

- Assess for underlying infectious or other noxious stimuli that may interfere with spasticity assessment.

- Evaluate for clinical progression of disease (i.e., multiple sclerosis [MS]).
- Consider new clinical diagnoses that may present as increased spasticity (i.e., syrinx).
- Assess for development of joint contracture and other rheological changes.

Medication related

- Determine if the patient is having an adverse effect or reaction that may limit treatment.
- Consider a primary or secondary non-response due to immunogenicity.

Immunoresistance

Neutralizing antibodies are antibodies that are thought to form against proteins within the molecule and may lead to a primary or secondary non-response.

Definitions

- Primary non-responders are those who receive no benefit from BoNT.
- Secondary non-responders are those who previously responded successfully to at least two cycles of BoNT therapy who now have an unsatisfactory response after two cycles.

Below are two objective ways to assess clinical immunoresistance to BoNT[25]

Frontalis Test

- Unilateral injection of BoNT into the frontalis muscle
  - Example dosing: 10 U onaBoNTA, 10 U incoBoNTA, or 30 U aboBoNTA
- Follow up response in 2 to 4 weeks by asking patient to raise eyebrows. It is recommended to take images to compare.
- Interpretations
  - Unilateral paralysis suggests that the BoNT is active.
  - Symmetrical facial movements with absence of paralysis indicates that the patient may have developed immunoresistance to the toxin.

Extensor Digitorum Brevis (EDB) Test With Electromyography (EMG)

- Unilateral injection into EDB muscle
  - Example dosing: 20 U onaBoNTA or 100 U aboBoNTA
- Use EMG to measure the compound motor action potential (CMAP) of the peroneal nerve.
- Repeat EMG in 2 weeks.
- Interpretations:
  - CMAP reduction by >50% with atrophy and weakness suggests that the BoNT is active.
  - CMAP reduction by 20% to 50% is equivocal and clinical correlation should be considered.
  - CMAP reduction by <20% suggests the presence of immunoresistance and the presence of neutralizing antibodies.

When immunoresistance is encountered, many clinicians may trial other BoNT formulations or may consider other treatment options for spasticity. Some BoNT manufacturers, such as incoBoNTA have attempted to reduce excess proteins in attempts to reduce the development of neutralizing antibodies. It is unknown if a drug holiday will provide a clinically positive response; however, it has been shown that neutralizing antibody titers may decrease over time when toxin cessation occurs.

Additional Considerations

Timing of Botulinum Toxin Therapy
The use of BoNT treatment for spasticity is often performed in the outpatient setting due to limitations on cost and reimbursement as well as timeline for the treatment to take effect. Although BoNT therapy therefore generally occurs in the subacute or chronic phase of a disease process, positive effects have been shown when poststroke spasticity is treated within the first 3 months following stroke.[26] Continued research looking into the earlier use of BoNT is ongoing and should be considered in order to optimize long-term outcomes.

Adjuvant Treatments
Adjuvant treatments such as physical and occupational therapy and modalities such as the use of e-stim may be considered to enhance outcomes following BoNT therapy.[27] E-stim has been hypothesized to boost the uptake of BoNTA at the presynaptic cholinergic nerve terminal; however, there is no clear consensus on the timing, frequency, or duration of recommended use.[28]

Clinicians should also consider the role for concomitant spasticity interventions such as orthotics, pharmacologic antispasmodics, neurolysis, or intrathecal therapy. Each treatment has specific indications for use and patients may benefit from a multimodal approach utilizing various interventions within their treatment plan.

KEY POINTS

- BoNTs have various clinical indications for use in those living with spasticity.
- Our understanding of the optimal dosing, timing, and adjunct treatment interventions continues to evolve as our understanding of the pathophysiology and safety of its use continues to grow.
- There is no recommended dose conversion between toxins as the potency of each toxin is dependent on the specific preparation and assay method used for each toxin.
- Adjuvant treatments may be considered to enhance BoNT outcomes.

REFERENCES

1. Palazón-García R, Benavente-Valdepeñas AM. Botulinum toxin: from poison to possible treatment for spasticity in spinal cord injury. *Int J Mol Sci.* 2021;22(9):4886. https://doi.org/10.3390/ijms22094886
2. Das TK, Park DM. Effect of treatment with botulinum toxin on spasticity. *Postgrad Med J.* 1989;65(762):208–210. https://doi.org/10.1136/pgmj.65.762.208

3. Samizadeh S, De Boulle K. Botulinum neurotoxin formulations: overcoming the confusion. *Clin Cosmet Investig Dermatol.* 2018;11:273–287. https://doi.org/10.2147/CCID.S156851

4. Zhang S, Masuyer G, Zhang J. et al. Identification and characterization of a novel botulinum neurotoxin. *Nat Commun.* 2017;8:14130. https://doi.org/10.1038/ncomms14130

5. Carr WW, Jain N, Sublett JW. Immunogenicity of botulinum toxin formulations: potential therapeutic implications. *Adv Ther.* 2021;38(10):5046–5064. https://doi.org/10.1007/s12325-021-01882-9. Epub 2021 Sep 13. PMID: 34515975; PMCID: PMC8478757.

6. Barnes M. Botulinum toxin--mechanisms of action and clinical use in spasticity. *J Rehabil Med.* 2003;(41 Suppl):56–9. https://doi.org/10.1080/16501960310010151. PMID: 12817658.

7. Scaglione F. Conversion ratio between Botox®, Dysport®, and Xeomin® in clinical practice. *Toxins (Basel).* 2016;8(3):65. https://doi.org.10.3390/toxins8030065

8. Lee J, Chun MH, Ko YJ, et al. Efficacy and safety of MT10107 (Coretox) in poststroke upper limb spasticity treatment: a randomized, double-blind, active drug-controlled, multicenter, phase III clinical trial. *Arch Phys Med Rehabil.* 2020;101(9):1485–1496. https://doi.org/10.1016/j.apmr.2020.03.025. Epub 2020 Jun 1. PMID: 32497599.

9. Botox [package insert]. Madison, NJ: Allergan USA, Inc; 2022.

10. Dysport [package insert]. Wrexham, UK: Ipsen Biopharmaceuticals, Inc; 2023.

11. Xeomin [package insert]. Frankfurt, Germany. Merz Pharmaceuticals, LLC; 2022.

12. Myobloc [package insert]. Rockville, MD. Solstice Neurosciences, LLC; 2019.

13. Daxxify [package insert]. Newark, CA. Revance Therapeutics, Inc; 2022.

14. Jeuveau [package insert]. Newport Beach, CA. Evolus, Inc; 2019

15. Spiegel LL, Ostrem JL, Bledsoe IO. FDA approvals and consensus guidelines for botulinum toxins in the treatment of dystonia. *Toxins (Basel).* 2020;12(5):332. https://doi.org/10.3390/toxins12050332. PMID: 32429600; PMCID: PMC7290737.

16. LaVallee J, Royer R, Smith G. Prevalence of bleeding complications following ultrasound-guided botulinum toxin injections in patients on anticoagulation or antiplatelet therapy. *PM R.* 2017;9(12):1217–1224. https://doi.org/10.1016/j.pmrj.2017.06.002

17. Tan YL, Wee TC. Botulinum toxin injection and electromyography in patients receiving anticoagulants: a systematic review. *PM R.* 2021;13(8):880–889. https://doi.org/10.1002/pmrj.12486

18. O'Dell MW, Brashear A, Jech R, et al. Dose-dependent effects of abobotulinumtoxina (Dysport) on spasticity and active movements in adults with upper limb spasticity: secondary analysis of a phase 3 study. *PM R.* 2018;10(1):1–10. https://doi.org/10.1016/j.pmrj.2017.06.008

19. Wissel J, Ward AB, Erztgaard P, et al. European consensus table on the use of botulinum toxin type a in adult spasticity. *J Rehabil Med.* 2009;41(1):13–25. https://doi.org/10.2340/16501977-0303

20. Kirshblum S, Solinsky R, Jasey N, et al. Adverse event profiles of high dose botulinum toxin injections for spasticity. *PM R.* 2020;12(4):349–355. https://doi.org/10.1002/pmrj.12240

21. Baricich A, Grana E, Carda S. et al. High doses of onabotulinumtoxinA in post-stroke spasticity: a retrospective analysis. *J Neural Transm.* 2015;122(9):1283–1287. https://doi.org/10.1007/s00702-015-1384-6

22. Intiso D, Simone V, Bartolo M, et al. High dosage of botulinum toxin type a in adult subjects with spasticity following acquired central nervous system damage: where are we at? *Toxins (Basel).* 2020;12(5):315. https://doi.org/10.3390/toxins12050315

23. Wissel J, Bensmail D, Ferreira JJ, et al. Safety and efficacy of incobotulinumtoxinA doses up to 800 U in limb spasticity: the TOWER study. *Neurology*. 2017;88(14):1321–1328. https://doi.org/10.1212/WNL.0000000000003789

24. Esquenazi A, Lee S, Mayer N, et al. Patient registry of spasticity care world: data analysis based on physician experience. *Am J Phys Med Rehabil*. 2017;96(12):881–888. https://doi.org/10.1097/PHM.0000000000000781

25. Marion M, Humberstone M, Grunewald R, et al. British neurotoxin network recommendations for managing cervical dystonia in patients with a poor response to botulinum toxin practical. *Pract Neurol*. 2016;16:288–295. https://doi.org/10.1136/practneurol-2015-001335

26. Picelli A, Santamato A, Cosma M, et al. Early botulinum toxin type A injection for post-stroke spasticity: a longitudinal cohort study. *Toxins (Basel)*. 2021;13(6):374. https://doi.org/10.3390/toxins13060374

27. Picelli A, Santamato A, Chemello E, et al. Adjuvant treatments associated with botulinum toxin injection for managing spasticity: an overview of the literature. *Ann Phys Rehabil Med*. 2019;62(4):291–296. https://doi.org/10.1016/j.rehab.2018.08.004

28. Picelli A, Filippetti M, Sandrini G, et al. Electrical stimulation of injected muscles to boost botulinum toxin effect on spasticity: rationale, systematic review and state of the art. *Toxins (Basel)*. 2021;13(5):303. https://doi.org/10.3390/toxins13050303

10 Neurolysis

Areerat Suputtitada, Heakyung Kim, Michael C. Munin, and Paul Winston

INTRODUCTION

Neurolysis

Neurolysis is the temporary denervation of a nerve or nerve plexus through chemical infiltration, cryoablation, or radiofrequency ablation. A nerve block occurs when nerve conduction is interfered by an induced process.[1] Peripheral nerves, saddle blockade, lumbar sympathetic blocks, the celiac plexus, and the neuraxis are all possible targets for neurolysis. Neurolytic techniques are more commonly recognized for the treatment of pain. Peripheral nerve blocks, by stopping the stretch reflex arc, have been demonstrated to be an effective technique of treating spasticity when it is localized to specific muscle targets. In the treatment of spasticity, motor or mixed nerves are targeted preferentially, which is a significant difference from neurolytic blocks for pain relief. This chapter focuses on the most common chemical injectable agents, phenol and alcohol, as well as the novel use of cryoneurolysis. To better understand the concept of nerve-targeted procedures for spasticity, it is essential to understand the relationship between the blood vessels and nerves (Figure 10.1(a),(b)) This can both improve the safety of the procedures and add a method for more rapid identification. As each nerve may innervate multiple muscles downstream, it is important to recognize that one can identify a single muscle branch versus a more proximal neurolysis to affect multiple muscles (Figure 10.2). As there is no large-scale controlled research on the use of neurolysis, the literature is limited to short retrospective studies, case series and reports, observations, and book chapters based on the opinions of experienced doctors. Despite the lack of consensus recommendations or indications, neurolysis can be used to treat spasticity if the right patient is picked for the right procedure. This requires an in-depth knowledge of the location of each nerve as it innervates the targeted muscle(s). Nerve-targeted procedures were once considered a last resort treatment. With better understanding and localization of nerves, they are becoming more common, whether surgical or with nonsurgical neurolytic techniques including chemoneurolysis and the novel cryoneurolysis.

Phenol

History
Doppler et al. first detailed the use of phenol as a neurolytic agent in 1926 for pain and gynecologic conditions.[2] Paravertebral injections for sympathectomies also date the 1920s.[3] In 1946, Haxton noted that proper patient selection was key for a good

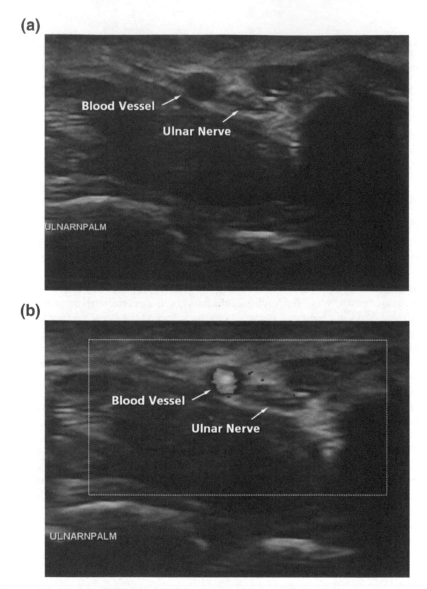

(a)

Blood Vessel

Ulnar Nerve

ULNARNPALM

(b)

Blood Vessel

Ulnar Nerve

ULNARNPALM

Figure 10.1 (a) The ulnar nerve in the palm is seen next to the blood vessel.
(b) Doppler flow enabled.

outcome and that complications were few.[3] Phenol is a chemical compound composed of carbolic acid, phenic acid, phenylic acid, phenyl hydroxide, hydroxybenzene, and oxybenzone.[4] The antiseptic plant and oil derivatives of benzene have been in use since the Egyptians employed them for embalming. Phenol or carbolic acid is a benzene ring with one hydroxyl group substituted for a hydrogen ion. It was first isolated in 1834 and used as an antiseptic by Lister in 1861.[2] Phenol has existed as a neurolytic agent since the 1930s for the purpose of sympathectomy to treat vascular

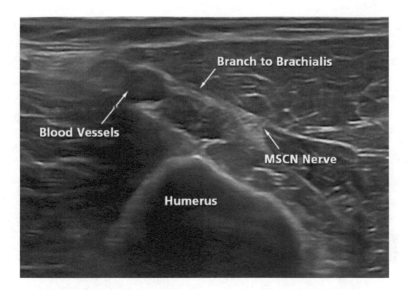

Figure 10.2 The musculocutaneous nerve branch to brachialis.

disease in humans by phenol infiltration along the paravertebral and perivascular sympathetic fibers.[5] The effects of phenol could be a mix of neurotoxicity and ischemia. With phenol injections, histologic specimens have shown nonselective nerve damage, muscular atrophy, and necrosis.[6] Phenol was first used to treat spasticity via intrathecal administration in patients with spastic paraplegia in 1959.[7] In 1965, the use of peripheral phenol injections to reduce spasticity was promoted as a novel rehabilitative method to avoid permanent nerve destruction.[8]

Mechanism of Neurolytic Action

Phenol causes protein denaturation and impairs nerve conduction when injected near neural structures by causing separation of the myelin sheath, axonal destruction resulting in loss of cellular lipid content, dissociation of the myelin sheath from the axon, and axonal edema and subsequent Wallerian degeneration. Phenol is used perineurally to create a mixed sensorimotor nerve block, or at the motor nerve branch termed motor point block[2] (Figure 10.3).

Phenol neurolysis has an immediate effect in reducing spasticity, with a peak effect around 1 week after injection. Wallerian degeneration will lead to longer-term improvement after repeated phenol injections. The effects of phenol injection can last for months or even years until axonal regrowth occurs and repeated as needed.[9,10] Concentration and dosing is found in Table 10.1.

Efficacy

Phenol works immediately after injection and lasts nearly twice as long compared to botulinum toxin: 6 months as opposed to 3.[10] Phenol is inexpensive and can be used more frequently than every 3 months if needed.[11] Multiple studies have demonstrated phenol has the potential to last longer with greater clinical efficacy as compared with botulinum toxin.[12,13,19,20]

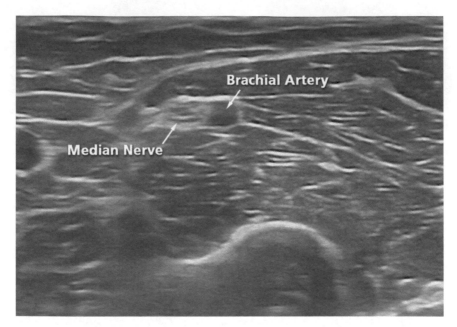

Figure 10.3 Median nerve above the elbow will cause a motor and sensory block.

Table 10.1 Concentration and Dosing of Phenol and Ethyl Alcohol

Phenol	Lethal Dose	Pediatric Dose	General Guidelines
Typically prepared as a sterile aqueous solution diluted to a 3%–6% concentration to induce Wallerian degeneration and reduce spasticity.[9,11–13] One study demonstrated successful treatment in nearly 90% of patients who received 4.5% phenol compared to less than 20% benefit in those who received 3% concentration.[14,15]	A lethal dose of 8.5 g has been reported in humans. The fatal dose for ingestion of phenol ranges from 1.0 g to 32 g.[3,16] A general rule for clinicians is to use no more than 1.0 g of phenol per session as 20 mL of 5% aqueous phenol solution, as 1.0 g of phenol delivered in this concentration equals approximately 1.0 mL of pure phenol.[9]	In children, a total dose of 30 mg/kg is considered safe. Similar to adults, the total dose should not exceed 1.0 g.[17] The dose for a pediatric patient could be calculated using a 60 kg adult patient and 20 mL of 5% phenol as the maximum dose. A child is 1/3 the body weight of an adult (1/3 of 60 kg = 20 kg body weight). The adult maximum of 20 mL should be downgraded to 7 mL in children (1/3 dose).	For specific phenol, injections range from 0.5 mL to 1.0 mL in motor points and 0.5 mL to 3.0 mL in peripheral nerves[17] as a comparison ratio of between 70 and 110 units of onabotulinumtoxinA to 1.0 mL of 5% phenol has been used in children but a relationship is unclear for adults.[18]

(continued)

Table 10.1 Concentration and Dosing of Phenol and Ethyl Alcohol *(continued)*

Ethyl Alcohol		Pediatric Dose	
The drug dilution most commonly used clinically ranges from 35% to 60%.[1] Studies with alcohol concentrations ranging from 48% to 95% found varying degrees of temporary paralysis and the concentration was not correlated with the degree of weakness.[1]		In children with cerebral palsy, multiple studies applied 45% alcohol to spastic muscles targeting the muscle bulk and motor point. Results showed a decrease in spasticity with preservation of motor strength with a reported duration of benefit from 6 to 12 months and sporadically up to 2–3 years.[1]	

Efficacy of Repeat Administration

There is limited data on repeated nerve blocks with phenol for chronic spasticity. Helweg-Larsen and Jacobsen achieved similar effects and duration of improvement with repeated phenol administration,[16] while in some patients, there is permanent reduction in spasticity after the third or fourth round of phenol neurolysis due to extensive fibrosis and necrosis preventing reinnervation.[21] This will obviously make the ability to stimulate motor nerve branches after multiple injections more difficult.[6] Ultrasound (US) guidance and electrical stimulation (E-stim) required a smaller volume due to improved accuracy in up to eight repeated injections in the musculocutaneous nerve.[17] US guidance is our recommended standard of care where available.

Adverse Effects

Mild side effects include pain on injection, bleeding, and bruising.[4] Phenol can cause dysesthesias when injected around mixed or sensory nerves, at rates reported between 2% and 32%.[17] Higher rates have been reported in the tibial nerve compared to the musculocutaneous or obturator nerves.[17] Nerve destruction and local muscle damage, myonecrosis, can occur near the site of injection and correlates with the concentration and dose applied.[22] Additionally, phenol can cause occlusion and fibrosis in the microcirculation around the nerve. Rare, but more serious effects include peripheral edema, skin slough, excessive motor weakness, and deep vein thrombosis. High systemic doses above 8.5 g can lead to toxicity that presents with convulsions, central nervous system (CNS) depression, and eventual cardiovascular collapse. Inadvertent intravascular injection can be catastrophic with arterial sclerosis and infarction of distal tissue.[18] To avoid this very rare complication, we recommend using an injection needle connected to anesthesia tubing. If there is a flash of blood in the tubing during aspiration, the needle should be promptly withdrawn. Phenol is generally avoided in patients with advanced liver disease due to reduced hepatic metabolism.[4] Overall, severe side effects are uncommon when using proper technique and dosing.[18]

Ethyl Alcohol

History

Ethyl alcohol (alcohol or ethanol) was the first alcohol compound to be studied on nerve cells and used for nerve blocks.[14] Phenol is more potent than alcohol, with 5% phenol corresponding to 40% alcohol in neurolytic strength.[15] Ethyl alcohol once had a range of applications, from treating trigeminal neuralgia and intractable carcinoma to performing sympathectomy. In the United Sates, the cost of ethyl alcohol significantly increased in 2020 due to a new indication in the treatment of hypertrophic cardiomyopathy.[23]

Mechanism of Action

Alcohol causes protein denaturation and tissue destruction including nerve coagulation and myonecrosis. At low concentrations of 5% to 10%, alcohol acts as a local anesthetic by decreasing sodium and potassium conductance. At higher concentrations, alcohol denatures proteins and causes cellular injury.[24] Lower concentrations cause inconsistent axonal destruction, whereas absolute alcohol produced neuronal degeneration with extensive fibrosis and partial regeneration. Concentration and dosing are found in Table 10.1. Studies with multiple alcohol concentrations ranging from 48% to 95% found varying degrees of temporary paralysis, and the concentration was not correlated with the degree of weakness.[25,26] There have been multiple studies comparing the efficacy of alcohol and phenol with varying results. A story by Kocabas et al, found them to be equally effective.[16]

Adverse Effects

Alcohol appears to be safe and efficient in treating spasticity when injected intramuscularly close to the motor point. Some studies show that alcohol has fewer systemic side effects compared to phenol.[4,27] These effects include burning pain with intramuscular injection, transient muscle discomfort, local hyperemia, and skin irritation if injected superficially. It is important to note that as most of the alcohol that enters the body is metabolized, patients receiving alcohol neurolysis could demonstrate acute intoxication in the immediate postinjection period.[28] If injected perineurally, there is risk of temporary sensory deficits and pain.

Injection Technique for Nerve Blocks, Chemical Neurolysis, and Motor Point Blocks

A nerve block arises when chemical neurolysis inflicts nerve damage preventing nerve conduction.[1]

Motor points are the location in a muscle belly where the motor branch of a nerve enters.[29] They represent the area of the muscle with a high concentration of motor end plates.[30] Cutaneous neuromuscular E-stim will identify motor points by applying the least intensity and shortest duration necessary to evoke a visible muscle contraction.[29,30]

Injection Technique

Phenol neurolysis can target numerous peripheral nerves in the upper and lower extremities. Historically, phenol and ethyl alcohol have been administered via percutaneous injection with E-stim guidance. Most children require sedation using general anesthesia or conscious sedation as this process is painful and requires the patient to remain still, while adolescents and adults may tolerate the procedure without

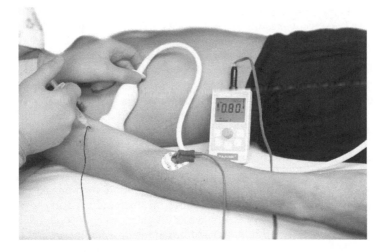

Figure 10.4 Stimulator setup. Set to 0.8 mA.

systemic anesthesia.[31] Typically, a hypodermic needle with Teflon insulation is used. The needle is on average 26 gauge and length ranges from 25 mm to 70 mm depending on the patient's body habitus. The tip of the needle is bare and serves as the stimulating electrode.

The needle is connected to either a peripheral nerve stimulator or conventional electromyography (EMG) machine and inserted through the skin to locate the nerve[10] (Figure 10.4). The nerve stimulator should have an adjustable current because some machines used for botulinum toxin do not have a fine adjustment capacity for low amplitude stimulation and are meant for muscle stimulation.

US can identify anatomic variation of nerves and/or muscles to improve accuracy and outcomes.[17] Combination techniques using E-stim with US guidance have been developed to improve nerve or motor point localization. High frequency US enables visualization of the muscle echotexture, motor and cutaneous nerves, and vasculature. With US, injectors can decrease the incidence of dysesthesias and/or phlebitis after neurolysis. In one study by Karri et al., phenol neurolysis of 139 nerves belonging to 57 patients were reviewed. All procedures utilized both E-stim and US guidance, and no dysesthesias were reported during the follow-up period of more than 40 days.[19] Matsumoto and colleagues evaluated 167 musculocutaneous nerve blocks comparing E-stim only versus E-stim plus US guidance. The results showed that the combination was associated with lower injected doses compared to E-stim alone (2.31 mL versus 3.69 mL, p <.001). With subsequent injections, the dose of phenol increased with E-stim guidance but not with E-stim and US guidance indicating that there was less scarring using combination techniques. Both methods had high technical success and low rates of adverse events.[18] Another advantage was that once the nerve was identified with the stimulation response, E-stim could be turned off and the injections completed using US alone, causing less discomfort for patients.

Phenol injection technique requires proficiency and new injectors may need 1 hour to complete the procedure. However, US can greatly facilitate nerve identification that may shorten procedural time. E-stim with probing is painful and requires the needle tip to be very close to the depolarizing nerve that can be technically difficult in some patients. For effective results, phenol must be injected circumferentially around the nerve termed hydrodissection. Without visualization, the physician cannot be certain where are the fluid layers (often away from the nerve), but with US visualization, the physician has a better chance of obtaining nerve hydrodissection.[31] Locating the target motor point or nerve and selecting the appropriate dose require experience to avoid adverse events. We recommend US guidance with E-stim, as muscle fibrosis from previous neurolysis may result in a poorly noticeable contraction with E-stim alone, whereby with US, the twitch is easier to observe.

Single Event Multilevel Chemoneurolysis

Single event multilevel chemoneurolysis (SEMLC) refers to combining procedures that treats various spastic limbs at multiple levels with more than one chemoneurolytic agent. Most commonly, phenol and botulinum toxin are used in combination. It can more efficaciously treat diffuse spasticity compared with one agent alone, especially in small children due to weight-based dosing limitations. The implementation of phenol or alcohol allows treatment to larger muscle groups during a single injection and spares botulinum toxin for other muscles in both children and adults. Ploypetch et al. showed that significantly more spastic muscles were treated in the SEMLC group compared to the botulinum toxin only group (15 muscles versus 8 muscles, respectively). They noted that 91.4% of patients in the SEMLC group attained injection goals versus 77.5% in the botulinum toxin only group with minimal adverse effects.[32] SEMLC is safe and effective in managing diffuse spasticity.[32,33] A further advantage of SEMLC over oral medications or intrathecal baclofen is the ability to selectively target affected muscles. It allows for better dose adjustment based on the severity of spasticity and functional contribution of the individual muscles.[32]

In general, botulinum toxin is injected into smaller muscles while phenol is reserved for motor nerves with a limited sensory component that are easily located. Ideal targets for phenol neurolysis include the musculocutaneous nerve supplying the elbow flexors and the obturator nerve targeting the hip adductors for relief of scissoring gait and difficulty with personal hygiene. Hamstring motor points and rectus femoris motor point blocks, motor point blocks to the brachialis, and motor point blocks to the gastrocnemius and tibialis posterior have also shown clinical utility. Botulinum toxin is traditionally the preferred choice for muscles such as wrist and finger flexors or intrinsic hand muscles, which are supplied by nerves that have many sensory axons that can be damaged and result in dysesthesias. Phenol is generally avoided for the tibial nerve, where botulinum toxin is preferred to treat equinus foot positioning to avoid dysesthesias via the tibial nerve.[34] However, with US guidance and a deep understanding of the anatomy, some clinicians are able to use phenol blocks in the distal upper extremity without causing dysesthesias.[19]

Cryoneurolysis

Introduction

It is possible to perform a neurolysis, without a chemical agent, as a treatment for spasticity. Cryoneurolysis is a nerve-targeted procedure for spasticity in which reduction of spasticity and improved range of motion can be achieved in the absence of the need for surgical lengthening.[35,36] Cryoneurolysis involves the freezing of a peripheral nerve branch or trunk at temperatures sufficient enough to cause a neurolysis via the percutaneous insertion of a cryoprobe through the skin and subsequent generation of an ice ball or oval. Though novel to spasticity, cryoneurolysis has been utilized in the practice of pain medicine for decades for peripheral nerve pain and neuromas.[37-40] Prior to our renewed interest by author PW's clinic, there was one published case report of using percutaneous cryoneurolysis to the obturator nerve in 1998 for the lower extremity.[41] For the upper limb, there was one published abstract that documented improvements in elbow spasticity using cryoneurolysis to the musculocutaneous nerve in 2015.[42]

History and Mechanism of Action

Lloyd first utilized liquid nitrogen in 1961 to cool a probe for percutaneous use. His group later utilized the term "cryoanalgesia" in 1976 and noted the absence of neuritis or neuralgia with their procedures.[43] Cryoneurolysis, the process of using cold to cause a neurolysis and Wallerian degeneration, is possible due to a rapid cooling with a percutaneous probe. The rapid cooling is possible due to the process of throttling a gas through an orifice from high to low pressure. This causes a rapid expansion of the gas and a rapid drop in temperature, known as the Joule–Thomson effect.[43] The change in temperature generates an ice ball/oval between 3.5 mm and 18 mm, depending on the device used, that is formed at the tip of the cryoprobe using closed circuit system with compressed gas (Figure 10.5a and 10.5b). The temperature at which the ice ball is formed is determined by the boiling point of the gas. Typically, a temperature between $-60°C$ and $-88°C$ (the boiling point of N_2O is $-88°C$[43]) is desired for cryoneurolysis. With cryoneurolysis, the ice ball becomes quickly fixed and tethers in place as it forms without any dispersion of fluids. There is resulting loss of axon continuity due to Wallerian degeneration extending outward from the lesion over a limited distance. The hallmark feature of cryoneurolysis is that the basal lamina, epineurium, and perineurium of the targeted nerve remain intact and serve as a tube for nerve regeneration.[44] The key advantage of cryoneurolysis is this selective property whereby Wallerian degeneration occurs, but the epineurium and perineurium, muscles, and vessels are not damaged, which is effectively a reversible secondary axonotmesis on the Sunderland Classification Scale.[39,44] Unlike alcohol or phenol chemodenervation, cryoneurolysis has not been shown to damage the surrounding structures and should not cause myonecrosis or perineural or muscular fibrosis. Therefore, it does not pose a challenge for subsequent US visualization. It is opined that the maintenance of the perineurium prevents the release of the chemical agent, neurotropin, which is implicated in the formation of painful neuromas and explains why Lloyd noted the absence of the neuritis or neuralgia formation.[45]

The use of cryoneurolysis produces an immediate effect on sensory and motor nerves mimicking that of the diagnostic nerve block (DNB) such that the target muscle can be easily identified as having had a successful block. Muscle relaxation will be instant. This results from the time- and temperature-dependent thermal disruption of neural conduction. The ice ball formation is under the control of the user and generates and melts in seconds. The process can be immediately aborted should any unwanted sensory disturbance be noted reducing the risk of permanent neural damage and the probe moved to a different spot. This would not be the case with chemoneurolysis where fluid is diffused. The immediate onset allows for one targeted muscle or group to be performed before selecting another. For example, after the musculocutaneous to the brachialis is completed, the decision to add in the biceps branch or the radial nerve to the brachioradialis can be made if those muscle bellies and tendons may now appear shortened or prominent after the brachialis is lengthened or shows reduced spasticity.

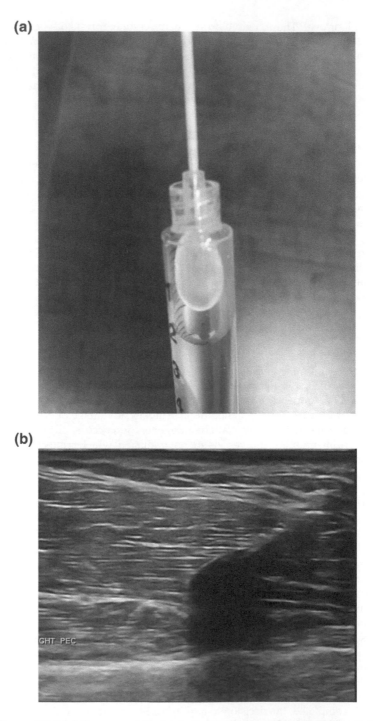

Figure 10.5 (a) Cryoneurolysis ice ball with the iovera® handheld (Pacira). (b) Cryoneurolysis ice ball to the lateral pectoral nerve.

Selecting the Patient

Diagnostic Nerve Blocks

Cryoneurolysis for spasticity is modelled on the long history of anesthetic DNBs.[46,47] It is imperative that a DNB is performed to target and select the desired nerve or nerve branch using a small amount of a short acting local anesthetic such as lido- caine (1mL–1.5 mL of 2% solution).[48] Targeted DNBs serve to isolate problematic spastic muscle groups and predict their response to spasticity treatment based on their response to cessation of nerve conduction.[48] The DNB offers a temporary block of electrical conduction and allows the muscle to relax. The DNB will distinguish between what is a fully reducible deformity and a fixed contracture. The fully reduc- ible deformity is a joint that can be stretched passively to full range at rest, with an accompanied reduction in spasticity. A fixed contracture will not improve to full range after a DNB, but many joints may gain many degrees of range after a DNB even after having undergone the administration of botulinum toxin.

The DNB may predict potential of adverse outcomes such as loss of function or sensory impairment. This is particularly important for the tibial nerve and ability to weight bear and walk, or for hand function. The preselection technique of DNB can be used for choosing the targets for all methods of focal spasticity management including botulinum toxin, phenol or ethyl alcohol, and surgery.[48]

After a successful DNB, cryoneurolysis can be performed onto the same targeted peripheral nerves. Cryoneurolysis is performed at a separate visit or after several hours when the DNB effects have worn off to allow for the nerve to be stimulated and the cryoneurolysis to be performed accurately.

Usually, these spastic muscle groups have previously received various combina- tions of botulinum toxin, chemoneurolysis (ethyl alcohol or phenol), physical thera- pies, and bracing but have reached a therapeutic plateau. Cryoneurolysis may also be the initial treatment, rather than botulinum toxin, provided the DNB identifies a reducible deformity and not a fixed contracture after DNB. The nerves that are best tailored for cryoneurolysis are found in Table 10.2.

Technique for Cryoneurolysis

We (author PW) currently use a device with N_2O (iovera® system, Pacira, Parsippany-Troy Hills, NJ, USA)[39] although there are multiple devices that perform cryoneurolysis that are sold around the world. Our procedural guideline is found in Table 10.3.

We strongly endorse US and E-stim as the only guidance techniques for cryo- neurolysis, for the reasons described for phenol and ethyl alcohol and to directly visualize and touch the desired nerve target. In most cases, the nerve will be found alongside or adjacent to a blood vessel (Figures 10.1(a),(b), 10.2, 10.3.). A nerve stim- ulator with an adjustable digital display of milliamp output is essential to identify and stimulate the targeted nerve. The cryoprobe should have either an internal nerve stimulator or an external stimulator attached that can conduct electricity along the exploring probe.

Cryoneurolysis delivered via a small cryoprobe (e.g., 20 gauge) can be safely used in a novel manner to perform selective thermal lesions of peripheral motor nerve branch(es) for the management of limb spasticity.[49,50] For E-stim, the threshold for muscle twitches should be less than 0.8 to 1.0 milliamps.[51] Cryoneurolysis involves touching the nerve. Once the ice ball has formed, it will "stick" to the nerve and be tethered into place until the ball melts. The optimal duration of the ice ball has not

Table 10.2 Recommended Nerve Targets for Cryoneurolysis

Shoulder Girdle
Lateral pectoral nerve to the pectoralis major muscle
Medial pectoral nerve to pectoralis minor muscle
Thoracodorsal nerve to latissimus dorsi
Suprascapular nerve for reducing pain

Elbow Flexors
Musculocutaneous to brachialis and/or biceps brachii
Radial to brachioradialis

Wrist and Fingers
Imperative to assure no sensory dysesthesia in this group
Stimulation required to find branches or whole trunk
Median nerve if no sensory dysesthesia with a DNB. Above elbow for the pronator
  teres and below elbow will target flexor carpi radialis, distal muscles, and the
  anterior interosseus nerve. It is possible to just target the flexor digitorum
  superficialis fascicles.
Ulnar nerve if no sensory dysesthesia with a DNB
Radial nerve for finger extensors

Hip
Obturator nerve anterior divisions: pectineus, adductor longus, gracilis, adductor
  brevis
Posterior divisions: obturator externus, adductor magnus, adductor brevis

Knee
Femoral to the rectus femoris
Sciatic nerve to hamstring groups

Foot and Ankle
Tibial nerve can be targeted to the trunk, and individual muscles, including medial
  and lateral gastrocnemius, soleus, tibialis posterior, and flexor digitorum longus.
At the ankle for the intrinsic muscle groups

been established; our current practice is approximately three cycles of 104 seconds at three spots along/around the nerve, a total of approximately 5 minutes per nerve. Sensory nerves that are smaller then may require less cycles.

Our cryoneurolysis protocol was initially primarily focused on targeting motor nerves; however, sensory branches and mixed nerves can also be treated. This includes the suprascapular nerve for shoulder pain, median and ulnar nerve (Figures 10.1(a),(b), 10.3) trunks for the painful fisted hand and wrist, or the tibial nerve. Like motor point blocks, with US guidance, one can track the nerve into a muscle, such as the median nerve into the pronator teres to avoid a sensory block or motor block to the digits or a femoral nerve block to the rectus femoris (Figure 10.6). As another example, patients with multiple sclerosis (MS) may have painful dysesthesias in their feet that can improve with cryoneurolysis of the tibial nerve trunk.

Outcome Measures

The goal of cryoneurolysis is to obtain a reduction in spasticity but also increased range of motion. Standardized outcome measures should be used to capture

Table 10.3 Procedural Guideline for Cryoneurolysis

1. Prepping the skin with sufficient antibacterial precautions, e.g., use of a sterile or bacteriostatic ultrasound gel

2. Small dose of local anesthesia for cutaneous and subcutaneous anesthesia to reduce pain at percutaneous entry site; less than 0.5 ml of 1% lidocaine to avoid diffusion and anesthetizing the nerve

3. There are specialized probes that allow for deeper injections without need for insulation and should be used with the manufacturer's guidance. If not available, then either a thermal insulating catheter (#16 or #18 angiocath) or similar gauge needle larger than the probe to serve as a guide and offer protection from cutaneous frostbite. The use of the catheter will act as an additional insulator to provide optimal low dose E-stim and assist in cryoprobe positioning.

4. Color Doppler can be enabled to ensure localization of the targeted nerve in the neurovascular bundle. We recommend an in-plane ultrasound approach for cryoneurolysis. This ensures the large needle is visualized as it approaches the targeted nerve, to minimize unnecessary repositioning. The probe is guided until it is juxtaposition to the motor nerve branch, with the tip of the probe clearly visualized and away from any vein or artery.

5. The stimulator should be engaged prior to needle or probe insertion to ensure that the muscle is responding at a low amperage of between 0.5 and 0.8 milliamps. Using ultrasound and E-stim, observe for the desired muscle movement and adjust the needle and probe depth to obtain the best muscle stimulation. Avoid excessive or repeated entries, and if in doubt, reexamine the ultrasound imagery to confirm best point of entry and depth. If there is a painful sensory stimulation along the sensory branch, the tip is moved.

6. If the patient experiences a painful sensation down the nerve during the cryoneurolysis, the device is immediately turned off, the cryoprobe is allowed to defrost, and the probe tip is then readjusted prior to resuming a subsequent lesion.

7. To ensure a complete neurolysis occurs, we suggest that two lesions are performed along the same nerve branch at least 1 cm apart or from opposite sides of a nerve. Each device will have a different protocol. At a temperature of $-60°C$ to $-88°C$, we recommend two to three lesions per large nerve for a total of 3 to 4.5 minutes. It is possible and typical to do multiple nerves in one setting. With 1-3 lesions per target. There is no maximal number of nerves per treatment.

8. In the upper extremity, we find that starting with a suprascapular nerve block can reduce shoulder pain and allow for better positioning for abduction. The lateral pectoral nerve can be done next. This will also allow for shoulder external rotation that will allow for better access to the musculocutaneous, median, and ulnar nerves.

9. After completion of the procedure, the percutaneous entry point is stabilized with pressure. An occlusive dressing can be used or in rare cases sealed with a skin glue.

10. There are no specific activity restrictions required.

11. Patients on systemic anticoagulants may proceed with DNBs or cryoneurolysis.

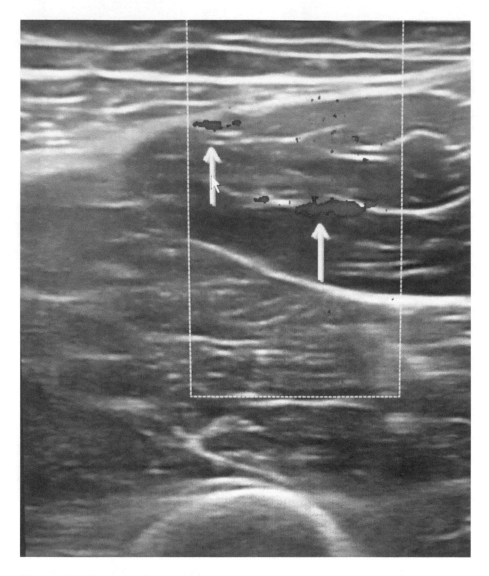

Figure 10.6 The femoral nerve branch to rectus femoris is indicated by arrows. The Doppler flow assists to localize.

outcomes of the DNB to ensure improvements. We recommend using the Modified Tardieu Scale, Modified Ashworth Scale (MAS), as well as video capture to compare before and after. Video capture is helpful in documenting nerve block efficacy and motor control. A goniometer is ideal for measuring range of motion. Inter-knee distance is used for obturator nerve interventions. For functional outcomes, the Goal Attainment Scale (GAS), the Disability of Shoulder Hand Arm (DASH), the Box and Block test, grip strength, and House Score are among the outcome measures that can track outcomes in the upper extremity, whereas for the lower extremity, walk tests can be implemented for ambulators.

A post-procedure reassessment of the patient is required to assess the relative benefits of the cryoneurolysis, alter the management strategy, and reassess expected goals. Redistribution of BoNT will likely occur in other muscle groups. Like phenol and alcohol, combination therapy is common. For example, finger flexor spasticity or dystonia with preserved active movements is best treated with BoNT, whereas a painful fisted hand is amenable to cryoneurolysis of the median and ulnar nerves. Long-term follow-up is needed due to potential for neural regrowth (typically at the 6-month mark) and changes in spastic patterns.

The clinical experience of author PW includes more than 150 patients and hundreds of nerves.[35,36,50] The outcomes and data are still under collection and have not yet been submitted for peer review (ClinicalTrials.gov Identifier: NCT04670783, NCT04907201, NCT04907201). The data to date has documented continual improvement in muscle tone and ROM with immediate onset but is most notable at 1 to 3 months post cryoneurolysis and then maintained.[35,50] With passive stretching, active movements, therapies, and bracing, further improvements have been documented over periods of several months.[7,8] To maximize the gains, rehabilitation of the antagonistic muscles is also recommended. The patient may now experience an increase in unopposed movements. For example, patient may be able to extend the wrist and fingers or abduct the shoulder after the flexors are overcome with cryoneurolysis. Physical therapies, bracing at full length, adjusting orthoses, and functional E-stim of the antagonist muscles are all forms of recommended adjuvant care.

Adverse Effects

Adverse effects include the failed therapeutic results, rare risk of infection, bleeding, and a sensory dysesthesia or pain from the sensory branches. This is typically short-lived but could last for a few weeks. Unwanted numbness can be reduced by ensuring DNB does not elicit this. A complex regional pain syndrome type II or neuritis is possible but is self-limiting and is treated using conservative measures. A 2023 review of 277 treated nerves in 113 patients found 96.75% of treatments had no reported side effects. Nearly one third of the nerves were mixed sensorimotor targets. Of nine cases of reported dysesthesia or pain, five required medical treatment and all resolved, with the tibial nerve trunk the most common.[52] No fluid is injected; thus, there is no risk of vascular injection unlike phenol or alcohol injections. The US guidance should confirm that the injection is perivascular or adjacent to vessels and not intravascular. It has also been noted in numerous studies that large blood vessels are "remarkably resistant to structural change after freezing and their function as a conduit of blood was not impaired."[53] Frostbite is possible and the use of a 16 to 18 gauge insulated catheter is suggested to protect the skin.

KEY POINTS

- Phenol and ethanol are used perineurally to create a mixed sensorimotor nerve block, or at the motor nerve branch to the muscle termed motor point block. Cryoneurolysis uses similar principles.
- Efficacy of phenol can last up to 6 months in many individuals. Cryoneurolysis in initial case studies is showing maintenance beyond 1 to 2 years.

- SEMLC with botulinum toxin and phenol/alcohol or cryoneurolysis is a single session procedure that enables the physician to treat multiple spastic muscles.
- The use of US can greatly facilitate nerve identification that may shorten procedural time of neurolysis.

REFERENCES

1. Escaldi S. Neurolysis: a brief review for a fading art. *Phys Med Rehabil Clin N Am.* 2018;29(3):519–527. http://www.embase.com/search/results?subaction=viewrecord&from=export&id=L2000821275%0A. https://.doi.org/10.1016/j.pmr.2018.03.005

2. Wood KM. The use of phenol as a neurolytic agent: a review. *Pain.* 1978;5(3):205–229. https://doi.org/10.1016/0304-3959(78)90009-X

3. Haxton HA. Chemical sympathectomy. *Br Med J.* 1949;1(4614):1026. https://doi.org/10.1136/BMJ.1.4614.1026

4. D'souza RS, Affilations NSW. *Phenol Nerve Block - StatPearls - NCBI Bookshelf.* https://www.ncbi.nlm.nih.gov/books/NBK525978. Accessed February 21, 2022.

5. Hughes-Davies DI, Redman IR. Chemical lumbar sympathectomy. *Anaesthesia.* 1976;31(8):1068–1075. https://doi.org/10.1111/j.1365-2044.1976.tb11946.x

6. Halpern D, Meelhuysen FE. Phenol motor point block in the management of muscular hypertonia. *Arch Phys Med Rehabil.* 1966;47(10):659–664.

7. Kelly RE, Smith PCG. Intrathecal phenol in the treatment of reflex spasms and spasticity. *Lancet.* 1959;274(7112):1102–1105. https://doi.org/10.1016/S0140-6736(59)90095-9

8. Feldman D, Knott L, Katz J. Peripheral phenol injections reduce spasticity. *JAMA J Am Med Assoc.* 1965;193(12):31. https://doi.org/10.1001/jama.1965.03090120093044

9. Okazaki A. [The effects of two and five percent aqueous phenol on the cat tibial nerve in situ--II: Effect on the circulation of the tibial nerve]. *Masui.* 1993;42(6):819–825. https://europepmc.org/article/med/8320797. Accessed February 19, 2022.

10. Halpern D, Meelhuysen FE. Duration of relaxation after intramuscular neurolysis with phenol. *JAMA J Am Med Assoc.* 1967;200(13):1152–1154. https://doi.org/10.1001/jama.1967.03120260048007

11. Karri J, Zhang B, Li S. Phenol neurolysis for management of focal spasticity in the distal upper extremity. *PM R.* 2020;12(3):246–250. https://doi.org/10.1002/pmrj.12217

12. Manca M, Merlo A, Ferraresi G, Cavazza S, Marchi P. Botulinum toxin type a versus phenol. A clinical and neurophysiological study in the treatment of ankle clonus. *Eur J Phys Rehabil Med.* 2010;46(1):11–18. https://www.researchgate.net/publication/42441114. Accessed February 21, 2022.

13. Kocabas H, Salli A, Demir AH, Ozerbil OM. Comparison of phenol and alcohol neurolysis of tibial nerve motor branches to the gastrocnemius muscle for treatment of spastic foot after stroke: a randomized controlled pilot study. *Eur J Phys Rehabil Med.* 2010;46(1):5–10. https://pubmed.ncbi.nlm.nih.gov/20332720. Accessed February 21, 2022.

14. May O. The functional and histological effects of intraneural and intraganglionic injections of alcohol. *Br Med J.* 1912;2(2696):465–470. https://doi.org/10.1136/bmj.2.2696.465

15. Histopathological lesions in the sciatic nerve of the rat following perineural application of phenol and alcohol solutions - PubMed. https://pubmed.ncbi.nlm.nih.gov/5377823/. Accessed February 19, 2022.

16. Helweg-Larsen J, Jacobsen E. Treatment of spasticity in cerebral palsy by means of phenol nerve block of peripheral nerves. *Dan Med Bull*. 1969;16(1):20–25. https://europepmc.org/article/med/5371940. Accessed February 21, 2022.

17. Matsumoto M E, Berry J, Yung H, Matsumoto M, Munin M C. Comparing electrical stimulation with and without ultrasound guidance for phenol neurolysis to the musculocutaneous nerve. *PM R*. 2017;10(4):357–364. https://doi.org/10.1016/j.pmrj.2017.09.006

18. Saeed K, Adams MCB, Hurley RW. Central and peripheral neurolysis. In: *Essentials of Pain Medicine*. Elsevier; 2018:655–662.e1. https://doi.org/10.1016/b978-0-323-40196-8.00072-3

19. Karri J, Mas MF, Francisco GE, Li S. Practice patterns for spasticity management with phenol neurolysis. *J Rehabil Med*. 2017. https://doi.org/10.2340/16501977-2239

20. Bakheit AMO, Badwan DAH, McLellan DL. The effectiveness of chemical neurolysis in the treatment of lower limb muscle spasticity. *Clini Rehabil*. 2016;10(1):40–43. https://doi.org/10.1177/026921559601000108

21. Awad E, Awad O. *Injection Techniques for Spasticity: A Practical Guide to Treatment of Cerebral Palsy, Hemiplegia, Multiple Sclerosis and Spinal Cord Injury*. Minneapolis, MN; 1993.

22. Zafonte RD, Munin MC. Phenol and alcohol blocks for the treatment of spasticity. *Phys Med Rehabil Clin N Am*. 2001;12(4):817–832, vii. http://www.ncbi.nlm.nih.gov/pubmed/11723866. Accessed June 5, 2018.

23. Savarimuthu S, Harky A. Alcohol septal ablation: a useful tool in our arsenal against hypertrophic obstructive cardiomyopathy. *J Card Surg*. 2020;35(8):2017–2024. https://doi.org/10.1111/jocs.14815

24. Ritchie J. The aliphatic alcohols. In: Gilman AG, Goodman LS, Rall TW, Murad F, eds. *The Pharmacologic Basis of Therapeutics*. 7th ed. New York: MacMillan; 1985.

25. Karen SG, Chua KHK. Clinical and functional outcome after alcohol neurolysis of the tibial nerve for ankle? foot spasticity. *Brain Inj*. 2001;15(8):733–739. https://doi.org/10.1080/02699050121181

26. Kong KH, Chua KSG. Intramuscular neurolysis with alcohol to treat poststroke finger flexor spasticity. *Clin Rehabil*. 2002;16(4):378–381. https://doi.org/10.1191/0269215502cr508oa

27. Kheder A, Nair KPS. Spasticity: pathophysiology, evaluation and management. *Pract Neurol*. 2012;12(5):289–298. https://doi.org/10.1136/practneurol-2011-000155

28. Andrew Koman L, Mooney JF, Smith BP. Neuromuscular blockade in the management of cerebral palsy. *J Child Neurol*. 1996;11(SUPPL. 1). https://doi.org/10.1177/0883073896011001s04

29. Botter A, Oprandi G, Lanfranco F, Allasia S, Maffiuletti NA, Minetto MA. Atlas of the muscle motor points for the lower limb: implications for electrical stimulation procedures and electrode positioning. *Eur J Appl Physiol*. 2011;111(10):2461–2471. https://doi.org/10.1007/S00421-011-2093-Y

30. Moon JY, Hwang TS, Sim SJ, Chun S Il, Kim M. Surface mapping of motor points in biceps brachii muscle. *Ann Rehabil Med*. 2012;36(2):187. https://doi.org/10.5535/ARM.2012.36.2.187

31. Gormley ME. The treatment of cerebral origin spasticity in children. *Neuro Rehabil*. 1999;12(2):93–103. https://doi.org/10.3233/nre-1999-12203

32. Ploypetch T, Kwon JY, Armstrong HF, Kim H. A retrospective review of unintended effects after single-event multi-level chemoneurolysis with botulinum toxin-a and

phenol in children with cerebral palsy. *PM&R*. 2015;7(10):1073–1080. https://doi.org/10.1016/J.PMRJ.2015.05.020

33. Gooch JL, Patton CP. Combining botulinum toxin and phenol to manage spasticity in children. *Arch Phys Med Rehabil*. 2004;85(7):1121–1124. https://doi.org/10.1016/j.apmr.2003.09.032

34. Picelli A, Battistuzzi E, Modenese A, et al. Diagnostic nerve block in prediction of outcome of botulinum toxin treatment for spastic equinovarus foot after stroke: a retrospective observational study. *J Rehabil Med*. 2020;52(6). https://doi.org/10.2340/16501977-2693

35. Winston P, Mills PB, Reebye R, Vincent D. Cryoneurotomy as a percutaneous mini-invasive therapy for the treatment of the spastic limb: case presentation, review of the literature and proposed approach for use. *Arch Rehabil Res Clin Transl*. 2019. https://doi.org/10.1016/j.arrct.2019.100030

36. Scobie J, Winston P. Case report: Perspective of a caregiver on functional outcomes following bilateral lateral pectoral nerve cryoneurotomy to treat spasticity in a pediatric patient with cerebral palsy. *Front Rehabil Sci*. 2021;0:35. https://doi.org/10.3389/FRESC.2021.719054

37. Trescot AM. Cryoanalgesia in interventional pain management. *Pain Physician*. 2003.

38. Ilfeld BM, Preciado J, Trescot AM. Novel cryoneurolysis device for the treatment of sensory and motor peripheral nerves. *Expert Rev Med Devices*. 2016;13(8):713–725. https://doi.org/10.1080/17434440.2016.1204229

39. Cheng JG. Cryoanalgesia for refractory neuralgia. *J Perioper Sci Cheng J Perioper Sci*. 2015;2(2). http://www.perioperative-science.com/content/02/02

40. Gekht G, Nottmeier EW, Lamer TJ. Painful medial branch neuroma treated with minimally invasive medial branch neurectomy. *Pain Med (United States)*. 2010;11(8):1179–1182. https://doi.org/10.1111/j.1526-4637.2010.00851.x

41. Kim PS, Ferrante FM. Cryoanalgesia: a novel treatment for hip adductor spasticity and obturator neuralgia. *Anesthesiology*. 1998;89(2):534–536. https://doi.org/10.1097/00000542-199808000-00036

42. Paulin MH, Patel AT. Cryodenervation for the treatment of upper limb spasticity: a prospective open proof-of-concept study. *Am J Phys Med*. 2015;94(3):12.

43. Ilfeld BM, Gabriel RA, Trescot AM. Ultrasound-guided percutaneous cryoneurolysis for treatment of acute pain: could cryoanalgesia replace continuous peripheral nerve blocks? *Br J Anaesth*. 2017;119(4):709–712. https://doi.org/10.1093/bja/aex142

44. Hsu M, Stevenson FF. Wallerian degeneration and recovery of motor nerves after multiple focused cold therapies. *Muscle and Nerve*. 2015;51(2):268-275. https://doi.org/10.1002/mus.24306

45. Trescot AM, ed. *Peripheral Nerve Entrapments*. Cham: Springer International Publishing; 2016. https://doi.org/10.1007/978-3-319-27482-9

46. Tardieu G, Hariga J. [Treatment of muscular rigidity of cerebral origin by infiltration of dilute alcohol. (RESULTS of 500 injections)]. *Arch Fr Pediatr*. 1964;21:25–41. http://www.ncbi.nlm.nih.gov/pubmed/14135061. Accessed July 16, 2019.

47. Deltombe T, De Wispelaere JF, Gustin T, Jamart J, Hanson P. Selective blocks of the motor nerve branches to the soleus and tibialis posterior muscles in the management of the spastic equinovarus foot 11No commercial party having a direct financial interest in the results of the research supporting this article has. *Arch Phys Med Rehabil*. 2003;85(1):54–58. https://doi.org/10.1016/s0003-9993(03)00405-2

48. Yelnik AP, Hentzen C, Cuvillon P, et al. French clinical guidelines for peripheral motor nerve blocks in a PRM setting. *Ann Phys Rehabil Med*. 2019. https://doi.org.10.1016/j.rehab.2019.06.001

49. Winston P, Mills P, Ganzert C, Reebye R, Vincent D. Cryoneurotomy as a novel adjunct to botulinum toxin treatment for the spastic elbow: a case study. *Toxicon*. 2019;156(2018):S114–S115. https://doi.org/10.1016/j.toxicon.2010.11.273

50. Rubenstein J, Harvey AW, Vincent D, Winston P. Cryoneurotomy to reduce spasticity and improve range of motion in spastic flexed elbow. A visual vignette. *Am J Phys Med Rehabil*. 2020; Publish Ah(5):100030. https://doi.org/10.1097/phm.0000000000001624

51. Winston P, Hashemi M, Vincent D. Ultrasound with e-stimulation diagnostic nerve blocks for targeted muscle selection in spasticity. *Am J Phys Med Rehabil*. 2021; Publish Ah. https://doi.org/10.1097/PHM.0000000000001801

52. Winston P, MacRae F, Rajapakshe S, Morrissey I, Boissonnault È, Vincent D, Hashemi M. Analysis of side effects of cryoneurolysis for the treatment of spasticity. *Am J Phys Med Rehabil*. 2023 Apr 25. doi: 10.1097/PHM.0000000000002267.

53. Gage AA, Baust JM, Baust JG. Experimental cryosurgery investigations in vivo. *Cryobiology*. 2009;59(3):229–243. https://doi.org/10.1016/J.CRYOBIOL.2009.10.001

11 Diagnostic Anesthetic Blocks: Differentiating Contracture From Spasticity

Jessica Mulhern, Shivani Gupta, and Kimberly Heckert

INTRODUCTION

Both neural and nonneural forces play a role in the diversity of movement patterns seen in patients with an upper motor neuron syndrome (UMNS). Nonneural forces include the changes in the rheological factors of soft tissues. Evidence suggests actual intrinsic changes in the properties of muscles including both the muscle cell and the extracellular matrix (ECM). These changes can lead to muscle contractures, an invariant physical state of fixed tissue shortening. Muscle contractures would not respond to oral antispasmodic agents that are meant for dynamic muscle movement only. Neural forces are those that involve alterations in the afferent and/or efferent signals between the brain/spinal cord and the muscle. These neural forces can be further divided into positive signs, which involve involuntary muscle overactivity, and negative signs, such as voluntary muscle underactivity. There are several available objective measures of spasticity; however, most do not distinguish between the neural and nonneural effects of muscle forces across a joint.

A diagnostic selective motor nerve block (DSMNB) is the use of an anesthetic agent at the branch of a motor nerve innervating a muscle to temporarily decrease signals to that muscle. With a low-risk profile, this procedure can serve as a diagnostic tool as well as a prelude to treatment with chemodenervation or neurolysis. DSMNB can help differentiate between static rheological tension, such as a muscle contracture, from dynamic tension of muscle overactivity or spasticity. For instance, a common finding in patients with UMNS is excessive flexion of the finger metacarpophalangeal and proximal interphalangeal joints. On physical examination, when passively moving the finger joints into extension, a Modified Ashworth Scale (MAS) score of 4 suggests the joints are rigid in flexion. Rigidity, however, could be secondary to neural or nonneural forces, or both. After performing a DSMNB to the motor nerves innervating the flexor digitorum superficialis, any additional movement eludes that muscle overactivity is playing a role in finger flexion and bodes well for the use of chemodenervation or neurolysis for spasticity treatment. However, if no additional finger extension was obtained after the DSMNB, the majority of the rigidity is secondary to nonneural causes and further interventions involving chemodenervation and neurolysis may no longer be as appropriate. Surgical procedures may offer more benefit in these instances. DSMNB serves the purpose of allowing both the physician and the patient to visualize expected outcomes after the contribution of spasticity is diminished. This can help with realistic goal setting for the patient and caregivers. DSMNB is particularly useful as a prelude to neurolysis with ethyl alcohol or phenol. The procedural component of DSMNB, described later in this chapter, is very similar to that of neurolysis; however, the effects of DSMNB are temporary, lasting up to several hours, where neurolysis can last months to years. Performing DSMNB prior to neurolysis would allow evaluation for anatomic variants that can lead to sensory nerve involvement and thus resultant increased risk of dysesthesias post chemoneurolysis. If patients experience any neuropathic abnormalities (i.e., tingling, burning, or shock sensations in the concentrated distribution) following the DSMNB, that particular region can be avoided or the patient and caregiver can be counseled regarding the potential for dysesthesia with chemoneurolysis in that region.[1]

Pre-Procedure

Prior to the procedure, the patient and caregiver should be informed regarding all aspects of the proposed interventions. When discussing DSMNB, one should discuss what can be expected following completion of the procedure including potential benefits, potential adverse events and side effects, and post-procedural instructions.

One of the benefits, as well as a potential negative aspect, of DSMNBs is the temporary nature of the medication used for the block. A patient and/or caregiver may be comforted knowing that any effects of the procedure will be short-lived, lasting only several hours post procedure. This may be seen as a benefit if a patient or caregiver is concerned about potential excessive weakness occurring as a result of the selective motor nerve blocks. The temporary effects of the procedure may be perceived as a negative aspect as the patient will only obtain relief or improvement in range of motion (ROM) or mobility for a relatively short time. Having a candid discussion regarding the various perceptions of the temporary effects will ensure patients and caregivers enter the procedure with the proper expectations.

Reasons for performing the procedure should be understood by patients and caregiver. These reasons may include definitive determination of suspected muscles involved in the patient's presentation, evaluation of the presence or degree of contracture, and the provision of a temporary trial period during which the patient can experience what it may feel like to have the treated areas addressed with longer-lasting interventions such as chemodenervation with botulinum toxin (BoNT) or chemoneurolysis with phenol or alcohol.

Risks of bleeding, infection, neurovascular injury, and potential for intravascular injection of anesthetic agent and its complications should be disclosed and understood by patients and caregivers and written and verbal consent obtained. Measures taken to reduce these risks (such as skin preparation, guidance methods, and technical skills applied) may also be discussed.

Post-procedure instructions should be discussed, including mitigation of local discomfort caused by the procedure with ice application or use of over-the-counter analgesics. The patient and/or caregiver should also be counseled that while the patient may resume regular activities, the patient should refrain from excessive and prolonged stretching and use of the treated area. In these authors' experience, patients may be tempted to complete tasks and activities they previously were unable to perform secondary to limitations from spasticity. However, the patient should be educated that immediate and aggressive ROM may result in injury as the muscles and soft tissues are unaccustomed to these activities. Once the longer-lasting interventions are performed, the patients and caregivers should be educated on how they may safely incorporate these activities and stretching routines. Allot time to discuss any questions the patients and caregivers raise and consider asking them to summarize their understanding.

Equipment

Equipment required for a DSMNB can be acquired from most medical supply companies. One will need a surface stimulator, peripheral nerve stimulator, surface electrodes, betadine, alcohol swabs, gloves, surgical marker, 30-gauge needle, 3-mL syringe, peripheral nerve block needle (gauge and length determined according to physician preference; these authors typically use 24 G x 25 mm for cervical region, 22 G x 40 mm for pectoral and forearm regions, and 22 G x 80 mm for arm, thigh, and leg regions), 10-mL syringe, band-aids, and gauze (Figure 11.1).

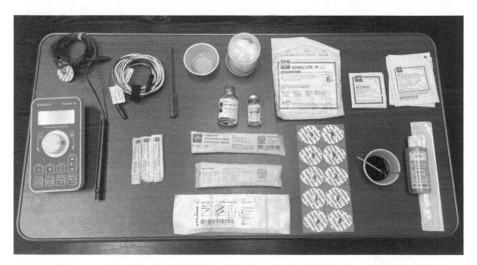

Figure 11.1 Procedural equipment table.

Medications

There are a variety of anesthetic agents available for use, each with their own benefit as well as risk. The anesthetic agents most frequently used by the authors, and the ones that were discussed, are 1% lidocaine and 0.25% bupivacaine. Both of these medications are in the amide class of anesthetics, which act as voltage-gated sodium channel blockers. The onset of action of lidocaine is typically 1 to 2 minutes, while bupivacaine is more often 5 to 10 minutes. Duration of action of lidocaine is about 2 hours or less, whereas bupivacaine is longer-lasting, approximately 4 to 8 hours depending on concentration and amount used.[2] With onset and duration of action taken into consideration, these authors prefer to use 1% lidocaine for local skin anesthesia to the skin overlying the motor nerve branches, and 0.25% bupivacaine for diagnostic block of motor nerve branches. The risk of systemic effects and/or toxicity is minimal due to the concentration and amount used for DSMNBs. The injecting physician should be aware of all the potential side effects and adverse events, including necessary actions to mitigate adverse effects, of medications utilized. The entire scope regarding the said adverse events and management will not be discussed in this text.

The Procedure

Once the patient has been evaluated and consent obtained, all supplies and equipment should be placed on the procedural table. This includes anesthetic agents drawn up into their proper syringes. These authors draw up 3 mL of 1% lidocaine into a 3-mL syringe, and 10 ml of 0.25% bupivacaine into a 10-mL syringe. These syringes should be labeled appropriately to avoid confusion during the procedure. A 30-gauge needle is placed on the syringe with lidocaine, and this will be used for local skin anesthesia. The syringe with the bupivacaine is connected to the nerve block needle, and the tubing is primed with bupivacaine to expel air present in the tubing. The surface nerve mapping probe and ground electrode should be connected to the peripheral nerve stimulator. The peripheral nerve stimulator should be turned on, stimulation intensity set to 0 mA, and placed on twitch setting at 1 Hz frequency.

One of the most important aspects of the procedure is positioning the patient. Extra time and attention should be dedicated to proper position for both patient comfort and physician comfort. Once the patient is most optimally positioned, "time out" can occur to ensure the accuracy of all details prior to the start of the procedure, including patient information, laterality, appropriate limb, and procedure type. Once "time out" is complete, the ground electrode should be placed on a bony prominence away from the region to be treated and not directly overlying another peripheral nerve.

For localization of a motor nerve branch on an x- and y-axis, the surface stimulator will be placed on the skin, and stimulation intensity slowly increased from 0 mA to a max of 20 to 35 mA depending on the region. As stimulation intensity is increased, the physician should be looking for muscle contraction. Once muscle contraction is noted, stimulation may be decreased to the lowest amount at which muscle contraction occurs. The probe should be moved slightly (~1 cm) cephalad, caudad, medially, and laterally to assess if muscle contraction is stronger in any of these locations. The surgical marker is then used to mark the skin at the site of the probe where maximal muscle contraction at the lowest stimulation intensity is observed. The skin is then cleansed and prepped with an alcohol swab, with care taken to avoid excessive smudging of the skin mark. Next, the physician should provide local skin anesthesia using a 25-gauge needle and 1% lidocaine at all areas marked by injecting 0.25 to 0.50 mL to form a skin wheal at the mark. The skin should then be prepped again, but this time with betadine. The nerve block needle with tubing primed with bupivacaine should be connected to the peripheral nerve stimulator. This needle will be utilized to further localize the motor nerve branch along the z-axis. The nerve block needle is inserted perpendicular to the anesthetized skin mark. Once through the skin, the stimulation intensity on the peripheral nerve stimulator is increased to 2.5 to 3.5 mA. The needle is then advanced in small (~1 mm) increments while pausing to assess for muscle contraction. Once muscle contraction is noted, the needle hub can slightly be tilted cephalad, caudad, medially, and laterally, again to assess for maximal contraction. Once maximal contraction is achieved, and the patient denies paresthesias at current needle position, stimulation intensity is decreased to less than 1 mA. If the needle tip is in close proximity to the motor nerve branch, there should be slight muscle contraction at the reduced stimulation intensity. The physician then aspirates while observing the tubing closest to the needle hub for a flash of blood, which would indicate intravascular needle placement. If intravascular needle placement is suspected, the needle should immediately be withdrawn and attempts for re-localization can be performed according to physician's comfort. If negative aspiration is achieved, then 1 mL of 0.25% bupivacaine is injected. The injecting physician should warn the patient prior to injection that he/she may feel a burning or tingling sensation with injection of anesthetic agent. The process of needle insertion, localization, aspiration, and injection of anesthetic agent should be repeated at each skin mark identified with the surface stimulator.

All of the above steps are followed regardless of the region being treated. For the sake of brevity, these authors address in detail three most commonly treated muscle groups: the elbow flexors, knee flexors, and ankle plantar flexors. See also Tables 11.1 to 11.3 that summarize the anatomic localization landmarks for these muscle groups.

For the elbow flexors (biceps brachii, brachialis, and brachioradialis) (Figures 11.2 and 11.3), the patient would optimally be positioned in the supine position with the limb to be addressed on the edge closest to the physician. The arm and forearm should be exposed, and placed in anatomic positioning as much as able, with

Table 11.1 Anatomic Localization Guide for Muscle Branches of the Elbow Flexors

Elbow Flexors	Location Guide
Brachialis	Midline, at the junction of the middle and distal third of the biceps brachii muscle
Biceps Brachii	~3–4 cm cephalad of the brachialis location
Brachioradialis	~2–3 cm distal to the lateral margin of the antecubital crease, in a line from the lateral antecubital crease to the radial styloid

Table 11.2 Anatomic Localization Guide for Muscle Branches of the Knee Flexors

Knee Flexors	Location Guide
Long Head of Biceps Femoris	~¼ the distance of the femur from the ischial tuberosity, ~1 cm lateral of midline; ~ ⅓ the length along the femur from the ischial tuberosity, 1–2 cm lateral of midline
Semitendinosus	~¼ the distance of the femur from the ischial tuberosity, ~1 cm medial of midline; ~⅓ the length along the femur from the ischial tuberosity, 1–2 cm medial of midline
Semimembranosus	~⅓ the length along the femur from the ischial tuberosity, 1–3 cm medial of midline

Table 11.3 Anatomic Localization Guide for Muscle Branches of the Ankle Plantar Flexors

Ankle Plantar Flexors	Location Guide
Medial Head of Gastrocnemius	Junction of the proximal third and middle third of the calf, 2–3 cm medial of midline
Lateral Head of Gastrocnemius	Junction of the proximal third and middle third of the calf, 2–3 cm lateral of midline
Soleus	Midline, distal portion of the middle third of the calf

the elbow extended and the forearm supinated. The ground surface electrode is frequently placed on the acromion. Care should be taken to avoid placement close to the course of the musculocutaneous and radial nerves to avoid inadvertent stimulation by the ground electrode. With the arm in proper positioning, the following areas can be used as a starting point for motor nerve branch localization: For biceps brachii and brachialis, the first area is midline of the limb at the junction of the middle and distal third of the biceps brachii muscle and a second area approximately 3 to 4 cm cephalad of the first. For the brachioradialis, the area is approximately 2 to 3 cm distal to the lateral margin of the antecubital crease, in a line from the lateral antecubital crease to the radial styloid.[3]

For the knee flexors (hamstrings) (Figure 11.4), optimal positioning is prone with the limb to be addressed, again on the side of the table closest to the physician. The knee should be extended as much as possible and as tolerated by the patient. With the leg in optimal position, there are two general areas that can be used as a starting point for motor nerve branch localization. The first area is located about one fourth of the distance of the femur from the ischial tuberosity. Approximately 1 cm lateral of the midline of the limb, one may be able to locate a motor nerve branch to the long

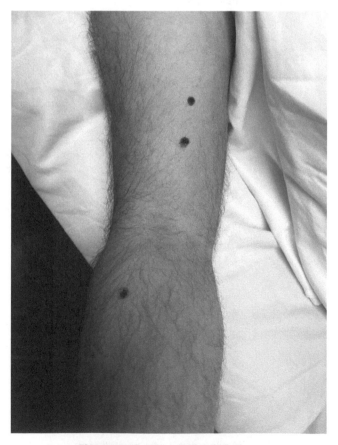

Figure 11.2 Elbow flexors AP view.

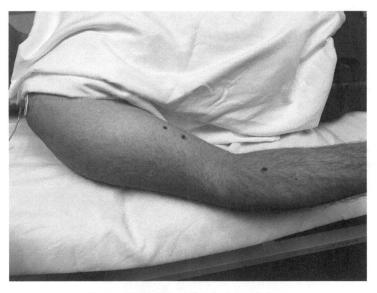

Figure 11.3 Elbow flexors lateral view.

head of the biceps femoris, and approximately 1 cm medial of midline, one may find a motor nerve branch to the semitendinosus. The second area is about one third of the length along the femur from the ischial tuberosity. By moving 1 to 2 cm laterally, additional motor nerve branches to the long head of the biceps femoris may be located. By moving 1 to 2 cm medially, a motor nerve branch to the semimembranosus may be found, as well as additional motor nerve branches to the semitendinosus.[4]

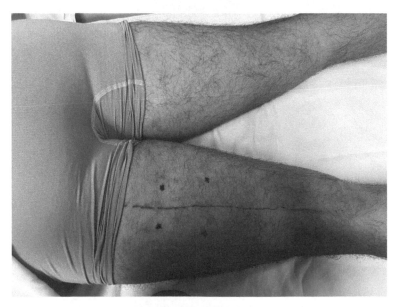

Figure 11.4 Hamstrings.

For the ankle plantar flexors (gastrocnemius and soleus) (Figures 11.5 and 11.6), optimal positioning is prone with the knee flexed 30 to 40 degrees with use of a wedge pillow, with the foot and ankle off the pillow to allow for dorsiflexion. The ground electrodes may be placed on the medial femoral condyle. Avoidance of placement over the lateral femoral condyle or fibular head is important as this may result in stimulation of the common, deep, and/or superficial fibular/peroneal nerve. While the muscles innervated by these nerves have different actions than that of the tibial innervated gastrocnemius and soleus, the repetitive muscular contractions and movement of the limb can be distracting to the performing physician. There are three general areas that may be used as a guide for localization of motor nerve branches to the medial and lateral heads of the gastrocnemius and the soleus. The junction

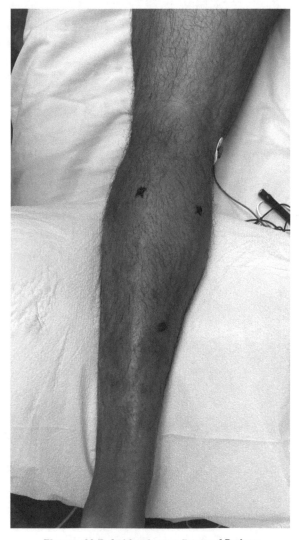

Figure 11.5 Ankle plantar flexors AP view.

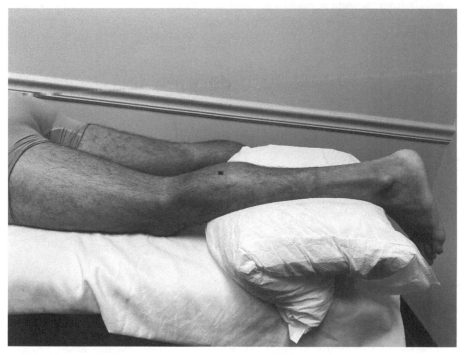

Figure 11.6 Ankle plantar flexors lateral view.

of the proximal third and middle third of the calf is an appropriate starting point when searching for motor nerve branches of the gastrocnemius. The probe should be positioned 2 to 3 cm medially and laterally from midline for each respective head of the gastrocnemius. An appropriate starting position for localization of the motor nerve branches to the soleus is the distal portion of the middle third of the calf in the midline.[5]

Pitfalls

If the surface stimulator is located within the recommended areas and the patient is placed in recommended positioning, and difficulty eliciting muscle contraction persists, the muscles being targeted may be placed in a position of gentle stretch. For example, gently dorsiflex the ankle to aid in localization of motor nerve branches to the gastrocnemius.

- Patience is required to allow for observance of muscle contraction between needle advancements. Advancing too hastily may result in bypassing targeted motor nerve branches, as well as unnecessary patient discomfort with increased needle positioning and movements.
- If a patient is unable to be placed in optimal positioning previously described, the performing physician must adapt and consider alternative positioning such as seated, lateral recumbent, or supine with the hip flexed and externally rotated.
- If a patient reports paresthesias with needle placement and minimal stimulation intensity despite needle relocation and repositioning attempts, it may be best to

refrain from injection of anesthetic agent and subsequent chemoneurolysis in this region as there may be increased risk for dysesthesias. The recommended starting locations are where motor nerve branches have been identified. However, anatomic variations may occur, and sensory fibers may be intertwined with motor nerve branches.

KEY POINTS

- DSMNB is a cost-effective, relatively low-risk procedure (with proper training) that has broad applications.
- DSMNB is a useful diagnostic tool with immediate and temporary effects that provide insight into the relative contributions of various muscle groups to the clinical picture and inform expectations for other longer-lasting treatment interventions (i.e., chemodenervation with BoNT or chemoneurolysis with alcohol or phenol).
- DSMNB allows a physician to differentiate between neural and nonneural etiologies prior to preceding with longer-lasting intervention with higher-risk side effect profiles.

REFERENCES

1. Deltombe T, Wautier D, De Cloedt P, et al. Assessment and treatment of spastic equinovarus foot after stroke: guidance from the Mont-Godinne interdisciplinary group. *J Rehabil Med*. 2017;49(6);461–468. https://doi.org/10.2340/16501977-2226
2. Collins JB, Song J, Mahabir R. Onset and duration of intradermal mixtures of bupivacaine and lidocaine with epinephrine. *Can J Plast Surg*. 2013 Spring;21(1):51–53. https://doi.org/10.1177/229255031302100112
3. Yang ZX, Pho RW, Kour AK, et al. The musculocutaneous nerve and its branches to the biceps and brachialis muscles. *J Hand Surg Am*. 1995;20(4):671–675. https://doi.org/10.1016/S0363-5023(05)80289-8. PMID: 7594300.
4. Seidel PM, Seidel GK, Gans BM, et al. Precise localization of the motor nerve branches to the hamstring muscles: an aid to the conduct of neurolytic procedures. *Arch Phys Med Rehabil*. 1996;77(11):1157–60. https://doi.org/10.1016/s0003-9993(96)90140-9. PMID: 8931528.
5. Yoo WK, Chung IH, Park CI. Anatomic motor point localization for the treatment of gastrocnemius muscle spasticity. *Yonsei Med J*. 2002;43(5):627–630. https://doi.org/10.3349/ymj.2002.43.5.627.

12 Intrathecal Baclofen Therapy

Cindy B. Ivanhoe and Abana Azariah

INTRODUCTION

ITB therapy has been an approved treatment for spasticity since the early 1990s when the FDA approved the Medtronic ITB pump for spinal—origin spasticity. The cerebral—origin indication followed in 1996. ITB therapy has become an established intervention for spasticity. Despite the need for surgery and recovery, comparisons suggest that the ITB delivery system improves the therapeutic effects when compared to traditional oral medications.[1] The administration of ITB was first proposed by Penn and Kroin in 1984. Baclofen (analog of the inhibitory GABA-B agonist) has been used for the treatment of spasticity for decades. The precise mechanism of action for baclofen is not fully understood; however, it inhibits both mono- and polysynaptic reflexes, predominantly at the spinal cord level. It is believed to reduce the release of excitatory neurotransmitters in the presynaptic neurons and stimulate inhibitory neuronal signals in the postsynaptic neurons with resultant relief of spasticity.[2]

Pharmacodynamics

When baclofen is administered orally, only a small portion of the original dose crosses the blood–brain barrier to enter the cerebrospinal fluid (CSF), the site of action. Orally, it is dosed 3 to 4 times a day due to a short half-life. Delivering baclofen intrathecally allows for microgram dosing of the medication with less than 100th of an oral dose. There is approximately 1% systemic passage of the medication when delivered intrathecally.[3]

Through the intrathecal pump, the medication is delivered continuously and can be dosed in different ways through the course of the day via programming of the implanted pump. The intrathecal baclofen (ITB) dose is programmed via an external programmer. Recommended dose adjustments can be made by 5% to 20 % at a time, depending on the clinical presentation and the dose at the time of adjustment. For example, there would be a significant difference if programming a 25% increase in a dose of 600 mcg a day as opposed to a dose of 100 mcg a day. Patients may receive bolus doses over the course of the day with or without a continuous release of ITB baseline.

While there is concern and the possibility of tolerance to ITB, there have also been a fair amount of mechanical/catheter issues noted that have sometimes led to the perception of tolerance. In the pharmacologic literature, there appears to be improved effectiveness with periodic bolus of ITB in limited studies versus continuous mode of drug delivery.[4]

Catheter tip location, mode of drug infusion, bolus infusion, drug concentration and infusion speed, position, baricity, and tolerance are all factors that can affect clinical response to ITB therapy. Little is understood about the interplay of these factors or the impact of ventriculoperitoneal (VP) shunts. If a patient presents with the need for a change in ITB dosing that had previously been stable for an extended period, aside from considering tolerance, one should first consider medical or mechanical changes, remembering that any noxious stimulus can cause a significant increase in one's spasticity.[3]

Patient Selection

Candidates for ITB therapy may have any diagnosis associated with the upper motor neuron syndrome (UMNS). Spasticity is often associated with other movement and reflex patterns that on the secondary level may also respond to ITB therapy.[5]

Per labeling, ITB therapy is considered appropriate for the treatment of "severe" spasticity, but it is increasingly prescribed for the use of "significant" spasticity.[6] It is also found to be effective when treating children and adults with cerebral palsy (CP) and the other associated movement disorders that can be seen with CP.[7] This includes secondary dystonias.

ITB therapy is the most dramatic way to reduce spasticity and associated movement disorders, particularly in the lower limbs. Hemiplegic ambulatory patients are also candidates for ITB. It does not affect the uninvolved side.[8]

Effects on the upper limbs and trunk are more unpredictable but present. Very often, candidates who are referred for ITB therapy are patients who have "failed" oral medications and injections or have more diffuse spasticity. There is a misconception that candidates need to go through some stepwise stratification of interventions before being referred for ITB therapy. Comparing oral baclofen and ITB is a false comparison, as they are not comparable therapies. Many patients are clearly candidates whether they have tried oral medications or not. For some patients, the potential benefit for ITB therapy is obvious. This may be based on the distribution of their spasticity and/or the interference of spasticity with their function and progress. In many cases, ITB would be the starting place in managing tone, even if it will be combined with other therapies and interventions. Delaying this intervention may delay a potentially life-changing intervention and limit access to neuroplasticity. This can contribute to the development of compensatory movement patterns, contractures, risk of skin breakdown, and other complications.

The question of appropriateness of ITB therapy for a particular patient is influenced by the treatment goals, distribution of hypertonicity, willingness to responsibly keep appointments for the baclofen pump refills once implanted, funding considerations, and the expectations and vision of the treating medical professionals. "Storming" or dysautonomia that may accompany brain injury can be well managed with ITB in the absence of the cognitive and sedating considerations associated with use of enteral medications. Dysautonomia presents with increased posturing, temperature, blood pressure, and pulse.[9,10]

Often, oral medications can be weaned or decreased, which may be a potential goal of ITB therapy as well. Whether spasticity is a new finding or whether someone has had spasticity all their lives, ITB can still lead to functional improvements. As with any other medical intervention, the risks and benefits should be weighed and discussed so that an appropriate decision can be made for each individual. Patients need to be educated about what this therapy can and cannot bring. They need to understand and decide if the benefits outweigh the risks. It is important for the prescribing or managing physician to understand the degree of disability created by the spasticity, the potential risks of intervening, and the potential risks of not intervening. The ITB trial is one way to understand what a patient might expect from the therapy.

The Process

Intrathecal Baclofen Trial

A baclofen trial is performed in a setting that provides safe monitoring and ability to evaluate the patient after the injection has occurred. This could be an inpatient or ambulatory center or outpatient clinic. Fluoroscopy should be available in case guidance is needed for injection. Some centers prefer to do a catheter trial. This involves admitting the patient to a hospital and titrating the dose over several days.

The purpose of the ITB trial is to answer the question; yes or no, the patient responds to the treatment. Once a patient is identified as a potential candidate for ITB therapy, the trial is planned. It is also important to inform the patient prior to the trial that they may feel weak after they receive the intrathecal injection of baclofen. That would indicate a highly positive trial. Many patients and clinicians become reluctant to proceed with implant at this point, missing that the actual degree of spasticity reduction after implant will not be immediately as dramatic.

Prior to the trial, certain measures and assessments are performed. These may be done the same day as the trial or a short period of time prior.

Measures such as the Ashworth Scale (AS), Modified Ashworth Scale (MAS), Tardieu Scale, Spasm Frequency Scale, Barry–Albright Scale (BAD; used for dystonia measures), clonus, and range of motion (ROM) are taken prior to the trial. The MAS, Tardieu Scale, and ROM are most frequently used. Their gait may take longer as the biomechanics and gait pattern may change during the trial. Quality of ambulation may also be considered in interpretation of the trial outcome. Video recording of the pretrial and trial assessments is highly recommended. Many facilities will record patients performing functional tasks that can be repeated once the patient is reassessed after the intrathecal bolus. Quality of movement, posture, donning, and doffing an article of clothing or other functional considerations might be noted.

Table 12.1   Suggested Outcome Measures for ITB Screening Trial (Pretrial and During Trial)

Modified Ashworth Scale
Range of motion
Tardieu Scale
Spasm Frequency Scale
Berry–Albright Scale
Clonus
6-Minute walk

On the day of the baclofen trial, the patient receives a 50, 75, or 100 mcg bolus of ITB via lumbar puncture. If the initial trial with a 50 mcg bolus is not convincing, the general recommendation is to repeat the trial at a higher dose. Patients with multiple sclerosis (MS) or significant weakness may receive a smaller bolus, for example, 25 mcg.

Approximately 4 hours after the bolus administration, the patient is reassessed. Possible side effects noted during a trial include light-headedness, weakness, hypotension, vomiting, and a CSF leak leading to a spinal headache.[11]

The purpose of the ITB trial is to see if there is a positive response to the bolus, making the patient a candidate for the therapy. The trial does not determine what a patient would look like in several months or future dose requirements. The interpretation of the trial can usually be made from the 50 mcg bolus. A one point drop in MAS is considered a positive trial. If the patient has gegenhalten (motor negativism) or contractures, it can be difficult to use the MAS as the only measure of a positive or negative trial. The potential benefits of proceeding to implant may be extrapolated from the trial. It may help distinguish spasticity from contracture and may even unmask underlying volitional movement when the constraints of synergy patterns and hypertonicity are removed.

Ultimate outcome will be influenced by many other medical and psychosocial factors once the pump is implanted. The primary question answered by an ITB trial is, does this patient respond to the intervention? The trial does not necessarily predict the impact of ITB on the patient's life.

Implant/Surgery

Baclofen pump implant is performed under general anesthesia in the lateral decubitus position. Both the abdomen and lumbar region of the spine are prepped. The pump is placed in the subcutaneous pocket in the abdominal area. A tract is tunneled between the abdomen and the lumbar insertion area. The catheter is threaded within the intrathecal space under fluoroscopy. It is important for patients to understand that they will have two incisions. There are additional considerations regarding catheter level. Many physicians choose to have the catheter tip placed at higher levels of the spinal cord when trying to capture a greater effect in the upper extremities.[12] The pump itself is usually placed in the lower abdomen though there are certainly instances where it may be placed in other areas of the body. It is usually subcutaneous. Some prefer the pump to be implanted subfascially. This can make pump refills a bit more challenging but more aesthetically acceptable. It has become common practice to place vancomycin powder within the surgical sites.[13]

The catheter tip is traditionally positioned in the midthoracic area, though there is interest in placing it at a higher level, such as the upper thoracic or lower cervical area.[14] This is done in hope of gaining more control of upper limb spasticity.[15] There are cases of the catheter being intentionally placed in the cerebral ventricles and pre-brainstem as well.[16] At the time of this printing, there is not sufficient evidence to support this. There are no published randomized controlled trials on cervical ITB catheter placement.

The literature contains retrospective studies and case reports of higher catheter placement. There are small retrospective reports of unquantified improvement and variable effects with higher catheter placement versus midthoracic placement. There are also variable degrees of unquantified effect on the upper extremities even with

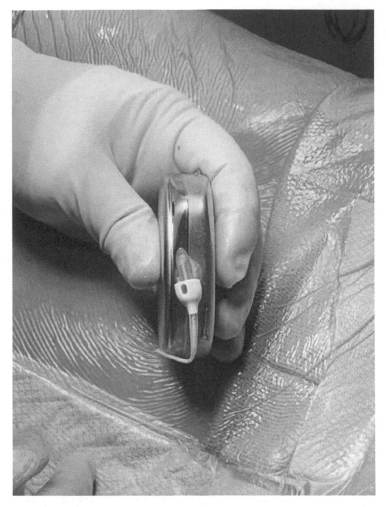

Figure 12.1 Catheter connection and insertion of ITB pump in the lower abdomen. Note: Patient in lateral decubitus position.

lower catheter placement and concerns that some lower extremity spasticity control may be lost with higher catheter placement.

The baclofen pump is filled and started in the operating room with a 500 mcg per mL concentration of baclofen. It is tradition to start the pump dose at twice the dose to which the patient responded during the trial. Dose increases are generally allowable at 24-hour intervals. That means that the dose delivered at trial, over a few minutes, is doubled but delivered over 24 hours. Analgesia and wound care should be provided as with any other surgery. An abdominal binder is often recommended to be worn postoperatively. Depending on the patient's circumstances and surgeons' preferences, age, insurance, and timing, the patient may go to inpatient rehabilitation or home. It is good practice to inform the patient and family that dose and drug concentration adjustments can take time and can be managed both in an inpatient and outpatient setting.

Contraindications

Some of the primary contraindications to ITB therapy include body weight not large enough to support the 20 mL or 40 mL pump. This is more common in children though it is not uncommon for some patients to gain weight once their spasticity is decreased. Some patients may lose weight because they become more active and mobile.

ITB is contraindicated in patients with hypersensitivity to baclofen, which is rare, and may be related to additives in the enteric formulation. Relative contraindications include an inability to come off anticoagulation for surgery (mechanical heart valves), renal disease, psychiatric history, unmanageable mental health issues, psychosocial factors affecting compliance, and financial burden. VP shunts for hydrocephalus are not a contraindication to ITB therapy, but consideration must be taken for the potential consequence of changing CSF volume in the setting of a malfunctioning VP shunt.[17] Seizures or prior abdominal or pelvic surgery should be discussed before proceeding to an ITB screening test.

Complications

Adverse effects of the ITB trial can be pain, hypotonia, infection, and vomiting, which are potentially due to a spinal headache from a CSF leak. Acute complications post ITB pump implant can include a CSF leak and spinal headache, infection, pain, seroma, and disconnection.[18] CSF may accumulate in the pump pocket or a seroma may develop. For this reason, abdominal binders are often recommended if not surgeons' choice.

In patients with cognitive communication deficits, look for other signs of CSF leak such as vomiting, agitation, or tachycardia. If symptoms do not resolve with bed rest and fluids, a blood patch can rapidly repair the leak.

When a complication of ITB therapy arises later after implant, it is most frequently related to a problem with the catheter. This can include a disconnect, a microfracture, a kink, an intermittent kink, and an obstruction by tissue. Human error is the next most common cause of programming errors. The pump is reprogrammed at the time of refill. No matter which model pump the patient has, the concentration, medication, and pump refill volume should be checked in the pump. Pumps can also be checked for any alarms that may have indicated a low pump volume. The amount of baclofen removed from the pump at the time of refill should be close to what is predicted by the pump.

Withdrawal Versus Overdose

Baclofen withdrawal, whether it is administered orally or intrathecally, can present with an initial complaint of itching or a feeling of ants crawling on one's body. This may be followed by agitation, insomnia, confusion, delusions, hallucinations, seizures, visual changes, psychosis, dyskinesias, hyperthermia, and increased spasticity with rhabdomyolysis. Withdrawal may need to be distinguished from neuroleptic malignant syndrome, autonomic dysreflexia, serotonin syndrome, sepsis, and malignant hyperthermia. Withdrawal from ITB is a medical emergency and potentially life-threatening. Large doses of oral baclofen, cyproheptadine, and intrathecal doses of baclofen can be used to try to manage withdrawal. Antiepileptics can also be used for seizure prevention. These interventions should be instituted immediately when withdrawal is suspected.

An ITB overdose presents with hypotonia, lethargy, and weakness and leads to respiratory depression and decreased consciousness. Management includes lowering or stopping the ITB delivery and supportive measures including ventilator, if necessary.

Surgical complications include catheter-related disconnection, migration, and pump flipping. Catheter-related complications include disconnection, occlusion, fracture, or kinks.

Underdosing may create an impression of a problem with the ITB system. Depending on the history and presentation of a lack or limited response to the therapy, the lack of response may just be due to inadequate dosing. This is particularly true in the early stage after pump implant.

Pump Replacement

The average battery life of an ITB pump is 6 to 7 years for a Synchromed II pump and 9 to 10 years for the Prometra II pump. If there is no suspicion of a problem with dosing, a replacement pump can be started at the same dose as the pump it is replacing. Each company makes its own catheter and that should be considered when the pump is exchanged. If a catheter issue is suspected, the best way to decide where to start the next pump dose is based on clinical judgment.

Intrathecal Baclofen Pump Maintenance

MRI Scans

There are some differences related to the compatibility of the two currently available pumps when it comes to MRI scans. The Synchromed II needs to be checked for restarting after an MRI. It generally restarts within a few hours of an MRI, but if it does not, it can be reprogrammed. While the Prometra II can go through an MRI scanner if an emergent situation arises, the FDA approval requires the emptying and refilling of the pump before and after an MRI, respectively.

Dose Adjustments

Patients should not expect that their spasticity would be reduced immediately following surgery as it was potentially at the ITB trial. It takes time, based on logistics and clinical changes, for them to reach their ultimate and most functional dose. Ultimate dosing may be affected by the pump chosen for implant, finances, refill schedule, and access to physical and occupational therapy. Dosing may be continuous or there may be boluses throughout the day, or both. Some patients may choose to maintain more spasticity so that they do not have to come for refills as frequently. Patients may be referred to outpatient therapies or get admitted for inpatient rehabilitation. Some patients may develop more potential isolated movement across particular joints and increased access to strength. There may be a balance between raising the dose and lowering their spasticity while maintaining some active movement. It is not unusual for some patients to become more lethargic if the dose is increased too rapidly. The concentration of medication in the pump is usually increased as the dose escalates. Most commonly, the initial 500 concentration may be increased to a 2,000 concentration or a 1,000 concentration depending on the manufacturer of the drug and the dose. There is evidence that the lower concentration may lead to a greater decrease in spasticity, at least neurophysiologically.[19]

Intrathecal Medication

There are currently two manufacturers of ITB: Amneal Pharmaceuticals (Lioresal) and Piramal Critical Care (Gablofen). Other companies have ITB products in development at the time of this writing. Additionally, many clinicians opt for compounded baclofen. It is important to monitor the consistency and purity of the medication in the pump. Additionally, many patients' pain in spasticity coexist and it may be difficult to tease out which is driving the other. Managing mixed medication in the pump can become a balancing act when mixing both analgesic medication and baclofen. Having mixed compounded medication in the pump does void the manufacturer's warranty. Morphine and other opiates are associated with granuloma formation at the tip of the catheter that can lead to withdrawal or, at the very least, inconsistent delivery of medication.[20,21]

Troubleshooting

There are times where clinical benefit is not as expected or is lost. Of note, all approaches to working up a potential malfunction have their value and limitations.

If a patient presents with a very high ITB dose or a need for an increase in ITB dosing that had previously been stable, aside from considering tolerance, one should first consider medical or mechanical changes. Any noxious stimulus can cause a significant increase in one's spasticity. At a minimum, basics of bladder, bowel, and skin should be considered. In patients with spinal cord injury (SCI), a syrinx should also be ruled out. In cases of brain injury, delayed post-traumatic hydrocephalus should be ruled out, though patients may need a VP shunt as well as a pump.

Troubleshooting is done differently in different programs and hospitals, partly due to a true lack of consensus, logistics, and clinical judgment. This is covered in more depth elsewhere in this text.

Considerations in Specific Patient Populations

Disorders of Consciousness

Patients with severe traumatic brain injuries (TBIs) may be classified as having a disorder of consciousness (DoC). A DoC can be subdivided into two broad states: states of consciousness (minimally conscious state [MCS]) and states of unconsciousness (coma and unwakeful responsiveness state [UWS]). In addition to addressing impaired consciousness, patients with a DoC often present with severe spasticity. A 2017 systematic review found the prevalence of spasticity in patients with DoC ranged from 59% to 89%.[22] A 2021 retrospective chart review of a large DoC rehabilitation program ($N = 146$ patients) found that 95% of patients were affected by spasticity and 52% had spasticity affecting all four limbs.[23] Not only did ITB show improvement in motor impairments, but also several case studies and reports found improvement in level of consciousness after treatment with ITB.[24] The pathophysiology explaining the relationship between ITB and improvements in awareness and cognition continues to be studied. Current theories suggest two possible mechanisms. First theory suggests ITB modulates dysregulated sleep–wake cycles while the second suggests ITB modulates afferent impulses at the spinal level leading to a reduction of overload within the cortical–thalamo–cortical connections that interfere with awareness.[25]

While ITB has been approved for the treatment of spasticity, it has been shown to be effective in the treatment of severe autonomic dysfunction. Paroxysmal sympathetic hyperactivity (i.e., autonomic dysfunction, storming, autonomic storming) is a common sequela of severe brain injury and is often seen in patients with a DoC. Several case reports have been published demonstrating stabilization of cardiocirculatory instability following introduction of ITB. GABA-B receptors are distributed throughout the central nervous system (CNS) (spinal cord, cerebellum, hippocampus) and are involved in blood pressure control at the rostral ventrolateral medulla (RVLM) of the rat and sympathetic activity of cats. Sympathetic activity studied in cats and rats demonstrated blood pressure control via GABA-B receptors; therefore, it is hypothesized that ITB is highly effective in reducing autonomic dysfunction.[25–27]

Untreated spasticity can essentially "lock in" a patient, preventing them from interacting with their environment. Additionally, oral antispasmodic medication can further impair cognition and interaction. An accurate determination of level of consciousness remains a fundamental goal, making it imperative to identify and treat spasticity.

A Tale of Two Pumps

Currently, the most used baclofen intrathecal pump is manufactured by Medtronic— the Synchromed II. Prometra II, manufactured by Flowonix, was approved for spasticity in 2020. Both pumps have indications for "severe" spasticity and pain. There are pros and cons to each of the two currently available intrathecal drug delivery systems. The baclofen trial (discussed previously) is performed the same way regardless of which pump a patient or implanter may choose. There are differences between the delivery systems though they both deliver medication directly into the CSF via the intrathecal space. The Prometra II pump delivers medication via a pressure-driven, valve-gated delivery system. Synchromed II pumps utilize motors and gears for drug delivery. The Synchromed II always delivers at least a basal rate or continuous dose of baclofen. The Prometra II delivers micro boluses continuously. When it comes to refills, both pumps are accessed the same; however, the Prometra II pumps are designed so that once the needle enters the pump, the drug automatically fills the syringe and no extra effort is needed from the provider. The Synchromed II has larger visibility and accessible support. It is also available internationally. Studies comparing the efficacy of ITB dose between the two pumps are currently in process and awaiting completion.

Table 12.2 Intrathecal Pump Comparison, Per FDA Information

Synchromed II	Prometra II
Battery life 4–7 years	Battery life 7–10 years
Weight 165/175 g	Weight 150.154 g
Indented septum	Raised palpable septum
Catheter not visible on x-ray	Catheter visible on x-ray
Peristaltic mechanism of delivery	Valve-gated mechanism of delivery
Re-interrogate after MRI	Empty before and refill after MRI

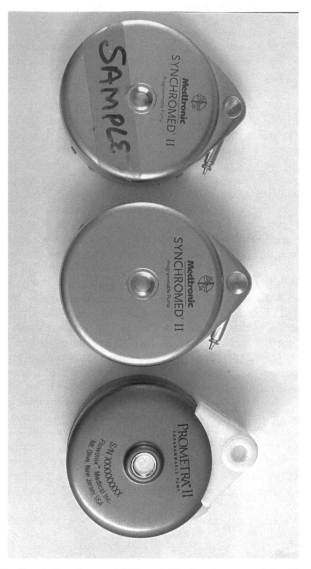

Figure 12.2 Medtronic Synchromed II 20 and 40 mL volumes and the Flowonix Prometra II 40 mL.

The average life expectancy of the Synchromed II pump battery is reportedly 6.5 to 7 years. The Prometra II pump has a potential battery life of 7 to 10 years. The battery life of each respective pump is contingent on dosing. Higher doses drain the battery more readily than lower doses. Nonetheless, the dosing should be adjusted appropriately to the patient's presentation and needs. The intrathecal catheter is visible on x-ray and the center port for filling of the pump is palpable. During a pump refill, the negative pressure in the pump allows the tubing to fill automatically once the pump is entered. This makes a pocket fill particularly rare. The greatest shortcoming to the use of the Prometra II pump is that currently, it must be emptied and refilled in the event of a non-emergent MRI. Arrangements are generally made to provide clinical support to address this need.

Closing Considerations

ITB therapy is a well-accepted intervention for the treatment of spasticity. ITB therapy has significant advantages for the management of spasticity and spastic dystonia. ITB allows for relative ease of titration without significant sedation and cognitive impairment. Spasticity across multiple joints can be managed simultaneously, particularly in the lower limbs and trunk.

Decision to proceed with ITB therapy should be preceded by careful patient selection, ITB trial, posttrial assessment, and implantation. One should be aware of the complications that can occur post trial and implant. Troubleshooting and pump maintenance are key to a successful outcome.

There are two pumps commercially available in the United States, but the overwhelming bulk of literature is based on the Synchromed II. The Prometra II was FDA approved in 2020. As more research is done, consideration should be given to catheter tip placement, as well as the type of dosing the patient is receiving. The mode of drug delivery via pump is different between the two pumps and there are additional differing characteristics to consider.

Many physicians are reluctant to offer ITB therapy to patients out of their own concerns for a complication, the potential for an emergency, and/or a lack of understanding as to the benefits of ITB therapy. Successful management of patients with ITB requires a team and coordination, coordination of assessments, trials, referrals, and associated therapies.

KEY POINTS

- The use of enteral baclofen is not a comparable trial to determine the effectiveness of ITB therapy, nor is it as effective.
- It is important to prepare patients prior to the trial; they may feel "weak" after they receive the intrathecal injection. The trial does not directly reflect their outcome after pump implant.
- Spasticity can contribute to the mischaracterization of someone as "vegetative/ DoC" as well as limit potential. Oral medications for spasticity can contribute to cognitive impairment and are not as effective.
- ITB may play a role in improvement in level of consciousness.
- ITB can be effective in the treatment and management of paroxysmal sympathetic hyperactivity.
- The primary purpose of an ITB trial is to determine if there is or is not a response to ITB.
- Every precaution should be taken to be sure that patients do not miss their baclofen pump refills.
- Patients should not need to fail other interventions prior to an ITB trial and implant.

- Hemiplegic and ambulatory patients are also candidates for ITB therapy and will not develop weakness on the uninvolved side.

REFERENCES

1. Creamer M, Cloud G, Kossmehl P, et al. "Intrathecal baclofen therapy versus conventional medical management for severe poststroke spasticity: results from a multicentre, randomised, controlled, open-label trial (SISTERS)." *J Neurol, Neurosurg Psychiatry.* 2018;89(6):642–650. https://doi.org/10.1136/jnnp-2017-317021

2. Gracies JM, Nance P, Elovic E, et al. "Traditional pharmacological treatments for spasticity part II: general and regional treatments." *Muscle Nerve Suppl.* 1997;6:S92–120.

3. Heetla HW, Staal MJ, Proost JH, et al. "Clinical relevance of pharmacological and physiological data in intrathecal baclofen therapy." *Arch Phys Med Rehabil.* 2014;95(5):2199–2206. https://doi.org/10.1016/j.apmr.2014.04.030

4. Heetla HW, Staal MJ, Kliphuis C, et al. "The incidence and management of tolerance in intrathecal baclofen therapy." *Spinal Cord.* 2009;47(10):751–756. https://doi.org/10.1038/sc.2009.34

5. Abboud H, Macaron G, Yu XX, et al. "Defining the spectrum of spasticity-associated involuntary movements." *Parkinsonism Relat Disord.* 2019;65:79–85. https://doi.org/10.1016/j.parkreldis.2019.05.007

6. Saulino M, Ivanhoe CB, McGuire JR, et al. "Best practices for intrathecal baclofen therapy: patient selection." *Neuromodulation.* 2016;19(6):607–615. https://doi.org/10.1111/ner.12447

7. Bonouvrié LA, Becher JG, Vles JSH, et al. "The effect of intrathecal baclofen in dyskinetic cerebral palsy: the IDYS trial." *Ann Neurol.* 2019;86(1):79–90. https://doi.org/10.1002/ana.25498

8. Ivanhoe CB, Francisco GE, McGuire JR, et al. "Intrathecal baclofen management of poststroke spastic hypertonia: implications for function and quality of life." *Arch Phys Med Rehabil.* 2006;87(11):1509–1515. https://doi.org/10.1002/ana.25498

9. Cuny E, Richer E, Castel JP. "Dysautonomia syndrome in the acute recovery phase after traumatic brain injury: relief with intrathecal Baclofen therapy." *Brain Injury.* 2001;15(10):917–925. https://doi.org/10.1080/02699050110065277

10. Becker R, Benes L, Sure U, et al. "Intrathecal baclofen alleviates autonomic dysfunction in severe brain injury." *J Clinl Neurosci.* 2000;7(4):316–319. https://doi.org/ 10.1054/jocn.1999.0227

11. Boster AL, Bennett SE, Bilsky GS, et al. "Best practices for intrathecal baclofen therapy: screening test." *Neuromodulation.* 2016;19(6): 616–622. https://doi.org/10.1111/ner.12437

12. Jacobs NW, Maas EM, Brusse-Keizer M, et al. "Effectiveness and safety of cervical catheter tip placement in intrathecal baclofen treatment of spasticity: a systematic review." *J Rehabil Med.* 2021;53(7):jrm00215. https://doi.org/10.2340/16501977-2857

13. McCall TD, MacDonald JD. "Cervical catheter tip placement for intrathecal baclofen administration." *Neurosurgery.* 2006;59(3):634–640. https://doi.org/10.1227/01.NEU.0000227570.40402.77

14. Chang, Eric Yao, and Amirpasha Ehsan. "Placement of baclofen pump catheter tip for upper extremity spasticity management." *Neuromodulation.* 2018;21(7):714–716. https://doi.org/10.1111/ner.12768

15. Hugenholtz H, Nelson RF, Dehoux E. "Intrathecal baclofen–the importance of catheter position." *Can J Neurol Sci.*1993;20(2):165–167. https://doi.org/10.1017/s0317167100047776

16. Saenz A, Grijalba M, Mengide JP, et al. "Baclofen pump with pre-brainstem catheter tip placement: technical note and case series." *Child's Nerv Syst.* 2021;37(1):203–210. https://doi.org/10.1007/s00381-020-04679-3

17. Turner MS. Assessing syndromes of catheter malfunction with SynchroMed infusion systems: the value of spiral computed tomography with contrast injection. *PM&R.* 2010;2(8):757–766. https://doi.org/10.1016/j.pmrj.2010.05.011

18. Imerci A, Rogers KJ, Miller F, et al. "Evaluation of risk factors for cerebrospinal leakage in pediatric patients with cerebral palsy treated with intrathecal baclofen." *J Pediatr Orthop.* 2020;40(6):e522–e526. https://doi.org/10.1097/BPO.0000000000001472

19. Stokic DS, Yablon SA. "Effect of concentration and mode of intrathecal baclofen administration on soleus H-reflex in patients with muscle hypertonia." *Clin Neurophysiol.* 2012;123(11):2200–2204. https://doi.org/10.1016/j.clinph.2012.04.007

20. Miele VJ, Price KO, Bloomfield S, et al. "A review of intrathecal morphine therapy related granulomas." *Eur J Pain.* 2006;10(3):251–261. https://doi.org/10.1016/j.ejpain.2005.05.002

21. Delhaas EM, Huygen FJPM. Complications associated with intrathecal drug delivery systems. *BJA Educ.* 2020;20(2):51–57. https://doi.org/10.1016/j.bjae.2019.11.002

22. Martens G, Laureys S, Thibaut A. "Spasticity management in disorders of consciousness." *Brain Sci.* 2017;7(12):162. https://doi.org/10.3390/brainsci7120162

23. Zhang B, Karri J, O'Brien K, et al. "Spasticity management in persons with disorders of consciousness." *PM&R.* 2021;13(7):657–665. https://doi.org/10.1002/pmrj.12458

24. Formisano R, Aloisi M, Contrada M, et al. "Late recovery of responsiveness after intra-thecal baclofen pump implantation and the role of diffuse pain and severe spasticity: a case report." *Acta Neurochir.* 2019;161(9);1965–1967. https://doi.org/10.1007/s00701-019-03994-2

25. Bowery NG. "GABAB receptor pharmacology." *Ann Rev of Pharmacol Toxicol.* 1993;33:109–147. https://doi.org/10.1146/annurev.pa.33.040193.000545

26. Amano M, Kubo T. "Involvement of both GABAA and GABAB receptors in tonic inhibitory control of blood pressure at the rostral ventrolateral medulla of the rat." *Naunyn-Schmiedeberg's Arch Pharmacol.* 1993;348(2):146–153. https://doi.org/10.1007/BF00164791

27. Stanovnik L, Huchet AM, Schmitt H. "The action of baclofen on blood pressure and sympathetic activity." *7th Int. Congr. Pharmac.* 1978.

13 Surgical Treatments and Neuro-Orthopedics

Christina K. Hardesty

INTRODUCTION

Surgical treatment for management of spasticity is often thought of as a "last resort." Spasticity has usually been present for a long time before deformity becomes progressive, significant, or concerning enough to require surgery. In some cases, such as traumatic brain injuries (TBIs), spasticity can be so severe that deformity begins to occur early, requiring more aggressive intervention. Chronic or congenital disorders may be associated with deformity that develops over a longer period. In both circumstances, spasticity is the underlying cause and requires a multidisciplinary approach. As the team evaluates each patient to determine the most appropriate treatment plan, consideration for the severity of the spasticity, the level of function, and the potential for improvement is critical. Secondarily, the team must evaluate the extent of spasticity and its manifestations, determining if the problem is generalized or focal. Both nonsurgical and surgical options exist for each type of problem.

A number of nonsurgical options include physical or occupational therapy, stretching, massage, botulinum toxin (BoNT) or other chemodenervation, casting, or bracing. These can be used to treat spasticity at any stage and can often be used as both preventative and therapeutic measures. Nonsurgical management can address both generalized and focal problems with tone. When these fail or deformity progresses beyond the extent treatable by conservative management, surgical options can be considered.

Surgery for spasticity can be divided into two categories: procedures meant to prevent deformity and procedures necessary to treat the manifestations of spasticity.

Preventing deformity includes tendon lengthenings, tendon or muscle releases, casting, or neurectomy. Selective dorsal rhizotomy (SDR) is another technique used to manage spasticity by dividing selective sensory nerve roots within the spinal canal. It is irreversible and must be followed by intensive therapy. It is intended to improve the lower extremity gross motor function of children who function at GMFCS level II or III. Results have been mixed and SDR should be considered one tool available for treatment, not an all-encompassing solution.[1]

The manifestations of spasticity include shortened muscle or tendon units; deformity at joints including angular deformity, subluxation, or dislocation; contractures; or spinal deformity. These are often treated with tendon releases or transfers, osteotomies, joint reductions or reconstructions, or arthrodesis. Spinal deformity is corrected surgically with segmental instrumentation and arthrodesis. As surgical treatment options are considered, it is essential to consider patient needs and expectations as well as goals. Surgery can achieve changes, but they are usually irreversible, can be accompanied by weakness postoperatively, and should only be considered if the end result will actually improve the life of the patient or caregiver. Spastic muscles are inherently weak, and surgery is known to exacerbate that weakness. Furthermore, surgeons must pay very close attention to the length of the musculotendinous unit and be careful not to overlengthen a muscle, since loss of tension will also produce weakness and worse outcomes. It is also relevant to understand that surgery must usually be followed by therapy to support the goals of the surgical intervention.

Evaluation of any candidate for surgery should also be done in a systematic way. Consider the diagnosis, the locations of tone, previous treatment, and concurrent treatment options. Approach each patient by considering all options, including both operative and non-operative. Do not undertake any surgical procedure without a full understanding of their medical and surgical history; the function of their extremities, trunk, and neck; as well as the support they will have postoperatively.

UPPER EXTREMITY SURGERY

The manifestations of spasticity in the upper extremity result in more limitations of function than difficulty with positioning or pain. Hygiene problems can occur because of fingers or thumbs tucked into the palm, wrist or elbow contractures limit the ease of getting dressed, and shoulder contractures cause problems with both. In addition, limitations of any upper extremity joint means that the hand and arm are not able to grasp and deliver to the body things a typical upper extremity would do.

Tone management must be in place first for any subsequent treatment to be effective. Oral, enteral, injectable, and intrathecal medications can assist with this. Neurectomies have also been considered as a surgical option for management of spasticity, both to reduce tone and to address potential deformity.[1,2] While they have

Table 13.1 Manifestations of Upper Extremity Spasticity by Region	
Shoulder	Rotator cuff injury
	Subluxation or dislocation
	Adduction contracture
	Adhesive capsulitis
	Fractures
	Brachial plexopathy
	Internal rotation contracture
Elbow	Biceps and brachialis contractures
	Triceps contracture
	Joint contracture
	Ulnar neuropathy
	Fractures
	Elbow dislocation

(continued)

Table 13.1 Manifestations of Upper Extremity Spasticity by Region *(continued)*

Forearm	Pronation contractures
	Biceps spasticity causing supination
	Proximal synostosis
Wrist	Wrist flexion contractures
	Ulnar or radial deviation
	Ulnar positive deformity
	Subluxation
	Wrist extension contractures
Thumb	Thumb-in-palm deformity
	Adduction contracture
Fingers	Clenched fist
	Ulnar clawing (Benediction sign)
	Finger contractures
	Swan neck deformity
	Boutonniere deformity

been very popular in Europe, they have been less popular in the United States and are most often considered for non-functional upper extremities. Problems can occur at multiple levels throughout the upper extremity, causing different limitations and requiring a wide variety of treatment options.

Shoulder

Shoulder problems, detailed in Table 13.1, may or may not be painful, but many of them can limit function. Many patients with lower extremity limitations will become more dependent on their upper extremities, including using them for primary weight-bearing, locomotion, or transfers. This results in rotator cuff pathology and arthritis at an early and high rate. Rotator cuff sprains can be managed symptomatically, but larger tears may require repair or arthroplasty procedures. Unfortunately, the continued use of the shoulder for load-bearing tasks means that good outcomes can be difficult to achieve. Adhesive capsulitis or tendonitis pathologies can be managed with anti-inflammatory medications (oral, topical, or intra-articular) and therapy. Adduction and internal rotation contractures tend to be the most common deformity with spasticity and can be managed with medications or releases. Untreated, this can make hygiene and activities of daily living (ADLs; such as getting dressed, feeding, washing or combing hair, two-handed tasks) difficult. For those with flaccid or weak muscles around the shoulder, subluxations and dislocations can occur. If the humeral head subluxes inferiorly, pressure can be applied on the brachial plexus, leading to brachial plexopathy and additional upper extremity impairment. Support from a sling may be helpful. Surgical intervention for contractures, such as releases, tendon lengthenings, or transfers, are more likely to be successful than surgical treatment for instability, since the muscle tension is not there to keep the head located postoperatively.[14]

Elbow

Elbow flexion deformities are the most common and are due to spasticity of the brachialis, biceps, and brachioradialis muscles. Oral and injectable medications can be helpful to treat this problem early, but surgery may be helpful for advanced deformity in a patient who could potentially use their elbow or is unable to perform hygiene tasks. Shortening of the muscles can be treated with fractional lengthening at the myotendinous junction, which is near the shoulder for the biceps, near the elbow for the brachialis, and in the forearm for the brachioradialis.[15,16] If the contracture is severe, with anterior tightening of the joint capsule, the muscles can be released, but the capsule will need to be released as well. Most patients are unlikely to achieve complete lengthening with a single surgical procedure, so expectations should be set that serial casting and therapy will follow. The neurovascular bundle has usually also shortened and cannot be lengthened surgically. Spontaneous elbow fractures and dislocations are not common but can occur with trauma. Similarly, elbow extension contractures are not common, but triceps lengthening can be considered.

Forearm

The most common forearm deformity is pronation due to spasticity of the pronator teres and quadratus. Supination deformity is occasionally seen. Surgical management of pronation deformity is rare but consists of releasing both the pronator teres and quadratus off the radius. The interosseus membrane contributes to the pronation but cannot be released. Surgical management of a supination deformity may be achieved by releasing the distal attachment of the biceps or transferring it to the lateral border of the radial neck. A proximal synostosis can occur in cases of ankylosis or heterotopic ossification (HO).

Wrist

Wrist deformity can occur in multiple planes. Flexion is most common followed by radial or ulnar deviation. Wrist extension contractures are less common but can be seen. Flexed wrists are a little less likely to have concomitant finger flexion contractures due to the intrinsic muscles of the hand, but wrist extension deformity is usually associated with flexed fingers. Multiple muscles contribute to wrist flexion deformities, including the flexor carpi radialis (FCR), flexor carpi ulnaris (FCU), flexor digitorum superficialis (FDS), and flexor digitorum profundus (FDP). For wrist deformities, there is often a tendency to think about surgical procedures without considering the patient's ability to move their own wrist. Surgical procedures, as stated above, weaken muscles and should only be considered if there is enough strength present to have successful function following surgery. Options include fractional lengthening, tendon releases, or tendon transfers. If the desire is to simply establish a fixed position for the hand, the proximal row carpectomies or wrist fusions can be performed. One other consideration for patients who have progressive wrist flexion is that they are at high risk of carpal tunnel syndrome. Those who are symptomatic may benefit from a carpal tunnel release. Wrist extension is treated in similar fashion to wrist flexion.

Thumb

Spasticity of the thenar musculature can cause thumb adduction and spasticity of the flexor pollicis longus (FPL) can cause flexion at the interphalangeal (IP) joint or metacarpophalangeal (MCP) joint. This results in a "thumb-in-palm" position that causes problems with function, skin breakdown, and hygiene. As with other upper extremity muscles, any consideration of surgery is based on the ability of the patient to use their thumb. Attempts to release contractures may be considered, but it is rare that a significant contracture can be treated with a single surgery alone and additional stretching or casting may be indicated. Fusion is also a rarely employed option.

Fingers

Treatment of finger deformities can be quite challenging. The muscles are difficult to treat with injectable neurotoxins. Neurectomies can play a role in treating the spasticity. Releases, transfers, fractional lengthenings, or thenar slide procedures can be useful in very specific circumstances, often following a brain injury or stroke compared to children or adults with cerebral palsy (CP). Once again, some level of function must be established as well as very specific goals and a commitment to therapy before surgery is performed. Finally, ulnar nerve pathology around the elbow can occur with deformity or flexion contractures and this can result in hand deformity.[3] If caught early, the ulnar nerve can be decompressed or transferred at the level of the elbow.

LOWER EXTREMITY SURGERY

Lower extremity spasticity can cause pain or limit function as well as affect the ability to perform standard hygiene tasks. Contractures develop easily and any increased tone can limit the ability to walk. The most common problem is ankle contractures, followed by angular foot deformity, knee contractures, and spastic hip dysplasia. Tone management must be in place first for any subsequent treatment to be effective. In addition to (or in place of) general tone management, focal tone management plays a significant role in reducing lower extremity tone. This can include therapeutic massage or manipulation, chemodenervation, or other methods. Toxins are a common choice, but alcohol blocks play a large role as well. In the lower extremity, there have been a few studies showing improved Modified Ashworth Scale (MAS) and improved patient satisfaction at 2-year follow-up for selective peripheral neurectomies.[4] Improvement in the soleus muscle sensory afferents without motor denervation was noted in a study looking at the reduction of H max following selective tibial neurotomy.[5]

Lengthening tendons or performing fractional lengthenings at the musculotendinous junction must be done cautiously with great attention paid to the length achieved by the surgery. Overlengthening can result in worse postoperative function and weakness due to iatrogenic lever arm dysfunction.

Table 13.2 Manifestations of Lower Extremity Spasticity by Region	
Hip	Adductor spasticity
	Subluxation or dislocation
	Femoral torsion
	Hip flexor spasticity
	Hip extensor spasticity
Knee	Hamstring spasticity
	Knee extensor spasticity
	Knee contracture

(continued)

Table 13.2 Manifestations of Lower Extremity Spasticity by Region *(continued)*

Ankle	Equinus contracture
	Equinovarus deformity
	Equinovalgus deformity
	Tibial torsion
	Varus deformity
	Valgus deformity
Foot	Cavus deformity
	Valgus deformity
	Varus deformity
Toes	Claw toes
	Hallux valgus
	Dorsal bunion

Hip

Hip problems can develop early following injury or in cases of CP. Close monitoring of hips has become the standard of care in many places. Spasticity of the muscles around the hip can be painful; can limit function, positioning, hygiene, and ambulation; and leads to joint deformity. The adductors tend to contract, which leads to scissoring with gait, can make it difficult to sit in a wheelchair, and limits the ability to do perineal care. The adductors can be managed with stretching or bracing combined with tone medications initially, but more severe cases require chemodenervation using toxins or phenol, surgical tenotomy of the adductors, obturator neurectomy, or release. In young children, the iliopsoas spasticity will occur concurrently and can be addressed in a similar manner. The deforming forces of the adductors and iliopsoas in combination can cause hip dysplasia in the growing child. As the femoral head moves superiorly and laterally, the acetabulum becomes dysplastic and shallow. Prevention of hip dislocation should consist of a screening program during early childhood. Aggressive bracing and management of spasticity can be used as first steps, but adductor tenotomies should be considered early along with an abduction program once subluxation is noted. Further subluxation may require reconstruction of the hip using a varus derotational osteotomy of the proximal femur, with or without acetabuloplasty and adductor tenotomy. If the acetabulum remains shallow and the femoral head is still at risk of subluxation, the acetabulum should be addressed. Older patients, such as those with closed growth plates, are less likely to develop a dysplastic acetabulum at this age, but if the deformity occurred earlier and was not addressed, then redirectional pelvic osteotomies or salvage procedures may be required in place of an acetabuloplasty. For patients with type IV hemiplegia, torsional deformities of the proximal femur can cause internal rotation of the hip that may require a proximal femoral derotational osteotomy. Hip extensor spasticity is uncommon but can make it difficult for patients to sit. Isolated hip flexor spasticity may manifest as a crouch or jump gait pattern, but consider whether lordosis is present and is affecting the overall sagittal profile. Hip flexor deformities will also often occur in tandem with knee flexion deformities and must be addressed simultaneously, as well.

Knee

The most common knee deformity comes from spasticity of the hamstrings. This can lead to knee flexion deformity or contractures. Hamstrings spasticity can initially be treated with oral medications, stretching, bracing, injectable medications, chemodenervation, or neurectomies. If this progresses, hamstring lengthenings may be considered, but timing is critical and tone management must be in place first to make this successful. Post-surgical bracing can also be helpful to prevent recurrence. Once a contracture develops, hamstring lengthening alone may not be enough and the patient may also need capsular release or a distal femoral extension osteotomy. In a child with sufficient growth remaining in the distal femoral physis, anterior distal femoral epiphysiodesis may be considered as well. If the extensor mechanism becomes too long by effectively shortening the anterior aspect of the knee, then patellar tendon advancement may be necessary. Spasticity of the rectus muscle in isolation can sometimes cause a "rectus firing out of phase" phenomenon in which the rectus muscle fires during swing phase and forces the toe to strike the ground when it should be clearing. This can sometimes be managed with stretching or toxins, but release or transfer of the rectus may be considered more permanent options.

Ankle

The most common problem in the ankle is spasticity of the gastrocnemius muscle, with or without soleus spasticity, that causes an equinus deformity in the ankle. This is exceptionally common in CP and develops as one of the first manifestations of a brain injury or strike. Early recognition of this problem is essential and prophylactic bracing after injury should be considered for most patients. As with other areas of spasticity, tone management through enteral or intrathecal medications should be part of the treatment plan. Toxins are widely used, sometimes combined with stretching, stretch casting, or dynamic bracing. Selective neurectomies can also be useful to manage very specific problems. When evaluating a patient for surgical intervention, the Silverskiold test should be performed. Isolated gastrocnemius shortening can be treated with a myofascial lengthening such as a Strayer or Vulpius procedure. If both the gastrocnemius and soleus are tight, then an Achilles lengthening can be performed. In very young children, a tenotomy may be utilized, but older children or adults are more appropriate to have a three-cut percutaneous lengthening or an open z-lengthening. Overlengthening of the soleus when it is not short can have devastating consequences for gait. The primary job of the soleus, in addition to plantar flexion, is to maintain extension of the tibia, and a patient will fall into an irreversible crouch gait if the soleus lever arm is compromised. Ankle varus and valgus may occur as a consequence of overpull from the tibialis anterior, tibialis posterior, or peroneals. These may be managed with similar non-operative methods or may require tendon releases or transfers. Tibial torsion does not respond well to non-operative management, so derotational osteotomies must be utilized if the problem is significant enough to require treatment.

Foot

Deforming forces in the feet are numerous and sometimes difficult to manage. Bracing can be a very effective method of managing the foot position, although it is not always a definitive treatment. Some disorders are also associated with progressive deformity such as Charcot–Marie–Tooth disease. Cavus deformity involves plantar flexion of the first ray followed by progressive varus of the hindfoot. When this deformity is still flexible, soft tissue procedures may be appropriate. When the deformity becomes fixed, first metatarsal osteotomy with or without calcaneus osteotomy may be considered. Isolated midfoot plantar flexion may be treated with a plantar fascia release. If the forefoot abducts, an abductor hallucis release may be useful. When varus or valgus is perceived in the foot, it is helpful to look for spasticity proximally. For example, a tight Achilles will often create a valgus deformity in the foot. Feet that are both flat and in valgus should be evaluated for tarsal coalition as well. For deformities that become significantly advanced and simple procedures are not expected to be successful, consider the ambulatory status of the patient and the level of pain. A painless plantigrade foot can be achieved with substantial releases, while some feet just need to be positioned to fit into a shoe and this might be achieved with arthrodesis procedures.

Toes

Flexion deformities, including curly toes, hammer toes, and claw toes often develop with spasticity. The great toe is at risk for a dorsal bunion if long-standing flexion is present. Hallux valgus can also occur in the great toes. In cases of spasticity, tone is still the underlying problem, so most cases of hallux valgus cannot be treated with typical methods and great toe MP fusion must be considered. Similarly, releasing toe flexors alone has a lower success rate compared to tendon transfers, intramedullary pinning, and arthrodesis of the joints.

SPINE DEFORMITY

Spinal deformity occurs as a result of spasticity or flaccid muscles. Coronal and sagittal deformity can be minimal or can be severe. Hypertonic muscles in the trunk tend to cause more severe deformity and can be harder to treat. Flaccid trunks can be supported with braces or positioning devices. Hypertonic trunks do not respond well to bracing or wheelchair positioning over time because the curves tend to be more progressive. Surgical intervention must address coronal and sagittal deformity as well as axial rotation. Many patients need to have their pelvis included in the levels of fixation and fusion. Seating balance is a priority for patients who sit, while preservation of ambulation may be more important for those who walk. Most caregivers find that spinal fusion surgery makes it easier to transfer and care for patients. The surgical procedures are often complex and should involve a multidisciplinary evaluation preoperatively.

DIAGNOSIS-SPECIFIC CONSIDERATIONS

Spinal Cord Injury

Spinal cord injuries (SCIs), which occur from a variety of etiologies, cannot be fully evaluated until spinal shock resolves. Spasticity is then likely to progress over a course of weeks to months following the injury. Early intervention should include non-operative methods at preventing contractures or deformity. The multidisciplinary team must be cognizant of the risk of pressure sores as well. Secondary musculoskeletal effects can occur later, such as shoulder arthritis or rotator cuff tears in people who use a wheelchair for primary mobility. Exercise can help prevent deterioration and the ability to perform exercise will vary over the first 1 to 5 years following injury but eventually stabilize.[6]

Stroke

Strokes can affect the brain unilaterally or bilaterally. Unilateral strokes are more common, so the manifestations tend to affect one side of the body more frequently than affecting both sides. Spasticity and weakness are common outcomes following a stroke, followed by limited use of extremities, joint contractures, subluxations, or dislocations.[7] Weak muscles are more susceptible to damage and adjacent pathology. In the shoulder, for example, a patient may experience adhesive capsulitis, rotator cuff tears, impingement, subluxation, or dislocation following a stroke.[8–10] The manifestations of spasticity can also be quite painful, so decision-making should focus on both pain management and potential for improvement in function.

TRAUMATIC BRAIN INJURY

TBI, unlike SCI and stroke, have a much higher incidence of cognitive and mental status changes that can also have emotional, behavioral, and psychosocial implications. This can make evaluation and decisions about treatment more challenging. In addition, a TBI puts patients at a much greater risk of HO following any fracture or surgical procedure, but it can also form spontaneously between muscles and joint capsules or in any area of tension.[11–13] In cases where occurrence is spontaneous, it may be diagnosed by a loss of motion or by the presence of a mass, which can be painless or painful. Patients with CP who have chronically dislocated hips sometimes undergo proximal femoral resections, which also have an increased risk of HO postoperatively.

KEY POINTS

- Treating spasticity and the manifestations of spasticity require a thoughtful approach.
- Both surgical and nonsurgical treatment options exist, but tone management should be in place before surgery occurs.
- Spasticity treatment options should not be thought of as linear. Doing so means that necessary preventative treatment might be delayed and more significant deformity may occur.
- Operative intervention should be considered early in neurologic injury if it can prevent larger problems later, but neurologic recovery is variable.
- A thorough assessment of the patient and their goals can guide decision-making at all stages to ensure the best outcomes.

REFERENCES

1. Summers J, Coker B, Eddy S, et al. Selective dorsal rhizotomy in ambulatory children with cerebral palsy: an observational cohort study. *Lancet.* 2019;3(7):455–64. https://doi.org/10.1016/S2352-4642(19)30119-1
2. Gras M, Leclerq C. Spasticity and hyperselective neurectomy in the upper limb. *Hand Surg Rehabil.* 2017;36(6):391–401. https://doi.org/10.1016/j.hansur.2017.06.009

3. Keenan MA, Kaufmann DL, Garland DE, et al. Late ulnar neuropathy in the brain injured adult. *J Hand Surg.* 1988;13(1):120–4. https://doi.org/1016/0363-5023(88)90214-6

4. Mahan MA, Ilyas E, Hamrick F, et al. Highly selective partial neurectomies for spasticity: a single-center experience. *Neurosurg.* 2021;89(5):827–35. https://doi.org/10.1093/neuros/nyab303

5. Roujeau T, Lefaucheur JP, Slavov V, et al. Long term course of the h reflex after selective tibial neurotomy. *J Neurol Neurosurg Psychiatry.* 2003;74(7):913–7. https://doi.org/10.1136/jnnp.74.7.913

6. Van Koppenhagen CF, de Groot S, Post M, et al. Wheelchair exercise capacity in spinal cord injury up to five years after discharge from inpatient rehabilitation. *J Rehabil Med.* 2013;45(7):646–52. https://doi.org/10.2340/16501977-1149

7. Kendall R. Musculoskeletal problems in stroke survivors. *Top Stroke Rehabil.* 2010;17(3):173–8. https://doi.org/10.1310/tsr1703-173

8. Lindgren I, Jönsson AC, Norrving B, et al. Shoulder pain after stroke: a prospective population-based study. *Stroke.* 2007;38(2):343–8. https://doi.org/10.1161/01.str.0000254598.16739.4e

9. Chae J, Mascarenhas D, Yu DT, et al. Post-stroke shoulder pain: its relationship to motor impairment, activity limitation, and quality of life. *Arch Phys Med Rehabil.* 2007;88(3):298–301. https://doi.org/10.1016/j.apmr.2006.12.007

10. Adey-Wakeling Z, Liu E, Crotty M, et al. Hemiplegic shoulder pain reduces quality of life after acute stroke: a prospective population-based study. *Am J Phys Med Rehabil.* 2016;95(10):758–63.

11. Botte MJ, Keenan MA, Abrams RA, et al. Heterotopic ossification in neuromuscular disorders. *Orthopedics.* 1997;20(4):335–41. https://doi.org/10.3928/0147-7447-19970401-11

12. Cipriano CA, Pill SG, Keenan MA. Heterotopic ossification following traumatic brain and spinal cord injury. *J Am Acad Orthop Surg.* 2009;17(11):689–97. https://doi.org/10.5435/00124635-200911000-00003

13. Chan KT. Heterotopic ossification in traumatic brain injury. *Am J Phys Med Rehabil.* 2005;84(2):145–6. https://doi.org/10.1097/01.phm.0000151939.59660.b1

14. Leclercq C, Perruisseau-Carrier A, Gras M, et al. Hyperselective neurectomy for the treatment of upper limb spasticity in adults and children: a prospective study. *J Hand Surg Eur Vol.* 2021;46(7):708–16. https://doi.org/10.31177/17531934211027499

15. Namdari S, Horneff JG, Baldwin K, et al. Muscle releases to improve passive motion and relieve pain in patients with spastic hemiplegia and elbow flexion contractures. *J Shoulder Elbow Surg.* 2012;21(10):1357–62. https://doi.org/10.1016/j.jse.2011.09.029

16. Photopoulos CD, Namdari S, Baldwin KD, et al. Decision making in the treatment of the spastic shoulder and elbow: tendon release versus tendon lengthening. *JBJS Rev.* 2014;2(10):e3. https://doi.org/10.2106/JBJS.RVW.M.00132

14 Emerging Technologies

Manuel F. Mas and William A. Ramos Guasp

INTRODUCTION

Spasticity is one of the most physically debilitating and prevalent conditions that interferes with functional improvement.[1-4] A wide spectrum of evaluation and treatment options exist for the management of spasticity. Classically, spasticity is evaluated using physical examination with scales such as the Modified Ashworth Scale (MAS)[5] and Modified Tardieu Scale (MTS).[6] Mainstream therapies include both non-pharmacologic and pharmacologic options. However, despite these, the evaluation and treatment of spasticity remains challenging.

The quest to better serve patients has led to the emergence of technology to better assess and treat spasticity. Due to the MAS's dependency on subjective assessment,[7] other evaluation options have emerged based on technological advances. These include ultrasound elastography (USE) and magnetic resonance elastography, among others. Among emerging technological treatment options, neuromodulation using both peripheral and central electrical stimulation (e-stim) and central magnetic stimulation has robust data available for review. Other options with moderate evidence include extracorporeal shock wave therapy (ESWT) and whole-body vibration (WBV). This chapter focuses on available evidence for new technological options for both the evaluation and treatment of spasticity, with an attempt to subdivide treatment options among the more commonly studied neurologic diseases.

EVALUATION OF SPASTICITY

As described elsewhere, the MAS and MTS remain the most used clinical tools for the evaluation of spasticity. Despite their widespread use, the validity, reliability, and sensitivity of such clinical scales have been challenged.[8,9] Apart from their subjective and qualitative nature, a major limitation of such scales is their inability to distinguish between the neurogenic and mechanical components of spasticity.[10] To address some of these limitations, promising measurement tools have emerged that may lead to more accurate characterization of spasticity. In this chapter, we highlight some of these technologies.

ULTRASOUND ELASTOGRAPHY

Conventional grayscale ultrasound (B-mode US) has been established as a reliable, safe, and cost-effective imaging modality for the evaluation of the musculoskeletal system.[11] Despite remarkable advances in spatial resolution and dynamic imaging capabilities, the use of B-mode US for the evaluation of spasticity is limited, as it does not provide information about the biomechanical and structural properties of tissues. To this end, USE has emerged as a promising real-time imaging technique for assessing spasticity.[12] USE is based on the principle that tissues will undergo deformation when subject to a stress or force, which is intrinsically related to its elastic properties.[13] Two main elastography techniques will be discussed in this chapter: *compression elastography* (CE) and *shear wave elastography* (SWE).

Compression Elastography

CE is a qualitative technique that evaluates tissue elasticity by characterizing its response to a compressive force. The technique is performed by repeated manual compressions over the region of interest and comparing before and after sonographic images. The displacement is calculated and converted to a two-dimensional color-coded strain image (elastogram) that can be superimposed over a conventional B-mode image. By convention, red is used to represent softer tissues (more displacement), blue represents harder tissues (less displacement), and yellow-green depict intermediate tissues. A semi-quantitative measurement can be generated by calculating the strain ratio, which compares the relative elasticity between the tissue of interest and a reference tissue.[13–15]

Multiple studies demonstrated a statistically significant difference in strain parameters when comparing spastic versus non-spastic biceps brachii in patients with chronic stroke.[16–18] Similar results have been reported for the biceps brachii and gastrocnemius in patients with multiple sclerosis (MS).[19] Further, the intra-rater and inter-rater reliability of CE was shown to be good to excellent for the biceps brachii and gastrocnemius.[20] Overall, available literature suggests CE has adequate discriminatory capacity for identifying spastic muscles.

Shear Wave Elastography

SWE is a quantitative method whereby stress is applied via an acoustic radiation force to generate mechanical vibrations, which propagate perpendicular to the primary ultrasound (US) wave and cause shear tissue displacement. The displacement generated is tracked and used to estimate shear wave speed, which is used as a proxy for tissue stiffness. In this scenario, shear waves propagate faster through stiffer tissues. Similar to CE, a color-coded elastogram is generated.[12,21,22]

As with CE, the strongest evidence for SWE comes from studies evaluating chronic poststroke spasticity (PSS) of the biceps brachii. To this end, multiple studies have shown a statistically significant increase in SW speed in chronic poststroke spastic biceps brachii muscles compared to the non-spastic side.[17,23–25] Further, SW speed differences between the spastic and non-spastic side are augmented as time from the stroke increases.[23,25]

Available literature evaluating spastic muscles in the lower extremities is limited. A couple of studies showed that spastic gastrocnemius has greater SW speed compared to the non-spastic side.[26,27] However, the reliability of the shear elastic modulus is insufficient on the non-spastic side.[27]

Monitoring Therapeutic Response

The feasibility of USE for monitoring the effectiveness of therapeutic interventions has also been studied. A prospective study of seven patients with stroke with unilateral spasticity of the biceps brachii demonstrated significant improvement in both CE and SWE parameters after botulinum toxin A (BoNTA) treatment.[20] Similar results have been documented in patients with cerebral palsy (CP) and unilateral gastrocnemius spasticity.[28,29] Taken together, the findings of USE may aid in treatment planning and ongoing monitoring of therapeutic modalities.

Limitations

Despite encouraging results, USE has important limitations for the evaluation of spasticity in the clinical setting. Common limitations in studies evaluating USE include small sample size, inconsistencies with terminology and reported parameters, and lack of standardized protocols. For CE, the inability to quantify or control the force applied is a major obstacle for reproducibility. For SWE, the anisotropic, viscoelastic, and active nature of skeletal muscle—which is not accounted for in SWE—is a major limitation. Lastly, access to the equipment and necessary expertise to perform and interpret these tests may limit their widespread adoption.[12,21]

MAGNETIC RESONANCE ELASTROGRAPHY

Magnetic resonance elastography (MRE) is a noninvasive MRI-based technology that also measures tissue stiffness. It follows similar steps and principles to USE. Although it has been used to study tissue stiffness, correlation with spasticity has not been widely studied. In patients with spinal cord injury (SCI), vastus lateralis stiffness as measured by MRE was significantly higher when compared to able-bodied controls. However, stiffness measures did not correlate with MAS scores. As with USE, many more studies are needed to understand the use of MRE to evaluate spasticity.[30]

ROBOT-AIDED SYSTEMS

The application of rehabilitation robotics sound particularly promising for the evaluation of spasticity, as this would arguably eliminate (or reduce) the subjectivity of current assessment tools. Despite still being in the early stages, several robot-based systems have been developed for this purpose with encouraging results. For example, Seth and colleagues developed a robotic arm system able to detect and quantify velocity-dependent resistance in the upper extremity.[31] Dehem and colleagues developed another system (REAplan device) able to quantify resistance force (RF) of spastic elbow flexors. Further, they demonstrated an improvement in RF after musculocutaneous nerve block.[32]

CONCLUSION

Technology continues to advance and new techniques have emerged to better assess spasticity. USE and robot-aided systems provide compelling tools to more objectively assess spasticity over more classical and potentially subjective measures. The reliability of these techniques is still being debated. Current cost of these new devices may limit their adoption in clinical practice.

TREATMENT OF SPASTICITY

In the next section, a detailed account of the most recent emerging technologies for spasticity treatment will be provided focusing on the most common neurologic disorders cited in the literature.

PERIPHERAL ELECTRICAL STIMULATION

E-stim to produce movement was recognized as early as 1790 by Luigi Galvani and 1831 by Michael Faraday.[33,34] The most common types of peripheral e-stim include neuromuscular electrical stimulation (NMES), transcutaneous electrical nerve stimulation (TENS), and functional electrical stimulation (FES). NMES employs an electrical current of sufficient intensity to elicit muscle contraction. FES applies stimulation to a set of muscles involved in a task to facilitate a functional activity.[35] TENS consists of the application of a low-intensity continuous electrical current to the cutaneous nerve fibers with no apparent muscular stimulation.[36] Despite existing for centuries now, its application specifically for the treatment of spasticity is a more novel and emerging approach that has been recently studied in diverse populations.

Stroke

E-stim has been shown to be effective as an adjunct therapy for botulinum toxin (BoNT) in chronic upper limb spasticity[37] and to physical therapy in ankle plantar flexor spasticity.[38] In a recent case series, patients with stroke participated in treadmill walking with FES to the quadriceps, hamstrings, peroneals, and plantar flexor muscle groups bilaterally. After 10 interventions, there was no improvement in knee extensors or ankle plantar flexors spasticity as measured by the MAS. However, there was improvement in other functional measures.[39] Yang et al. reported that ankle plantar flexor static and dynamic spasticity significantly improved when applying NMES to the tibialis anterior prior to ambulation training. Interestingly, findings were significant when compared to patients who had NMES applied to the medial gastrocnemius or those who received stretching exercises prior to training.[40]

FES was applied to the wrist and finger extensors for wrist flexor spasticity in patients with stroke. Stimulation was applied for 30 minutes, 5 days a week for 20 sessions per patient. When compared to a control group receiving conventional treatment of stretching exercises, there was a significant improvement in spasticity as measured by MAS at the end of the treatment course. The researchers propose that reciprocal inhibition achieved this treatment effect.[41]

TENS as an adjunct therapy for spasticity reduction following stroke has been supported in literature, particularly for ankle plantar flexors.[42,43] TENS in the peroneal nerve followed by exercise was found to significantly improve spasticity as measured by the composite spasticity score. When combined with taping of the ankle plantar flexors, spasticity improved further. The addition of taping is proposed to have reduced cortical excitability when applied to an overexcited muscle group. However, small sample size and reliance of the composite spasticity score as an outcome measure makes comparisons with other studies difficult.[44] Similarly, TENS applied to the triceps and wrist extensors before occupational therapy improved elbow flexor spasticity as measured by the MAS when compared to placebo TENS. However, in this study, TENS was applied at an intensity that provoked muscle contraction.[45]

A recent systematic review concluded that TENS is effective in reducing lower limb spasticity when administered along with other forms of physical therapy interventions in survivors of chronic stroke. It is postulated that TENS can lead to presynaptic inhibition of hyperactive stretch reflexes and decrease in co-contraction of spastic muscle antagonists.[46] One of the intricacies of e-stim for spasticity reduction is the wide range of variables that can change between study and in clinical practice affecting results. These include length of e-stim, intensity, and electrode placement, among others. In a systematic review, it was concluded that TENS applied for more than 30 minutes could be more effective in spasticity reduction. Electrode placement along the nerve or muscle belly appeared to be more effective than when applied over acupuncture points. In general, the intervention appeared to be effective in patients with chronic stroke. However, this was usually the population selected for most studies included for review. These findings were echoed in another systematic review particularly the effectiveness of combining TENS with therapy for spasticity reduction in patients with chronic stroke.[47]

Thus, peripheral e-stim is a promising tool to decrease upper and lower extremity spasticity in survivors of stroke, although there has been a greater focus on lower extremity spasticity. There is, however, no consensus on the prescription guidelines of peripheral e-stim. The duration of treatment effect duration is also in question. Yet peripheral e-stim can be considered a safe adjunct to enhance the effect of physical and occupational therapy in the treatment of spastic movement disorder.

Spinal Cord Injury

Peripheral e-stim has been more commonly utilized in conjunction with functional training in SCI with studies focusing on this topic since the 1980s.[48–50] Generally, results have been more favorable in patients with incomplete SCI, since spasticity is more prevalent in this population. In a recent meta-analysis, FES in combination with cycling was found to produce a significant reduction in spasticity in patients with paraplegia and tetraplegia. The proposed mechanisms of action included restoration of post-activation depression, which is decreased in chronic SCI and can be a cause of spasticity, and inhibition of Renshaw cells.[51] A recent systematic review concluded that e-stim such as NMES and FES can be effective in managing spasticity symptoms after SCI. Most studies studied an acute effect on spasticity, within 24 hours of treatment.[52] However, there is heterogenicity in e-stim parameters that proves difficult when attempting to provide standardized recommendations or guidelines.

Recent literature on the benefits of TENS for spasticity reduction in patients with SCI is scarce. In a recent study comparing the effects of TENS and FES on hip adductors and knee extensors in a group of patients with mostly incomplete SCI, both muscle and cutaneous e-stim modalities had similar results on immediate spasticity that lasted for at least 4 hours post treatment.[53] Prior to this, TENS over the common peroneal nerve in patients with SCI was shown to be an effective way of reducing ankle plantar flexor spasticity.[54]

It appears that peripheral e-stim may reduce SCI-related spasticity, especially when it is combined with functional activities, particularly in incomplete SCI. As with stroke, spasticity was not equally assessed in all studies and different e-stim techniques were utilized. Yet FES and TENS can both be used as safe adjuncts to physical therapy for spasticity reduction.

Multiple Sclerosis

Peripheral e-stim in patients with MS has been studied for multiple domains including gait, neurogenic bladder, and functional improvement; however, recent literature specific to spasticity treatment is limited. A study analyzing the safety of an FES cycling protocol targeting bilateral lower extremities showed no change in spasticity after 36 sessions (3 per week for 12 weeks). However, it was deemed safe, aided in reducing fatigue and improving some measures of quality of life (QOL).[55,56] Earlier studies showed that TENS applied to the spastic plantar flexor muscles was effective in reducing spasticity.[57,58]

Thus, patients with MS suffering from spasticity could trial peripheral e-stim as a safe treatment alternative. However, its evidence is not as robust as with other populations.

Cerebral Palsy

As with MS, peripheral e-stim has not been studied extensively in the population with CP and was initially focused to wrist and finger spasticity.[59,60] In a recent study, patients with CP and lower extremity spasticity who received BoNT injections were divided into three groups to compare the effectiveness of FES cycling to sham and standard treatment. After 4 weeks of treatment, all groups had significant improvement in spasticity as measured by the MAS. However, there was no significant difference between the groups.[61] Recently, a 30-minute conventional TENS treatment protocol to the calf muscles showed a statistically significant reduction in spasticity of the ankle plantar flexors as measured by MAS.[62] Liu et al. studied the combined effects of TENS and transcranial pulsed current stimulation in spasticity. When compared to a control group receiving routine physiotherapy, the treatment group had a significant reduction in spasticity as measured by the MAS and MTS.[63] However, it is difficult to discern if improvement in spasticity was due to TENS, transcranial stimulation, or both. Also, TENS was applied to multiple regions including cervicothoracolumbar areas, knee extensors, and calf muscles. The amount of potentially unstudied variables makes these results harder to recommend or replicate in clinical practice.

In summary, the effects of peripheral e-stim on spasticity have been studied in several patient populations. Peripheral e-stim appears to work best in combination with conventional therapy and functional activities. There is still much to learn about the therapeutic details of e-stim including type of stimulation, stimulation intensity, treatment length, and how it may best be combined with other treatments.

SPINAL CORD STIMULATION

Spinal cord stimulation (SCS) consists of inserting a percutaneous or surgical paddle lead containing multiple stimulating electrodes typically into the epidural space.[64] SCS has emerged as a standard of care treatment for chronic neuropathic pain.[65] In the United States, it is routinely used for failed back surgery syndrome and complex regional pain syndrome.[66] Yet it remains a controversial treatment for severe spasticity.[64]

Recent studies have pointed that the effects of epidural stimulation are mainly attributable to activation of peripheral nerve roots, primarily afferent fibers. These same circuits are also engaged by transcutaneous spinal cord stimulation (tSCS), a noninvasive treatment modality.[67] Transcutaneous spinal stimulation delivered at 50 Hz for 15 minutes over the thoracic spine at T11 to T12 proved to be comparable to whole-body vibration in the reduction of quadriceps spasticity in patients with motor-incomplete SCI with high spasticity as measured by the pendulum test.[68] However, in a separate study, when compared to a sham group, tSCS in combination with locomotor training did not show significant reduction in spasticity after 4 weeks of treatment.[67] Patients with MS who received tSCS for one session of 30 minutes showed a statistically significant reduction in lower extremity spasticity as measured by the MAS, immediately following the treatment as well as 24 hours afterward.[69]

Taken together, there is limited evidence documenting the efficacy of SCS to decrease spasticity although some accounts appear promising. Clinicians and patients must consider the high cost of epidural SCS.[70] Also, the better safety profile and lower costs of tSCS may make it a far more reasonable treatment alternative for spasticity reduction, although evidence is limited.

TRANSCRANIAL DIRECT CURRENT STIMULATION

Transcranial direct current stimulation (tDCS) is a noninvasive technique that can induce sustained changes in excitability in the brain.[71] The components of tDCS are a constant current stimulator and surface electrodes. Current intensities vary between 1 and 2 mA and are commonly applied for 10 to 20 minutes. Stimulation can be either anodal or cathodal. Anodal stimulation increases cortical excitability while cathodal stimulation decreases it.[72] For motor cortical stimulation, the stimulating electrode is usually placed over the motor cortex and the reference electrode is placed over the contralateral supraorbital ridge.

Stroke

Most of the studies on tDCS have been conducted in the population with stroke. However, spasticity is not necessarily the primary outcome measure studied, as much as function. Its effectiveness on PSS varies. In a sham-controlled trial, patients with chronic stroke treated with tDCS combined with sensory modulation and passive movements on the paretic hand had limited immediate improvement of spasticity and no long-term effects.[73] Anodal tDCS to the damaged primary motor cortex of patients with stroke in combination with FES was effective in reducing wrist flexor spasticity when compared to sham treatment and FES only control groups after 1 month from intervention.[74] In a cross-over, double-blinded study, dual tDCS (anode over affected motor cortex [M1] and cathode over contralateral M1) and cathodal tDCS (cathode over contralateral M1) both decreased upper extremity spasticity. Although both tDCS paradigms decreased spasticity, cathodal tDCS had a larger effect on spasticity supported by changes in H-reflex modulation.[75]

Ehsani et al. studied the effects of anodal tDCS on the ankle muscles of patients with stroke. Patients were divided into an experimental, sham, or control group. All of them participated in physical therapy and a home exercise program. Patients participated in 10-session 20-minute anodal tDCS stimulation over the affected primary cortex. There was a significant reduction of spasticity in the ankle plantar flexors, as measured by the MAS, immediately following the intervention and 1 month later.[76] The effects of tDCS in patients with acute stroke have been shown to be effective up to a year following intervention. Bornheim et al. studied patients within the first month of stroke onset opposite to most studies following survivors of chronic stroke. Patients either received 20 sessions of anodal tDCS or sham tDCS in addition to conventional rehabilitation. Anodal tDCS was applied to the primary motor cortex of the affected hemisphere. Patients were evaluated periodically during the first year following stroke onset. There was noted improvement in functional motor outcomes up to a year following intervention. However, spasticity, as measured by the Tardieu Spasticity Scale, was similar for both groups throughout all tests.[77] The study did not go into much detail on the spasticity measures throughout the study's time frame.

Two emerging treatment technologies, tDCS and robotic therapy, have been combined to modulate neuronal activity after stroke. In a recent systematic review, this combined treatment showed a non-significant effect in improvement of upper limb function and a positive effect in lower limb function. However, there were no significant results in spasticity reduction. Most of the studies analyzed for this review had small sample sizes and variability of tDCS parameters and robotic therapy devices.[78] In a separate meta-analysis, anodal tDCS was suggested as an effective and safe adjunct to reduce upper limb PSS. Stimulation seemed to be more effective when applied for more than 20 minutes. Yet evidence was deemed low quality.[79]

Taken together, these studies suggest that tDCS may be a useful adjunct to active therapies in reducing PSS. As with other modalities, there are still many variables to study including timing and length of treatment, anodal versus cathodal stimulation, and area and side of stimulation.

Cerebral Palsy

Studies regarding tDCS use in patients with CP generally focus on motor function, development, and other cognitive functions. However, the literature is sparse on the use of tDCS for spasticity in CP. In 2014, a sham-controlled trial was performed to investigate the antispasticity effects of anodal tDCS in individuals with spastic CP. The left primary motor cortex was targeted for 5 consecutive days. Children who were exposed to tDCS had significantly greater reduction in spasticity on the MAS, but not in passive range of motion (ROM) after treatment that persisted in some joints for 48 hours.[80] Since then, no notable studies have been published focusing on spasticity measurements following tDCS in this population. Other recently published studies have focused on motor function with generally favorable results.[81,82] There is very limited evidence on the benefits of tDCS for spasticity in individuals with CP.

Multiple Sclerosis

As with CP, the literature on the use of tDCS for spasticity due to MS is limited. One randomized, sham-controlled study of anodal tDCS to the primary motor cortex of the more affected side for 5 days did not show a significant improvement in spasticity.[71] Yet tDCS has been more widely studied for other symptoms of MS such as fatigue, pain, and cognition.[83] It has also been used to somewhat positive effect in gait in MS.[84,85]

In summary, tDCS appears to be a safe and potentially effective adjunct therapy for spasticity reduction in the population with stroke while evidence for other populations is lacking.

REPETITIVE TRANSCRANIAL MAGNETIC STIMULATION

Repetitive transcranial magnetic stimulation (rTMS) is a noninvasive, transcranial intervention that stimulates the cerebral cortex via the principles of electromagnetic induction.[86] The setup consists of a coil connected to a pulse generator, or stimulator, that delivers a changing electrical current. This coil is usually shaped like the number eight ("8") and is placed over the scalp of the patient. Pulses are delivered at a set frequency and intensity to change cortical excitability, thus modulating brain function.[87]

Different frequencies can either inhibit or excite the stimulated area.[88] Generally, 1 Hz is an inhibitory frequency while 5 to 10 Hz is considered excitatory. The goal of interventions with rTMS is to re-establish interhemispheric balance by exciting the injured hemisphere and inhibiting the contralesional one.[89] However, this theory is designed around unilateral lesions such as those seen in stroke.

Stroke

rTMS has been widely studied in patients with stroke, including for spasticity management. The most common stimulation parameter is low frequency, 1 Hz, to the contralesional hemisphere. A recent meta-analysis concluded that rTMS is effective in improving spasticity and activities of daily living (ADLs) in patients with stroke suffering from lower limb spasticity.[90] However, other systematic reviews and meta-analysis do not support rTMS for spasticity reduction in patients with prior stroke when compared to sham interventions[91] concluding that there is limited evidence available to support its use due to low sample size, inadequate duration, and lack of control arms.[92]

Yet researchers continue to utilize this therapy modality to assess improvement in motor function and spasticity following stroke. In a randomized sham-controlled cross-over trial, lower extremity spasticity in patients with chronic stroke was assessed after treatment with 1 Hz of rTMS directed at the contralesional lower extremity motor area with 1-week follow-up. After 5 consecutive daily sessions, spasticity reduced by 1 point on the MAS in the rTMS group that was not observed in a sham rTMS group.[93] Lower extremity spasticity also improved after 5 consecutive, 1-Hz rTMS sessions of 20 minutes as measured by the MAS in a separate small uncontrolled study.[94] Upper limb spasticity was significantly reduced after inhibitory, low-frequency rTMS to the contralesional hemisphere when compared to a sham rTMS group.[95]

Li et al. combined low-frequency rTMS on the contralesional side and cerebellar continuous theta burst stimulation (cTBS) to study its effects on upper and lower limb PSS. After daily sessions for 4 weeks (6 days a week), combined treatment of both modalities yielded significant reduction in MAS scores when compared to either rTMS or cerebellar cTBS groups alone. All three groups, however, showed significant reduction in spasticity after 4 weeks of treatment. Cerebellar cTBS may affect spasticity by modulating corticospinal excitability.[96] Similarly, both rTMS and cTBS applied to the contralesional hemisphere showed statistically significant reduction in poststroke upper limb spasticity, as compared to sham interventions. Of note, both modalities were combined with physiotherapy.[97] Due to its shorter stimulation times, cTBS might be a more time-efficient alternative to rTMS for spasticity treatment. A different rTMS modality, intermittent theta burst stimulation (iTBS), was also found to be effective in reducing PSS after 10 daily sessions, when compared to a sham group.[98]

As with other interventions discussed previously, rTMS shows promise as an adjunct to conventional therapy for spasticity reduction in patients with stroke. More research with larger study samples might lead to stronger recommendations in the future. Yet clinicians should be aware that this is not a readily available intervention.

Spinal Cord Injury

Studies focusing on rTMS after SCI are less frequent when compared to population with prior stroke. In a randomized, double-blinded, sham-controlled study, subjects with incomplete cervical or thoracic SCI received 10 daily sessions of real or iTBS. Patients who received real iTBS had significant reduction in spasticity as measured by the MAS that persisted for 1 week. This was not observed in the sham group.[99] These findings were similar to an earlier study done by the same group, focusing on rTMS to the contralesional motor area.[100] After one session of rTMS to the primary motor cortex, a more recent study did not find any changes in spasticity, using the MAS, with either low (1 Hz) or high (10 H) frequencies when applied to patients with incomplete SCI. However, high-frequency rTMS did increase cortical excitability.[101] Other groups have proposed very high-frequency (20–25 Hz) rRTMS applied to bilateral motor cortex in patients with incomplete SCI for spasticity reduction; however, the treatment algorithm and spasticity assessment are not consistent with the rest of the literature.[102]

Although rTMS has slightly more evidence for motor function improvement following SCI, literature on the effects of SCI-related spasticity is limited. Compared to the population with stroke, rTMS studies in SCI more frequently employ high-frequency stimulation to either hemisphere. As with other modalities, details regarding frequency and location to direct rTMS need to be better studied.

Multiple Sclerosis

There are very few studies evaluating rTMS for spasticity due to MS. Recent meta-analysis and systematic reviews concluded that rTMS can be an effective treatment for spasticity in patients with MS.[103,104] However, there is marked heterogeneity in the stimulation protocols (i.e., frequency, stimulation location, combination with therapy), making it difficult to replicate in clinical practice. iTBS was not effective in reducing lower limb spasticity in patients with relapsing-remitting MS. In this study, stimulation was applied to the contralateral motor cortex, daily, for 2 weeks.[105] However, a separate study found positive effects on MS spasticity for either high-frequency rTMS or iTBS when compared to sham stimulation.[106] Stimulation was targeted at both primary motor cortices, 5 times a week for 2 weeks (10 total daily sessions). After 10 sessions of rTMS (5 Hz) to the lower extremity motor area, patients with MS had a significant reduction in hip adductor spasticity as measured by the MAS, lasting for 1 month after the interventions. rTMS was combined with physiotherapy and compared to a sham rTMS group.[107]

As with SCI, evidence for the use of rTMS to improve MS-related spasticity is limited. Protocol details vary between studies. In addition, MS is a condition that can affect multiple regions of the upper motor neuron system (UMNS), contrary to more focal lesions as seen in stroke. This may create an issue in determining the effective stimulation location and protocols for individuals with MS.

Cerebral Palsy

rTMS use in CP has recently gained more interest. In 2021, a combination of 5 Hz of rTMS to the affected hemisphere and acupuncture in spastic CP did not provide significant difference in spasticity as measured by the Tardieu Scale, although it did improve gross motor function.[108] Rajak et al. demonstrated that increasing the number of rTMS and physical therapy sessions led to greater reduction in spasticity. However, there was no control group.[109] A recent systematic review concluded that evidence for rTMS in spasticity reduction in this population was uncertain.[110]

In summary, the evidence to support the use of rTMS to reduce spasticity is limited but has been growing recently. Studies on the population with stroke used mostly low-frequency rTMS while other patient populations responded to high-frequency stimulation. rTMS was generally combined with another intervention, usually physical therapy. More mechanistic research is warranted if rTMS is to be used in the treatment of spasticity, especially because the treatment is more involved and expensive than other stimulation therapies.

WHOLE-BODY VIBRATION

WBV is another emerging treatment option recently studied in spasticity reduction. It activates large-diameter afferent fibers leading to activation of inhibitory mechanisms and reduction of spasticity. This is a similar mechanism to other forms of e-stim treatments discussed previously.[111] A single session of WBV improved quadriceps spasticity, as measured by the pendulum test, in patients with SCI.[111] WBV also improved ankle plantar flexor spasticity in patients with cervical SCI after 80 sessions throughout 8 weeks when combined with conventional physical therapy.[112] It was also effective in reducing spasticity in patients with CP. In this study, children participated in three 15-minute sessions of WBV per week for 8 weeks in combination with therapy. Spasticity significantly improved in both upper and lower extremities when compared to a control group.[113] Immediate significant effects of WBV in MAS reduction of lower limb muscles has also been reported in patients with stroke.[114]

A systematic review concluded that there was weak evidence for a positive effect of short-term WBV training on spasticity of lower limbs in varied neurologic disorders. However, as with other treatments, specific parameters for wider adoption as a viable treatment option remain unclear.[115] Yet it remains an interesting and promising adjunct treatment option for spasticity reduction in neurologic disorders.

EXTRACORPOREAL SHOCK WAVE THERAPY

ESWT is a noninvasive modality that applies high-pressure waves to different targeted parts of the body. It has emerged as a treatment option for musculoskeletal injuries. It does not require analgesia, sedation, or anesthesia. ESWT includes focused shock wave and radial shock wave. They differ in their physical properties, depth of penetration, and mode of generation.[116] Relevant mechanisms have been attributed to alterations in muscle elasticity and extensibility, as well as ability to induce nitric oxide to act on neuromuscular junctions.[117] It has also been combined with other invasive options such as BoNT.[118,119]

Interest in the effectiveness of ESWT for spasticity after stroke has increased in recent years. There are numerous studies for both upper and lower body stroke-related spasticity. A recent systematic review concluded that ESWT was comparable to BoNT injections for PSS, with radial ESWT (rESWT) potentially being superior to all interventions.[120] Stroke-related ankle plantar flexor spasticity significantly decreased after 2 sessions per week for 2 weeks of rESWT and physical therapy. This was compared to a sham and a control group. There was also significant improvement in walking times in the 6-meter timed walk test for those treated with rESWT.[121] In a separate study, both focal and rESWT showed significant improvement in ankle plantar flexor spasticity after stroke in both MAS and Tardieu Scale measurements. There was no difference between groups in any outcomes, except for ankle passive ROM in favor of rESWT.[122] After analysis of 16 randomized controlled trials, ESWT was concluded to be effective in reducing upper limb spasticity and improving upper limb function when combined with conventional physiotherapy.[123] rESWT to either agonist or antagonist elbow flexor muscles was effective in reducing spasticity after 4 weeks following the completion of treatment.[124] ESWT has also been proposed as a long-lasting effective treatment for spasticity, as defined by follow-up of 4 weeks and later.[125]

ESWT has been proposed as a safe, noninvasive and effective intervention for spasticity in patients with CP. However, other interventions such as intrathecal baclofen (ITB) and selective dorsal rhizotomy (SDR) had a larger body of evidence.[126] In a randomized, controlled, cross-over study, rESWT was comparable to BoNT injections to reduce ankle plantar flexor spasticity in patients with CP. Both interventions were combined with physical therapy and spasticity was measured by the Tardieu Scale. In fact, rESWT showed greater improvement in spasticity at 6 months from first intervention when compared to BoNT, signaling a carry-over effect when patients were switched between groups.[127] Systematic reviews conclude that although ESWT shows promise in patients with CP, there is still limited evidence available to fully support its use.[128,129]

Vagus Nerve Stimulation

Vagus nerve stimulation is a novel treatment option emerging as a potential treatment for after stroke chronic symptoms. It has been recently proven to significantly improve motor function and impairment when combined with physical therapy and home exercise when compared to sham stimulation. Interestingly, patients had moderate-to-severe upper extremity impairment and were, on average, 3 years after stroke. However, spasticity was not measured in this study.[130] Transcutaneous auricular vagus nerve stimulation has also been shown to be an effective way to improve motor function following stroke[131] and, in a separate study, did improve spasticity in the wrist and hand as measured by the Tardieu Scale when compared to a sham group.[132] Although it is a novel and promising treatment alternative, it yet needs more studies to assess its use for spasticity reduction in stroke and other patient populations.

Other Emerging Treatments

Robotic-assisted therapy is another promising emerging treatment for spasticity. There have been promising results in spasticity reduction after stroke,[133,134] MS,[135] and SCI.[136] However, most studies generally focus on function rather than specifically on spasticity. Also, robotic-assisted therapy is a wide and evolving field that includes different forms of interventions such as robot-assisted upper limb movement, robotic-assisted gait training in treadmills, and ground-level gait training with exoskeletons, which complicate general recommendations and guidelines difficult. Virtual reality has been combined with robotic-assisted therapy with promising outcomes in spasticity reduction for after stroke upper limb spasticity.[137] However, as with robotic-assisted therapy, virtual reality has been studied more in functional improvements, not necessarily on spasticity reduction. Yet these are interventions that could potentially show more robust evidence for spasticity reduction in the near future.

FUTURE DIRECTIONS

Spasticity continues to be a major disabling condition following multiple neurologic disorders. Thus, researchers continue to explore new evaluation and treatment options to better serve this population. Emerging technological advances, such as those discussed in this chapter, have been showing promise in the measurement and treatment of spasticity. Technology has focused on measuring muscle elasticity to assess stiffness and spasticity more objectively. Emerging technological treatments seem to better serve as adjuncts to conventional physical therapy. Dosing details still need further study to recommend them conclusively. These include ideal intensity and sites of stimulation, most effective length of treatment, best time to use them, and the benefits of combining them with other treatments. However, the same can be said of several of the more conventional treatments. Other factors that should be considered when choosing from these evaluation and treatment options include cost and coverage by insurance, which is not common for emerging, still unproven technologies. None of these emerging technologies can be recommended as the gold standard for spasticity evaluation or reduction. Yet their low side effect profile and increasing evidence make them reasonable adjuncts to conventional modalities and show immense promise warranting further study.

KEY POINTS

- USE may be a more objective way to measure muscle spasticity in neurologic disorders. More research is warranted though.
- Peripheral stimulation, including FES, NMES, and TENS, may be reasonable adjuncts to physical therapy for spasticity reduction.
- tDCS shows promise as an adjunct to conventional physiotherapy in PSS treatment. However, evidence for other populations is scarce.
- rTMS has been gaining steam as a somewhat effective therapy adjunct for spasticity reduction.
- Other emerging treatments for spasticity include WBV and ESWT that warrant further study.

REFERENCES

1. Wissel J, Manack A, Brainin M. Toward an epidemiology of poststroke spasticity. *Neurology*. 2013;80(3 Suppl 2):S13–9. https://doi.org/10.1212/WNL.0b013e3182762448

2. Dorňák T, Justanová M, Konvalinková R, et al. Prevalence and evolution of spasticity in patients suffering from first-ever stroke with carotid origin: a prospective, longitudinal study. *Eur J Neurol*. 2019;26(6):880–886. https://doi.org/10.1111/ene.13902

3. Martin A, Abogunrin S, Kurth H, et al. Epidemiological, humanistic, and economic burden of illness of lower limb spasticity in adults: a systematic review. *Neuropsychiatr Dis Treat*. 2014;10:111–122. https://doi.org/10.2147/NDT.S53913

4. Haisma JA, van der Woude LH, Stam HJ, et al. Complications following spinal cord injury: occurrence and risk factors in a longitudinal study during and after inpatient rehabilitation. *J Rehabil Med*. 2007;39(5):393–398. https://doi.org/10.2340/16501977-0067

5. Meseguer-Henarejos AB, Sánchez-Meca J, López-Pina JA, et al. Inter- and intra-rater reliability of the modified Ashworth scale: a systematic review and meta-analysis. *Eur J Phys Rehabil Med*. 2018;54(4):576–590. https://doi.org/10.23736/S1973-9087.17.04796-7

6. Akpinar P, Atici A, Ozkan FU, et al. Reliability of the modified Ashworth scale and modified Tardieu scale in patients with spinal cord injuries. *Spinal Cord*. 2017;55(10):944–949. https://doi.org/10.1038/SC.2017.48

7. Cao J, Xiao Y, Qiu W, et al. Reliability and diagnostic accuracy of corrected slack angle derived from 2D-SWE in quantitating muscle spasticity of stroke patients. *J Neuroeng Rehabil*. 2022;19(1):15. https://doi.org/10.1186/S12984-022-00995-8

8. Alibiglou L, Rymer WZ, Harvey RL, et al. The relation between Ashworth scores and neuromechanical measurements of spasticity following stroke. *J Neuroeng Rehabil.* 2008;5. https://doi.org/10.1186/1743-0003-5-18

9. Malhotra S, Cousins E, Ward A, et al. An investigation into the agreement between clinical, biomechanical and neurophysiological measures of spasticity. *Clin Rehabil.* 2008;22(12):1105–1115. https://doi.org/10.1177/0269215508095089

10. Luo Z, Lo WLA, Bian R, et al. Advanced quantitative estimation methods for spasticity: a literature review. *J Int Med Res.* 2020;48(3). https://doi.org/10.1177/0300060519888425

11. Sconfienza LM, Albano D, Allen G, et al. Clinical indications for musculoskeletal ultrasound updated in 2017 by European society of musculoskeletal radiology (ESSR) consensus. *Eur Radiol.* 2018;28(12):5338–5351. https://doi.org/10.1007/S00330-018-5474-3/FIGURES/4

12. Zúñiga LDO, López CAG, González ER. Ultrasound elastography in the assessment of the stiffness of spastic muscles: a systematic review. *Ultrasound Med Biol.* 2021;47(6):1448–1464. https://doi.org/10.1016/J.ULTRASMEDBIO.2021.01.031

13. Prado-Costa R, Rebelo J, Monteiro-Barroso J, et al. Ultrasound elastography: compression elastography and shear-wave elastography in the assessment of tendon injury. *Insights Imaging.* 2018;9(5):791–814. https://doi.org/10.1007/S13244-018-0642-1/FIGURES/6

14. Klauser AS, Miyamoto H, Bellmann-Weiler R, et al. Sonoelastography: musculoskeletal applications. *Radiology.* 2014;272(3):622–633. https://doi.org/10.1148/RADIOL.14121765

15. Brandenburg JE, Eby SF, Song P, et al. Ultrasound elastography: the new frontier in direct measurement of muscle stiffness. *Arch Phy Med Rehabil.* 2014;95(11):2207–2219. https://doi.org/10.1016/J.APMR.2014.07.007

16. Gao J, O'Dell M, Chen J, et al. Ultrasound strain elastography in assessment of chronic post-stroke spasticity of biceps brachii muscle. *IEEE International Ultrasonics Symposium, IUS.* 2017. https://doi.org/10.1109/ULTSYM.2017.8091938

17. Gao J, Chen J, O'Dell M, et al. Ultrasound strain imaging to assess the biceps brachii muscle in chronic poststroke spasticity. *J Ultrasound Med.* 2018;37(8):2043–2052. https://doi.org/10.1002/JUM.14558

18. Hong MJ, Park JB, Lee YJ, et al. Quantitative evaluation of post-stroke spasticity using neurophysiological and radiological tools: a pilot study. *Ann Rehabil Med.* 2018;42(3):384–395. https://doi.org/10.5535/ARM.2018.42.3.384

19. Gao J, Memmott B, Poulson J, et al. Quantitative ultrasound imaging to assess skeletal muscles in adults with multiple sclerosis: a feasibility study. *J Ultrasound Med.* 2019;38(11):2915–2923. https://doi.org/10.1002/JUM.14997

20. Gao J, Rubin JM, Chen J, et al. Ultrasound elastography to assess botulinum toxin a treatment for post-stroke spasticity: a feasibility study. *Ultrasound Med Biol.* 2019;45(5):1094–1102. https://doi.org/10.1016/J.ULTRASMEDBIO.2018.10.034

21. Lehoux MC, Sobczak S, Cloutier F, et al. Shear wave elastography potential to characterize spastic muscles in stroke survivors: literature review. *Clin Biomech (Bristol, Avon).* 2020;72:84–93. https://doi.org/10.1016/J.CLINBIOMECH.2019.11.025

22. Taljanovic MS, Gimber LH, Becker GW, et al. Shear-wave elastography: basic physics and musculoskeletal applications. *Radiographics.* 2017;37(3):855–870. https://doi.org/10.1148/RG.2017160116

23. Wu CH, Ho YC, Hsiao MY, Chen WS, et al. Evaluation of post-stroke spastic muscle stiffness using shear wave ultrasound elastography. *Ultrasound Biol.* 2017;43(6):1105–1111. https://doi.org/0.1016/J.ULTRASMEDBIO.2016.12.008

24. Rasool G, Wang AB, Rymer WZ, et al. Shear waves reveal viscoelastic changes in skeletal muscles after hemispheric stroke. *IEEE Trans Neural Syst Rehabil Eng.* 2018;26(10):2006–2014. https://doi.org/10.1109/TNSRE.2018.2870155

25. Lee SSM, Jakubowski KL, Spear SC, et al. Muscle material properties in passive and active stroke-impaired muscle. *J Biomech.* 2019;83:197–204. https://doi.org/10.1016/J.JBIOMECH.2018.11.043

26. Jakubowski KL, Terman A, Santana RVC, et al. Passive material properties of stroke-impaired plantarflexor and dorsiflexor muscles. *Clin Biomechs (Bristol, Avon).* 2017;49:48–55. https://doi.org/10.1016/J.CLINBIOMECH.2017.08.009

27. Mathevon L, Michel F, Aubry S, et al. Two-dimensional and shear wave elastography ultrasound: a reliable method to analyse spastic muscles? *Muscle & Nerve.* 2018;57(2):222–228. https://doi.org/10.1002/MUS.25716

28. Bertan H, Oncu J, Vanli E, et al. Use of Shear wave elastography for quantitative assessment of muscle stiffness after botulinum toxin injection in children with cerebral palsy. *J Ultrasound Med.* 2020;39(12):2327–2337. https://doi.org/10.1002/JUM.15342

29. Brandenburg JE, Eby SF, Song P, et al. Quantifying effect of onabotulinum toxin a on passive muscle stiffness in children with cerebral palsy using ultrasound shear wave elastography. *Am J Phys Med Rehabil.* 2018;97(7):500–506. https://doi.org/10.1097/PHM.0000000000000907

30. Ghatas MP, Khan MR, Gorgey AS. Skeletal muscle stiffness as measured by magnetic resonance elastography after chronic spinal cord injury: a cross-sectional pilot study. *Neural Regen Res.* 2021;16(12):2486–2493. https://doi.org/10.4103/1673-5374.313060

31. Seth N, Johnson D, Allen B, et al. Upper limb robotic assessment: pilot study comparing velocity dependent resistance in individuals with acquired brain injury to healthy controls. *J Rehabil Assist Technol Eng.* 2020;7:205566832092953. https://doi.org/10.1177/2055668320929535

32. Dehem S, Gilliaux M, Lejeune T, et al. Assessment of upper limb spasticity in stroke patients using the robotic device REAplan. *J Rehabil Med.* 2017;49(7):565–571. https://doi.org/10.2340/16501977-2248

33. Doucet BM, Lam A, Griffin L. Neuromuscular electrical stimulation for skeletal muscle function. *Yale J Biol Med.* 2012;85(2):201–215.

34. Cambridge NA. Electrical apparatus used in medicine before 1900. *Proc R Soc Med.* 1977;70(9):635–641.

35. Kerr C, McDowell B, McDonough S. Electrical stimulation in cerebral palsy: a review of effects on strength and motor function. *Dev Med Child Neurol.* 2004;46(3):205–213. https://doi.org/10.1017/s0012162204000349

36. Maffiuletti NA, Gondin J, Place N, et al. Clinical use of neuromuscular electrical stimulation for neuromuscular rehabilitation: what are we overlooking? *Arch Phys Med Rehabil.* 2017;99(4):806–812. https://doi.org/10.1016/j.apmr.2017.10.028

37. Hesse S, Reiter F, Konrad M. Botulinum toxin type a and short-term electrical stimulation in the treatment of upper limb flexor spasticity after stroke: a randomized, double-blind, placebo-controlled trial. *Clinl Rehabil.* 1998;12(5):381–388. https://doi.org/10.1191/026921598668275996

38. Bakhtiary AH, Fatemy E. Does electrical stimulation reduce spasticity after stroke? a randomized controlled study. *Clin Rehabil.* 2008;22(5):418–425. https://doi.org/10.1177/0269215507084008

39. Hakakzadeh A, Shariat A, Honarpishe R, et al. Concurrent impact of bilateral multiple joint functional electrical stimulation and treadmill walking on gait and spasticity in post-stroke survivors: a pilot study. *Physiother Theory Pract.* 2021;37(12):1368–1376. https://doi.org/10.1080/09593985.2019.1685035

40. Yang YR, Mi PL, Huang SF, et al. Effects of neuromuscular electrical stimulation on gait performance in chronic stroke with inadequate ankle control - a randomized controlled trial. *Plos One.* 2018;13(12):e0208609. https://doi.org/10.1371/journal. pone.0208609

41. Nakipoğlu Yuzer GF, Köse Dönmez B, Özgirgin N. A randomized controlled study: effectiveness of functional electrical stimulation on wrist and finger flexor spasticity in hemiplegia. *J Stroke and Cerebrovasc Dis.* 2017;26(7):1467–1471. https://doi. org/0.1016/J.JSTROKECEREBROVASDIS.2017.03.011

42. Kwong PW, Ng GY, Chung RC, et al. Transcutaneous electrical nerve stimulation improves walking capacity and reduces spasticity in stroke survivors: a systematic review and meta-analysis. *Clin Rehabil.* 2017:026921551774534. https://doi. org/10.1177/0269215517745349

43. Lin S, Sun Q, Wang H, et al. Influence of transcutaneous electrical nerve stimulation on spasticity, balance, and walking speed in stroke patients: a systematic review and meta-analysis. *J Rehabil Med.* 2018;50(1):3–7. https://doi.org/10.2340/16501977-2266

44. In TS, Jung JH, Jung KS, et al. Effectiveness of transcutaneous electrical nerve stimulation with taping for stroke rehabilitation. *Biomed Res Int.* 2021. https://doi. org/10.1155/2021/9912094

45. Moon JH, Cho HY, Hahm SC. Influence of electrotherapy with task-oriented training on spasticity, hand function, upper limb function, and activities of daily living in patients with subacute stroke: a double-blinded, randomized, controlled trial. *Helathcare (Basel).* 2021;9(8):987. https://doi.org/10.3390/healthcare9080987

46. Mahmood A, Veluswamy SK, Hombali A, et al. Effect of transcutaneous electrical nerve stimulation on spasticity in adults with stroke: a systematic review and meta-analysis. *Arch Physl Med Rehabil.* 2019;100(4):751–768. https://doi. org/10.1016/J.APMR.2018.10.016

47. Marcolino MAZ, Hauck M, Stein C, et al. Effects of transcutaneous electrical nerve stimulation alone or as additional therapy on chronic post-stroke spasticity: systematic review and meta-analysis of randomized controlled trials. *Disabil Rehabil.* 2020;42(5):623–635. https://doi.org/10.1080/09638288.2018.1503736

48. Bajd T, Gregoric M, Vodovnik L, et al. Electrical stimulation in treating spasticity resulting from spinal cord injury. *Arch Phys Med Rehabil.* 1985;66(8):515–517.

49. Robinson CJ, Kett NA, Bolam JM. Spasticity in spinal cord injured patients: 2. Initial measures and long-term effects of surface electrical stimulation. *Arch Phys Med Rehabil.* 1988;69(10):862–868. 2018. https://www.ncbi.nlm.nih.gov/pubmed/3263102

50. Robinson CJ, Kett NA, Bolam JM. Spasticity in spinal cord injured patients: 1. Short-term effects of surface electrical stimulation. *Arch Phys Med Rehabil.* 1988;69(8):598–604. https://www.ncbi.nlm.nih.gov/pubmed/3261577

51. Fang CY, Lien ASY, Tsai JL, et al. The effect and dose-response of functional electrical stimulation cycling training on spasticity in individuals with spinal cord injury: a systematic review with meta-analysis. *Front Physiol.* 2021;12. https://doi. org/10.3389/FPHYS.2021.756200

52. Bekhet AH, Bochkezanian V, Saab IM, et al. The effects of electrical stimulation parameters in managing spasticity after spinal cord injury: a systematic review. *Am J Phys Med Rehabil.* 2019;98(6):484–499. https://doi.org/10.1097/PHM.0000000000001064

53. Sivaramakrishnan A, Solomon JM, Manikandan N. Comparison of Transcutaneous Electrical Nerve Stimulation (TENS) and Functional Electrical Stimulation (FES) for

spasticity in spinal cord injury - a pilot randomized cross-over trial. *J Spinal Cord Med*. 2017:1–15. https://doi.org/10.1080/10790268.2017.1390930

54. Oo WM. Efficacy of addition of transcutaneous electrical nerve stimulation to standardized physical therapy in subacute spinal spasticity: a randomized controlled trial. *Arch Phys Med Rehabil*. 2014;95(11):2013–2020. https://doi.org/10.1016/j.apmr.2014.06.001

55. Backus D, Moldavskiy M, Sweatman WM. Effects of functional electrical stimulation cycling on fatigue and quality of life in people with multiple sclerosis who are nonambulatory. *Int J MS Care*. 2020;22(4):193–200. https://doi.org/10.7224/1537-2073.2019-101

56. Backus D, Burdett B, Hawkins L, et al. Outcomes after functional electrical stimulation cycle training in individuals with multiple sclerosis who are nonambulatory. *I J MS care*. 2017;19(3):113–121. https://doi.org/10.7224/1537-2073.2015-036

57. Armutlu K, Meriç A, Kirdi N, et al. The effect of transcutaneous electrical nerve stimulation on spasticity in multiple sclerosis patients: a pilot study. *Neurorehabil Neural Repair*. 2003;17(2):79–82. https://doi.org/10.1177/0888439003017002001

58. Shaygannejad V, Janghorbani M, Vaezi A, et al. Comparison of the effect of baclofen and transcutaneous electrical nerve stimulation for the treatment of spasticity in multiple sclerosis. *Neurol Res*. 2013;35(6):636–641. https://doi.org/10.1179/1743132813Y.0000000200

59. Scheker LR, Chesher SP, Ramirez S. Neuromuscular electrical stimulation and dynamic bracing as a treatment for upper-extremity spasticity in children with cerebral palsy. *J Hand Surg*. 1999;24(2):226–232. https://doi.org/10.1054/JHSB.1998.0002

60. Ozer K, Chesher SP, Scheker LR. Neuromuscular electrical stimulation and dynamic bracing for the management of upper-extremity spasticity in children with cerebral palsy. *Dev Med child Neurol*. 2006;48(7):559–563. https://doi.org/10.1017/S0012162206001186

61. Özen N, Unlu E, Karaahmet Z, et al. Effectiveness of FES-cycling treatment in cp 144-nc-nd license (http://creativecommons.org/licenses/by-nc-nd/4.0/) effectiveness of functional electrical stimulation-cycling treatment in children with cerebral palsy original research. *Malawi Med J*. 2021;33(3):144–152. https://doi.org/10.4314/mmj.v33i3.1

62. Logosu D, Tagoe TA, Adjei P. Transcutaneous electrical nerve stimulation in the management of calf muscle spasticity in cerebral palsy: a pilot study. *IBRO Neurosci Rep*. 2021;11:194–199. https://doi.org/10.1016/J.IBNEUR.2021.09.006

63. Liu Z, Dong S, Zhong S, et al. The effect of combined transcranial pulsed current stimulation and transcutaneous electrical nerve stimulation on lower limb spasticity in children with spastic cerebral palsy: a randomized and controlled clinical study. *BMC Pediatr*. 2021;24;21(1):141. https://doi.org/10.1186/s12887-021-02615-1

64. Thiriez C, Gurruchaga JM, Goujon C, et al. Spinal stimulation for movement disorders. *Neurotherapeutics*. 2014;11(3):543–552. https://doi.org/10.1007/s13311-014-0291-0

65. Shealy CN, Mortimer JT, Reswick JB. Electrical inhibition of pain by stimulation of the dorsal columns: preliminary clinical report. *Anesth Analg*. 46(4):489–491.

66. Nagel SJ, Wilson S, Johnson MD, et al. Spinal cord stimulation for spasticity: historical approaches, current status, and future directions. *Neuromodulation*. 2017;20(4):307–321. https://doi.org/10.1111/ner.12591.

67. Estes S, Zarkou A, Hope JM, et al. Clinical medicine combined transcutaneous spinal stimulation and locomotor training to improve walking function and reduce spasticity in subacute spinal cord injury: a randomized study of clinical feasibility and efficacy. *J Clin Med*. 2021;10:1167. https://doi.org/10.3390/jcm10061167

68. Sandler EB, Condon K, Field-Fote EC, et al. Clinical medicine efficacy of transcutaneous spinal stimulation versus whole body vibration for spasticity reduction in persons with spinal cord injury. *J Clin Med.* 2021;10(15):3267. https://doi.org/10.3390/jcm10153267

69. Hofstoetter US, Freundl B, Lackner P, et al. Transcutaneous spinal cord stimulation enhances walking performance and reduces spasticity in individuals with multiple sclerosis. *Brain Sci.* 2021;11(4):472. https://doi.org/10.3390/brainsci11040472

70. Midha M, Schmitt JK. Epidural spinal cord stimulation for the control of spasticity in spinal cord injury patients lacks long-term efficacy and is not cost-effective. *Spinal Cord.* 1998;36(3):190–192. https://doi.org/10.1038/sj.sc.3100532

71. Iodice R, Dubbioso R, Ruggiero L, et al. Anodal transcranial direct current stimulation of motor cortex does not ameliorate spasticity in multiple sclerosis. *Restor Neurol Neurosci.* 2015;33(4):487–492. https://doi.org/10.3233/RNN-150495

72. Stagg CJ, Nitsche MA. Physiological basis of transcranial direct current stimulation. *The Neuroscientist.* 2011;17(1):37–53. https://doi.org/10.1177/1073858410386614

73. Koh CL, Lin JH, Jeng JS, et al. Effects of transcranial direct current stimulation with sensory modulation on stroke motor rehabilitation: a randomized controlled trial. *Arch Phys Med Rehabil.* 2017;98(12):2477–2484. https://doi.org/10.1016/j.apmr.2017.05.025

74. Halakoo S, Ehsani F, Masoudian N, et al. Does anodal trans-cranial direct current stimulation of the damaged primary motor cortex affects wrist flexor muscle spasticity and also activity of the wrist flexor and extensor muscles in patients with stroke? a randomized clinical trial. *Neurol Sci.* 2021;42(7):2763-2773. https://doi.org/10.1007/s10072-020-04858-9/Published

75. Del Felice A, Daloli V, Masiero S, et al. Contralesional cathodal versus dual transcranial direct current stimulation for decreasing upper limb spasticity in chronic stroke individuals: a clinical and neurophysiological study. *J S Cerebrovasc Dis.* 2016;25(12):2932–2941. https://doi.org/10.1016/j.jstrokecerebrovasdis.2016.08.008

76. Ehsani F, Mortezanejad M, Hafez Yosephi M, et al. The effects of concurrent M1 anodal tDCS and physical therapy interventions on function of ankle muscles in patients with stroke: a randomized, double-blinded sham-controlled trial study. *Neurol Sci.* 2022;43(3):1893–1901. https://doi.org/10.1007/s10072-021-05503-9/Published

77. Bornheim S, Croisier JL, Maquet P, et al. Transcranial direct current stimulation associated with physical-therapy in acute stroke patients - a randomized, triple blind, sham-controlled study. *Brain Stimulation.* 2020;13(2):329–336. https://doi.org/10.1016/J.BRS.2019.10.019

78. Comino-Suárez N, Moreno JC, Gómez-Soriano J, et al. Transcranial direct current stimulation combined with robotic therapy for upper and lower limb function after stroke: a systematic review and meta-analysis of randomized control trials. *J Neuroeng Rehabil.* 2020;18:148. https://doi.org/10.1186/s12984-021-00941-0

79. Huang J, Qu Y, Liu L, et al. Efficacy and safety of transcranial direct current stimulation for post-stroke spasticity: a meta-analysis of randomised controlled trials. *Clin Rehabil.* 2022;36(2):158–171. https://doi.org/10.1177/02692155211038097

80. Aree-uea B, Auvichayapat N, Janyacharoen T, et al. Reduction of spasticity in cerebral palsy by anodal transcranial direct current stimulation. *J Med Assoc Thait.* 2014;97(9):954–962.

81. Moura RCF, Santos C, Collange Grecco L, et al. Effects of a single session of transcranial direct current stimulation on upper limb movements in children with cerebral palsy: a randomized, sham-controlled study. *Dev Neurorehabil.* 2017;20(6):368–375. https://doi.org/10.1080/17518423.2017.1282050

82. Gillick B, Rich T, Nemanich S, et al. Transcranial direct current stimulation and constraint-induced therapy in cerebral palsy: a randomized, blinded, sham-controlled clinical trial. *Eur J Paediatr Neuroly.* 2018;22(3):358–368. https://doi.org/10.1016/J.EJPN.2018.02.001

83. Hiew S, Nguemeni C, Zeller D. Efficacy of transcranial direct current stimulation in people with multiple sclerosis; a review. *Eur J Neurol.* 2022;29(2):648–664. https://doi.org/10.1111/ENE.15163

84. Antoine Chalah M, Rudroff T, Steinberg F, et al. Gait and functional mobility in multiple sclerosis: immediate effects of transcranial direct current stimulation (tdcs) paired with aerobic exercise. *Front Neurol.* 2020;11:310. https://doi.org/10.3389/fneur.2020.00310

85. Pilloni G, Choi C, Shaw MT, et al. Walking in multiple sclerosis improves with tDCS: a randomized, double-blind, sham-controlled study. *Ann Clin Transl Neurol.* 2020;7(11):2310–2319. https://doi.org/10.1002/acn3.51224

86. Li Y, Li K, Feng R, et al. Mechanisms of repetitive transcranial magnetic stimulation on post-stroke depression: a resting-state functional magnetic resonance imaging study. *Brain Topogr.* 2022;35(3):363-374. https://doi.org/10.1007/s10548-022-00894-0

87. Corti M, Patten C, Triggs W. Repetitive transcranial magnetic stimulation of motor cortex after stroke: a focused review. *Am J Phy Med Rehabil.* 2012;91(3):254–270. Https://doi.org/10.1097/PHM.0b013e318228bf0c

88. Kobayashi M, Pascual-Leone A. Transcranial magnetic stimulation in neurology. *Lancet Neurol.* 2003;2(3):145–156. https://doi.org/10.1016/S1474-4422(03)00321-1

89. Hoyer EH, Celnik PA. Understanding and enhancing motor recovery after stroke using transcranial magnetic stimulation. *Restor Neurol Neurosci.* 2011;29(6):395–409. https://doi.org/10.3233/RNN-2011-0611

90. Liu Y, Li H, Zhang J, et al. A meta-analysis: whether repetitive transcranial magnetic stimulation improves dysfunction caused by stroke with lower limb spasticity. *Evid Based Complement Alternat Med.* 2021:7219293. https://doi.org/10.1155/2021/7219293

91. Xu P, Huang Y, Wang J, et al. Repetitive transcranial magnetic stimulation as an alternative therapy for stroke with spasticity: a systematic review and meta-analysis. *J Neurol.* 2021;268(11):4013–4022. https://doi.org/10.1007/S00415-020-10058-4

92. McIntyre A, Mirkowski M, Thompson S, et al. A systematic review and meta-analysis on the use of repetitive transcranial magnetic stimulation for spasticity poststroke. *PM & R .* 2017;10(3):293–302. https://doi.org/10.1016/j.pmrj.2017.10.001

93. Rastgoo M, Naghdi S, Nakhostin Ansari N, et al. Effects of repetitive transcranial magnetic stimulation on lower extremity spasticity and motor function in stroke patients. *Disabil Rehabil.* 2016;38(19):1918–1926. https://doi.org/10.3109/09638288.2015.1107780

94. Naghdi S, Ansari NN, Rastgoo M, et al. A pilot study on the effects of low frequency repetitive transcranial magnetic stimulation on lower extremity spasticity and motor neuron excitability in patients after stroke. *J Bodyw Movt The.* 2015;19(4):616–623. https://doi.org/10.1016/j.jbmt.2014.10.001

95. Gottlieb A, Boltzmann M, Schmidt SB, et al. Treatment of upper limb spasticity with inhibitory repetitive transcranial magnetic stimulation: a randomized placebo-controlled trial. *Neuro Rehabil.* 2021;49(3):425–434. https://doi.org10.3233/NRE-210088

96. Li D, Cheng A, Zhang Z, et al. Effects of low-frequency repetitive transcranial magnetic stimulation combined with cerebellar continuous theta burst stimulation on spasticity and limb dyskinesia in patients with stroke. *BMC Neurol.* 2021;21(1):369. https://doi.org 10.1186/s12883-021-02406-2

97. Kuzu Ö, Adiguzel E, Kesikburun S, et al. The effect of sham controlled continuous theta burst stimulation and low frequency repetitive transcranial magnetic stimulation on upper extremity spasticity and functional recovery in chronic ischemic stroke patients. *J Stroke Cerebrovasc Di.* 2021;30(7):105795. https://doi.org 10.1016/J.JSTROKECEREBROVASDIS.2021.105795

98. Chen YJ, Huang YZ, Chen CY, et al. Intermittent theta burst stimulation enhances upper limb motor function in patients with chronic stroke: a pilot randomized controlled trial. *BMC Neurology.* 2019;19(1). https://doi.org 10.1186/S12883-019-1302-X

99. Nardone R, Langthaler PB, Orioli A, et al. Effects of intermittent theta burst stimulation on spasticity after spinal cord injury. *Restor Neurol Neurosci.* 2017;35(3):287–294. https://doi.org/10.3233/RNN-160701

100. Nardone R, Höller Y, Thomschewski A, et al. rTMS modulates reciprocal inhibition in patients with traumatic spinal cord injury. *Spinal Cord.* 2014;52(11):831–835. https://doi.org/10.1038/sc.2014.136

101. Mendonça T, Brito R, Luna P, et al. Repetitive transcranial magnetic stimulation on the modulation of cortical and spinal cord excitability in individuals with spinal cord injury. *Restor Neurol Neurosci.* 2021;39(4):291–301. https://doi.org/ 10.3233/RNN-211167

102. Wincek A, Huber J, Leszczyńska K, et al. The long-term effect of treatment using the transcranial magnetic stimulation RTMS in patients after incomplete cervical or thoracic spinal cord injury. *J Clin Med.* 2021;10(13):2975. https://doi.org/10.3390/JCM10132975

103. Chen X, Yin L, An Y, et al. Effects of repetitive transcranial magnetic stimulation in multiple sclerosis: A systematic review and meta-analysis. *Mult Scler Relat Dis.* 2022;59:103564. https://doi.org/10.1016/J.MSARD.2022.103564

104. Kan RLD, Xu GXJ, Shu KT, et al. Effects of non-invasive brain stimulation in multiple sclerosis: systematic review and meta-analysis. *Ther Adv Chronic Dis.* 2022;13. https://doi.org/10.1177/20406223211069198

105. Diéguez-Varela C, Lión-Vázquez S, Fraga-Bau A, et al. Intermittent theta-burst transcranial magnetic stimulation for the treatment of spasticity in patients with recurring multiple sclerosis: the results of a double-blind randomised clinical trial. *Revista de Neurologia.* 2019;69(2):45–52. https://doi.org/10.33588/RN.6902.2018275

106. Korzhova J, Bakulin I, Sinitsyn D, et al. High-frequency repetitive transcranial magnetic stimulation and intermittent theta-burst stimulation for spasticity management in secondary progressive multiple sclerosis. *Eur J Neurology.* 2019;26(4):680-e44. https://doi.org/10.1111/ENE.13877

107. Şan AU, Yılmaz B, Kesikburun S. The effect of repetitive transcranial magnetic stimulation on spasticity in patients with multiple sclerosis. *J Clin Neurol (Seoul, Korea).* 2019;15(4):461–467. https://doi.org/10.3988/JCN.2019.15.4.461

108. Li J, Chen C, Zhu S, et al. Evaluating the effects of 5-hz repetitive transcranial magnetic stimulation with and without wrist-ankle acupuncture on improving spasticity and motor function in children with cerebral palsy: a randomized controlled trial. *Front Neurosci.* 2021;15:1603. https://doi.org/10.3389/FNINS.2021.771064/FULL

109. Rajak B, Gupta M, Bhatia D, et al. Increasing number of therapy sessions of repetitive transcranial magnetic stimulation improves motor development by reducing muscle spasticity in cerebral palsy children. *Ann Indian Academy of Neurol.* 2019;22(3): 302–307. https://doi.org/10.4103/AIAN.AIAN_102_18

110. Elbanna ST, Elshennawy S, Ayad MN. Noninvasive brain stimulation for rehabilitation of pediatric motor disorders following brain injury: systematic review of randomized controlled trials. *Arch Phys Med Rehabil.* 2019;100(10):1945–1963. https://doi.org/10.1016/J.APMR.2019.04.009

111. Sandler EB, Condon K, Field-Fote EC, et al. Clinical medicine efficacy of transcutaneous spinal stimulation versus whole body vibration for spasticity reduction in persons with spinal cord injury. *J Clin Med.* 2021;10(15):3267. https://doi.org/10.3390/jcm10153267

112. In T, Jung K, Lee MG, et al. Whole-body vibration improves ankle spasticity, balance, and walking ability in individuals with incomplete cervical spinal cord injury. *Neuro Rehabil.* 2018;42(1):191–497. https://doi.org/10.3233/NRE-172333

113. Tekin F, Kavlak E. Short and long-term effects of whole-body vibration on spasticity and motor performance in children with hemiparetic cerebral palsy. *Percept Mot Skills.* 2021;128(3):1107–1129. https://doi.org/10.1177/0031512521991095

114. Miyara K, Matsumoto S, Uema T, et al. Effect of whole body vibration on spasticity in hemiplegic legs of patients with stroke. *Top Stroke Rehabil.* 2018;25(2):90–95. https://doi.org/10.1080/10749357.2017.1389055

115. Alashram AR, Padua E, Annino G. Effects of whole-body vibration on motor impairments in patients with neurological disorders: a systematic review. *Am J Phy Med Rehabilitation.* 2019;98(12):1084–1098. https://doi.org/10.1097/PHM.0000000000001252

116. Walewicz K, Taradaj J, Rajfur K, et al. The effectiveness of radial extracorporeal shock wave therapy in patients with chronic low back pain: a prospective, randomized, single-blinded pilot study. *Clin Interv Aging.* 2019;14:1859–1869. https://doi.org/10.2147/CIA.S224001

117. Hsu PC, Chang KV, Chiu YH, et al. Comparative effectiveness of botulinum toxin injections and extracorporeal shockwave therapy for post-stroke spasticity: A systematic review and network meta-analysis. *EClinicalMedicine.* 2021;43. https://doi.org/10.1016/J.ECLINM.2021.101222

118. Ip AH, Phadke CP, Boulias C, et al. Practice patterns of physicians using adjunct therapies with botulinum toxin injection for spasticity: a Canadian multicenter cross-sectional survey. *PM & R.* 2021;13(4):372–378. https://doi.org/10.1002/PMRJ.12442

119. Marinaro C, Costantino C, D'esposito O, et al. Synergic use of botulinum toxin injection and radial extracorporeal shockwave therapy in multiple sclerosis spasticity. *Acta Biomed.* 2021;92:2021076. https://doi.org/10.23750/abm.v92i1.11101

120. Hsu PC, Chang KV, Chiu YH, et al. Comparative effectiveness of botulinum toxin injections and extracorporeal shockwave therapy for post-stroke spasticity: a systematic review and network meta-analysis. *EClinicalMedicine.* 2022;43:101222. https://doi.org/10.1016/J.ECLINM.2021.101222

121. Yoldaş Aslan Ş, Kutlay S, Düsünceli Atman E, et al. Does extracorporeal shock wave therapy decrease spasticity of ankle plantar flexor muscles in patients with stroke: a randomized controlled trial. *Clin Rehabil.* 2021;35(10):1442–1453. https://doi.org/10.1177/02692155211011320

122. Wu YT, Chang CN, Chen YM, et al. Comparison of the effect of focused and radial extracorporeal shock waves on spastic equinus in patients with stroke: a randomized controlled trial. *Eur J Phy Rehabil Med.* 2018;54(4):518–525. https://doi.org/10.23736/S1973-9087.17.04801-8

123. Cabanas-Valdés R, Serra-Llobet P, Rodriguez-Rubio PR, et al. The effectiveness of extracorporeal shock wave therapy for improving upper limb spasticity and functionality in stroke patients: a systematic review and meta-analysis. *Clin Rehabil.* 2020;34(9):1141–1156. https://doi.org/10.1177/0269215520932196

124. Li G, Yuan W, Liu G, et al. Effects of radial extracorporeal shockwave therapy on spasticity of upper-limb agonist/antagonist muscles in patients affected by stroke: a randomized, single-blind clinical trial. *Age and Ageing.* 2020;49(2):246–252. https://doi.org/10.1093/AGEING/AFZ159

125. Jia G, Ma J, Wang S, et al. Long-term effects of extracorporeal shockwave therapy on post-stroke spasticity: a meta-analysis of randomized controlled trials. *J Stroke Cerebrovasc Dis.* 2020;29(3). https://doi.org/10.1016/J.JSTROKECEREBROVASDIS.2019.104591

126. Kudva A, Abraham ME, Gold J, et al. Intrathecal baclofen, selective dorsal rhizotomy, and extracorporeal shockwave therapy for the treatment of spasticity in cerebral palsy: a systematic review. *Neurosurgical Review.* 2021;44(6):3209–3228. https://doi.org/10.1007/S10143-021-01550-0

127. Vidal X, Martí-fàbregas J, Canet O, et al. Efficacy of radial extracorporeal shock wave therapy compared with botulinum toxin type A injection in treatment of lower extremity spasticity in subjects with cerebral palsy: a randomized controlled cross-over study. *J Rehabil Med.* 2020;52:76. https://doi.org/10.2340/16501977-2703

128. Corrado B, di Luise C, Servodio Iammarrone C. Management of muscle spasticity in children with cerebral palsy by means of extracorporeal shockwave therapy: a systematic review of the literature. *Develop Neurorehabil.* 2021;24(1):1–7. https://doi.org/10.1080/17518423.2019.1683908

129. Kim HJ, Park JW, Nam K. Effect of extracorporeal shockwave therapy on muscle spasticity in patients with cerebral palsy: meta-analysis and systematic review. *Eur J Physical Rehabil Med.* 2019;55(6):761–771. https://doi.org/10.23736/S1973-9087.19.05888-X

130. Dawson J, Liu CY, Francisco GE, et al. Vagus nerve stimulation paired with rehabilitation for upper limb motor function after ischaemic stroke (VNS-REHAB): a randomised, blinded, pivotal, device trial. *Lancet (London, England).* 2021;397(10284):1545–1553. https://doi.org/10.1016/S0140-6736(21)00475-X

131. Li JN, Xie CC, Li CQ, et al. Efficacy and safety of transcutaneous auricular vagus nerve stimulation combined with conventional rehabilitation training in acute stroke patients: a randomized controlled trial conducted for 1 year involving 60 patients. *Neural Regen Res.* 2022;17(8):1809–1813. https://doi.org/10.4103/1673-5374.332155

132. Chang JL, Coggins AN, Saul M, et al. Transcutaneous auricular vagus nerve stimulation (TAVNS) delivered during upper limb interactive robotic training demonstrates novel antagonist control for reaching movements following stroke. *Front Neuroscience.* 2021;15. https://doi.org/10.3389/FNINS.2021.767302

133. Zhao M, Wang G, Wang A, et al. Robot-assisted distal training improves upper limb dexterity and function after stroke: a systematic review and meta-regression. *Neurological Sci.* 2022;43(3):1641–1657. https://doi.org/10.1007/S10072-022-05913-3

134. Zhai X, Wu Q, Li X, et al. Effects of robot-aided rehabilitation on the ankle joint properties and balance function in stroke survivors: a randomized controlled trial. *Front Neurol.* 2021;12. https://doi.org/10.3389/FNEUR.2021.719305

135. Calabrò RS, Cassio A, Mazzoli D, et al. What does evidence tell us about the use of gait robotic devices in patients with multiple sclerosis? a comprehensive systematic review on functional outcomes and clinical recommendations. *Euro J Phys Rehabil Med.* 2021;57(5):841–849. https://doi.org/10.23736/S1973-9087.21.06915-X

136. Tamburella F, Lorusso M, Tramontano M, et al. Overground robotic training effects on walking and secondary health conditions in individuals with spinal cord injury: systematic review. *J Neuroeng Rehabil.* 2022;19(1):27. https://doi.org/10.1186/S12984-022-01003-9

137. Abd El-Kafy EM, Alshehri MA, El-Fiky AAR, et al. The effect of robot-mediated virtual reality gaming on upper limb spasticity poststroke: a randomized-controlled trial. *Games Health J.* 2022;11(2):93–103. https://doi.org/10.1089/G4H.2021.0197

15 Imaging Guidance for Chemodenervation Procedures

Kristen A. Harris and Michael C. Munin

INTRODUCTION

Chemodenervation and neurolytic procedures for spasticity are optimized by precise localization, and there are several techniques that can improve injection accuracy. These localization techniques include surface anatomy and palpation, electromyographic (EMG) guidance, electrical stimulation (E-stim), ultrasound (US) guidance, and combination techniques. Rarely, other image-based guidance like fluoroscopy, computerized tomography (CT), or magnetic resonance imaging (MRI) may be used. Improved localization has several benefits that are implicit and clinical efficacy has been highlighted in small, randomized trials. Animal model studies demonstrate that specific targeting to the motor end plate zone during chemodenervation injections improves efficacy.[1,2] Instrumental guidance can be useful when full range of motion (ROM) within the injected limb is restricted, since torsional changes due to positioning will move targets away from standard anatomic positions documented on cadavers. Accurate localization will also allow the physician to safely inject the target while avoiding adjacent structures like major nerves and arteries, as well as improve patient tolerance of the procedure by avoiding small vessels and tendons.

Types of Guidance for Neurolytic and Chemodenervation Procedures

Anatomic Surface Landmarks

Identification of surface landmarks is a long-standing technique for chemodenervation procedures since physicians have training in gross anatomy and no special equipment is required. There are several well-known reference guides for use of surface landmarks, like those by Delagi and subsequently Perotto et al., as well as Geringer.[3-5] These texts utilize fingerbreadth measurements or proportion of limb length, and often provide instructions for angle and depth of needle insertion. Many physicians are familiar with these texts and may utilize training experience in combination with a reference text to help localize muscle targets. Additionally, anatomists have identified motor end plate bands in commonly injected muscles, such as the biceps and hamstrings, which can be targeted utilizing described landmark techniques.[6-8] A validated surface anatomy technique using more precise measurements has also been described by Bickerton et al. to localize each of the optimal injection sites for the four muscle bellies of the flexor digitorum superficialis.[9,10] A landmark line (LL) can be drawn from the medial epicondyle proximally to the pisiform bone distally. Flexor digitorum superficialis 2 (FDS2) can be localized at 70% of the LL measuring from the medical epicondyle and 14 mm lateral. Similarly, FDS3 can be localized 17 mm lateral to the 55% LL point, FDS4 is localized 7 mm lateral to the 50% LL point, and FDS5 6 mm lateral to the 75% LL point.[9,10] Surface localization does not require additional equipment or specialized injectable needles and can be performed quickly, which may be beneficial in patients with agitation, active spasms, or significant dystonia.

However, identification of target muscles utilizing anatomic landmarks is not always accurate, which may lead to unintended weakness. A cadaver study evaluated established surface anatomy techniques used to identify 36 muscles of the lower limb by tracing needle path and final resting place, and found that only 57% of needle insertions penetrated the intended muscle with accuracy ranging between 0% and 100%.[11] Seventeen percent penetrated or passed within 5 mm of an adjacent important structure such as a nerve, tendon, artery, vein, or joint. When muscles are layered and especially when there is prominent adipose soft tissue, it may be difficult to accurately target muscles. While some physicians believe that surface landmark techniques alone are sufficient for localization of large, superficial muscles like the gastrocnemius, Schnitzler et al. found that when 121 practitioners (mostly physiatrists) were asked to inject the gastrocnemius on cadavers using surface landmarks alone, only 43% of injections were successful with 37% too deep in the soleus and 20% in superficial fat.[12] Lastly, fingerbreadth measurements are based on cadavers that can be placed in the anatomic neutral position. However, for many patients with upper limb spasticity, full elbow extension and forearm supination may not be feasible, which can lead to further injection inaccuracies. Advantages and limitations of muscle localization by anatomic surface landmarks are summarized in Table 15.1.

Table 15.1 Advantages and Limitations of Localization by Anatomic Surface Landmarks

Advantages	Limitations
Decreased procedure time due to lack of specialized equipment and setup	Contractures and deformity may make neutral positioning challenging that may limit accurate target identification
Cost-effective due to lack of specialized equipment	Cannot assess muscle bulk or atrophy that may limit accurate target identification; injections often too deep especially with layered muscles such as in the forearm

Electromyographic Guidance
EMG localization detects muscle electrical activity to determine where to place botulinum toxin in patients with spasticity. For chemodenervation, a specialized hollow monopolar needle allows muscle EMG signals to be recorded at the tip simultaneously with the injection. Separate ground and surface electrodes must also be attached to the patient. Muscle tissue is electrically active and will show insertional activity or motor unit potentials. Fat or fibrotic tissue will not have any electrical activity, and this principle alerts the physician not to inject the medication into these tissues. As the needle electrode is advanced into the spastic muscle, motor unit action potentials (MUAPs) can be audible and/or visible, depending on the equipment used. To help confirm placement, the physician can ask the patient to activate the muscle (if the patient has voluntary control) or can passively range the muscle to listen for spastic MUAP activity generated by rapid stretch. Physicians who have completed

electrodiagnostic training during residency should be comfortable with EMG equipment. Targeting neurotoxin to the motor end plate or an area where there is a high concentration of MUAPs may increase the uptake of botulinum toxin into the nerve terminal and thereby increase efficacy.[13–16] Initially as the needle electrode is advanced into a muscle, MUAPs will sound dull and muffled but become sharper as the needle is advanced closer to the depolarizing MUAPs. Alternatively, the physician can observe miniature end plate potentials within the end plate zone signaling an optimal position for injection. For management of cervical dystonia, EMG can be particularly useful to note grouped, rhythmic MUAP firing to indicate muscle involvement.

There are several limitations with EMG guidance. While targeting end plate zones theoretically improves neurotoxin uptake, in practice repeatedly redirecting the needle electrode to search for miniature end plate potentials can be cumbersome, and very few use this approach. Although EMG guidance will help the physician identify spastic muscle by locating areas with MUAPs, this does not ensure that the needle is in the targeted muscle. In patients with upper motor neuron syndrome (UMNS), many adjacent muscles show increased MUAPs and the physician may not know if they are injecting the targeted muscle. While secondary techniques like voluntary activation or passive ROM can be useful, the risk of injecting muscles other than the target remains especially for deep or overlapping muscles. If patients are densely plegic, this overflow into adjacent muscles will not be problematic. However, if patients maintain some degree of voluntary control, misplaced chemodenervation can create muscle imbalance (i.e., injecting too much dose into the flexor digitorum profundus and missing the flexor digitorum superficialis) or unintended weakness that causes patients to stop treatment. Advantages and limitations of muscle localization by electromyographic guidance are summarized in Table 15.2.

Table 15.2 Advantages and Limitations of Localization by EMG

Advantages	Limitations
Useful for focal dystonia, especially cervical dystonia, where rhythmically firing grouped motor unit potentials can be seen	Cost of needle electrode and EMG amplifier
Can quickly identify muscle tissue for intramuscular injections	May be difficult to accurately localize target muscle if nearby muscle is also spastic
EMG machines or auditory feedback instruments are accessible in many practice settings	Targeting motor end plate may be uncomfortable for patient and time-consuming for physician

Electrical Stimulation Guidance

E-stim guidance can be used by electrically stimulating a mixed nerve or motor nerve branch, which will cause muscle contraction in the targeted muscle. A portable electrical stimulator or the stimulation mode of an EMG machine can be used with a hollow monopolar needle electrode. A separate ground and surface electrode are also required. E-stim guidance can be used for both intramuscular and perineural neurolytic injections.

When utilizing E-stim, the needle electrode should be moved in small increments to localize the targeted nerve. Small movements in needle position will have major effects on the delivered current based on Coulomb's law ($E = K(Q/R^2)$), where E is the required stimulating charge, K is constant, Q is minimal required simulating current, and R is distance to the nerve. The difference in energy reaching the nerve decreases with distance by a factor squared, such that 1 mA stimulation at 1 mm distance from the nerve (1 mA/1 mm^2) yields 100 times more energy compared to using the same intensity at 1 cm away (1 mA/10 mm^2). Movements, therefore, must be fine and steady to achieve optimal position. The physician may start using repetitive stimulation at 0.8 to 1 Hz with a higher intensity stimulus (5 mAmp) and slowly decrease the stimulation intensity, ideally maintaining target muscle contraction with a low stimulus intensity (1 mA).[13] After the target threshold is reached with visible muscle contraction, the phenol or alcohol is injected perineurally.[17] A strong understanding of nerve anatomy is necessary to avoid stimulating the wrong nerve, as the physician should observe that the desired gross motor function is occurring with stimulation.

E-stim provides accurate localization but can be time-consuming and requires more training than other localization techniques. Furthermore, repetitive E-stim may be uncomfortable for the patient. In patients with contracture or severe spasticity, it may be difficult to assess individual muscle contractions. If patients are having active spasms during the procedure, it may be difficult to achieve accurate E-stim. Advantages and limitations of target localization by electrical stimulation are summarized in Table 15.3.

Table 15.3 Advantages and Limitations of Localization by E-Stim

Advantages	Limitations
Useful for identifying optimal location for phenol or alcohol neurolysis	Cost of equipment, including portable electrical stimulator and needle electrode
Can provide accurate localization, especially when using low stimulation intensity	Repetitive E-stim may be uncomfortable for patient and time-consuming for physician
	Individual muscle contraction may be difficult to assess in cases of severe spasticity, active spasms, or deformity

Ultrasound Guidance

US guidance allows direct visualization of the muscle or nerve target and ensures that the injectate diffuses within the fascia of the targeted muscle or hydrodissects the targeted nerve. A US machine utilizes sound waves transmitted by the transducer through the soft tissues, with waves reflected to the transducer and sent to the computer processing unit, generating an image on the monitor. US transducers can be high or low frequency. Transducers >12 MHz are best utilized for superficial structures to provide high-resolution imagery, with many high-quality US machines offering linear array transducers ≥15 MHz. Lower-frequency, curvilinear transducers are useful to visualize structures more than 6 cm in depth. In most instances for spasticity management, it is appropriate to use a linear array transducer. The ultrasonographer should be comfortable identifying skeletal muscle, tendons, nerves, vessels bones, and glands, which each have a different echogenicity and therefore display with varying intensities on the monitor (see Table 15.4).[18] Because US visualization can be obtained in either longitudinal or transverse view, injections can be performed either in plane (needle inserted across long axis of transducer) or out of plane (across short axis of transducer). Adjacent vessels and nerves are best visualized in the transverse view, and out-of-plane injections often provide the most direct path to a target. In-plane injections allow the entire needle and its tip to be visualized which can be useful, for example, during pectoralis muscle injections where the pleura must be avoided. Dedicated US training is required for physician proficiency, which may be obtained through residency training, or dedicated courses and hands-on practice.

Table 15.4 Sonographic Characteristics of Key Structures

Structure	Appearance
Skeletal muscle	Mix of hyperechoic intramuscular connective tissue and hypoechoic contractile fascicles, separated by hyperechoic fascial planes
Tendons	Hyperechoic, fibrillar
Nerves	Less hyperechoic than tendon; can have appearance of railroad track in longitudinal view and a honeycomb in transverse view
Vessels	Anechoic; veins easily sonographically compressed in contrast to arteries that can be highlighted with Doppler flow
Bone	Hyperechoic with posterior acoustic shadowing

Source: From Alter KE, Karp BI. Ultrasound guidance for botulinum neurotoxin chemodenervation procedures. *Toxins (Basel).* 2017;10(1). https://doi.org.10.3390/toxins10010018

Spastic muscles may have increased echo intensity as compared to the sonographic appearance of normal muscle, decreased muscle thickness, and a posterior pennation angle.[19] The Modified Heckmatt Scale can grade muscle echogenicity with good inter- and intra-rater reliability and is useful for any ultrasonographer managing spasticity (see Figure 15.1).[20,21] Picelli et al. demonstrated that increased muscle echogenicity and fibrotic change is associated with decreased response to botulinum toxin A (BoNTA) in equinus spasticity.[22] It is therefore useful for the physician to observe any Modified Heckmatt changes under US guidance and consider injection protocols that target more normal-appearing muscle tissue.[20]

US allows for highly accurate localization and avoidance of neurovascular structures. In addition, visualization allows assessment of muscle tissue depth to ensure that deeper structures are not over-injected since physicians can misjudge depth of superficial muscles. Research has demonstrated that without US guidance, needle placement is significantly less accurate with the physician often going deeper than the intended muscle.[23] US guidance may lessen the risk of dysphagia when using botulinum toxin for management of cervical dystonia. With EMG guidance alone, Hong et al. found a 34% incidence of dysphagia after botulinum toxin injection, likely due to inadvertent injection through the sternocleidomastoid (SCM) with toxin spreading to deeper structures, as the SCM was measured to be <1.1 cm thick.[24] In children, US guidance for injections has been demonstrated to be less painful than E-stim.[25] US has also been described as a useful tool for challenging intrathecal baclofen pump refills, with direct visualization of the pump port as well

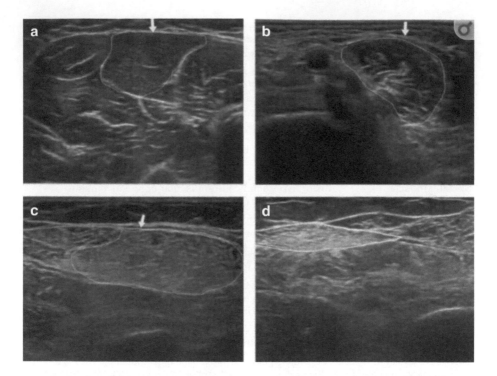

Figure 15.1 Traced muscles demonstrating the Modified Heckmatt grades. (a) Grade 1: normal echogenicity in more than 90% of the muscle that is distinct from bone echo. (b) Grade 2: increased muscle echogenicity in 10% to 50% of the tissue, but with distinct bone echo and some areas of normal muscle echo. (c) Grade 3: marked increase in muscle echogenicity between 50% and 90% of the tissue with reduced distinction of bone echo from the muscle. (d) Grade 4: very strong muscle echogenicity, with near complete loss of distinct bone echo from the muscle in more than 90% of the tissue.
Source: Reprinted with permission from Elsevier from Archives of Rehabilitation Research and Clinical Translation, Vol. 2 Issue 4, Moreta MC, Fleet A, Reebye R, McKernan G, Berger M, Farag J, Munin MC. Reliability and Validity of the Modified Heckmatt Scale in Valuating Muscle Changes with Ultrasound in Spasticity, 100071. 2020

as post-procedure visualization of the pump and overlying subcutaneous tissue to ensure there has been no mistaken pocket fill.[26] Research has demonstrated that instrument-guided techniques provide superior accuracy and outcomes to the use of surface anatomy landmarks alone.[27–30] While evidence distinguishing efficacy of different instrument-guided techniques is limited, several randomized control trials have demonstrated improved patient outcomes using US guidance. Kwon et al. compared techniques using E-stim to US guidance in pediatric patients with spastic equinus and found improved Physician's Rating Scale scores and gait pattern when using US.[31] In adults, Picelli et al. compared botulinum toxin injections to the gastrocnemius using surface landmarks, E-stim, and US in 49 patients and found better improvement in the Modified Ashworth Scale and ankle passive ROM in the

US group.[32] A later systematic review concluded chemodenervation procedures utilizing US guidance appear to be more effective for management of spastic equinus in adults with poststroke spasticity.[27] Use of US guidance for procedures is operator dependent and is associated with a significant learning curve. US education can be obtained through courses, and exposure is becoming increasingly common during residency training, but repetition and practice is paramount for comfort utilizing US guidance for procedures. Furthermore, high-quality US machines can be expensive, which may be a barrier although cheaper, portable units that can attach to smartphones have been developed. Simultaneous operation of the US transducer and syringe may require the presence of an assistant to help with equipment management. US guidance is not appropriate for agitated patients or those with ballistic limb movements who cannot remain still easily. Advantages and limitations of target localization by ultrasound are summarized in Table 15.5.

Table 15.5 Advantages and Limitations of Localization by Ultrasound

Advantages	Limitations
Direct needle and target visualization allows for accurate injection	Requires training and practice for proficiency
Direct visualization of neurovascular bundle can minimize risks of injection	Ultrasound equipment availability and cost
Potential use of smaller needle for injection that may minimize patient discomfort	May require an assistant to help manage equipment

Combination Techniques

Ultrasound and EMG

US and EMG guidance utilize an EMG amplifier, US machine, and hollow monopolar needle electrode during the procedure. This combination can be particularly useful for management of cervical dystonia and when practicing spasticity management in a training environment. When visualizing a muscle under US that has Modified Heckmatt grade 3, it can be useful to identify if there is reduced insertional or EMG activity that may signify fibrosis. For management of cervical dystonia, US visualization ensures that the injectate is not placed deep to the targeted structure, while EMG provides simultaneous identification of dystonic MUAP activity. This combination can also be helpful when learning spasticity management in a training environment, as it offers the supervising physician multiple opportunities to assess the practicing physician's technique. Dual instrument localization is an added cost, and in the United States, insurers only reimburse for one guidance technique for most spasticity procedures.

Ultrasound and E-Stim

US and E-stim utilizes a portable electrical stimulator, US machine, and hollow monopolar needle electrode during a procedure. This combination technique can be particularly useful for neurolytic procedures using phenol or for simultaneous identification of the motor point for intramuscular procedures. When performing phenol or alcohol neurolysis, precise injections using dual localization may limit painful myoneural scarring or serious adverse events rather than having the drug spread indiscriminately. Under US and E-stim combined guidance, the physician can hydrodissect the nerve target striving for the "target" sign. Matsumoto et al. demonstrated that the addition of US- to E-stim-guided phenol neurolysis of the musculocutaneous nerve was associated with lower volumes of phenol injected compared to E-stim alone.[17] The combination may also allow the physician to more quickly identify a target area, minimizing time spent on the procedure, when compared to using E-stim alone.[33] Like US and EMG combined guidance, dual instrument localization can be an added cost.

Other Techniques
Other imaging techniques may be available to the physician, including fluoroscopy, CT, and MRI. These techniques are less commonly used due to multiple factors including cost, difficulty accessing equipment due to availability or scheduling barriers, and time. However, if traditional localization or combination techniques are ineffective due to patient factors or deep and difficult to isolate muscles, fluoroscopy, CT, or MRI may be used.[13] Fluoroscopy, in particular, has been reported as a useful tool to access difficult intrathecal baclofen pumps.[34]

ADDITIONAL CONSIDERATIONS

Torsional Anatomy
Most anatomic references use surface landmarks in neutral position; however, many patients with spasticity are difficult or impossible to examine in the anatomic neutral position. Internal torsion secondary to spasticity can cause targets to be compressed and stretched to different degrees. Literature demonstrates differences in muscle location compared to cadaver landmarks secondary to torsional changes from spasticity in both the upper and lower limbs.[35,36] With torsion, many muscles become oblique, yet not all structures move equally for the same positional movement, and that which was anterior may now be posterior.[35] US guidance can be useful to ensure that a target is accurately identified and that neurovascular bundles are avoided. The sonographer should maintain an orthogonal plane by aiming the needle to the mid-transducer to keep a perpendicular approach to the muscle under torsion.[36,37]

Ergonomics
Optimizing workplace ergonomics is important to minimize risk of physician injury and improve procedural efficiency. Studies suggest that as many as 80% of sonographers develop musculoskeletal pain.[38] International expert consensus opinion of 10 physical medicine and rehabilitation specialists and one neurologist has identified ideal physician and patient ergonomics when performing US-guided procedures for spasticity (see Table 15.6).[39] Consensus opinion concluded that there are often ergonomic errors among trainees due to inadequate transducer grip, inadequate visualization of nearby structures, and poor posture during injection.[39] Of note, barriers to performing ergonomic scanning techniques can include patient factors like limited mobility, which is highly prevalent in the affected patient population.[40]

Table 15.6 International Expert Consensus: Ergonomic Recommendations for Ultrasound-Guided Chemodenervation

Workstation Ergonomics	Physician Ergonomics	Patient Ergonomics	Visual Ergonomics
Room of adequate dimensions to facilitate equipment maneuverability	Maintenance of neutral posture, with neck flexed and forearm horizontal	Comfortable and well-supported positioning for injections	Adequate field of view and depth
Use of height-adjustable table and comfortable chair	Injections should be performed seated when able	Ability for patient to visualize the screen when feasible	Appropriate ultrasound transducer selection
Maintain ultrasound screen at eye level and within arm's reach	Keep ultrasound screen in the same line of sight as target injection	Presence of an assistant when possible to help optimize positioning	Appropriate notch positioning to maintain orientation
Use of a small portable surface, like a mobile tray	Physician on same side as injected limb to avoid excessive reaching		
	Transducer handling placing the index and middle finger with thumb grip, and use fourth and fifth digits for stabilization on the patient		

Source: From Lagnau P, Lo A, Sandarage R, et al. Ergonomic recommendations in ultrasound-guided botulinum neurotoxin chemodenervation for spasticity: an international expert group opinion. *Toxins (Basel)*. 2021;13(4). https://doi.org.10.3390/toxins13040249

KEY POINTS

- Accurate localization is important for management of spasticity by chemodenervation and neurolytic procedures.
- Instrument-guided injections have improved accuracy compared to surface anatomy alone.
- EMG, E-stim, and US techniques have specific advantages and disadvantages that may influence selection.
- US can identify targets accurately and better visualize torsional or distorted anatomy while avoiding neurovascular structures.

- US guidance is associated with decreased pain during injections, lessened dysphagia in cervical dystonia, and appears to offer improved functional outcomes for adults and children with spastic equinus.
- Localization techniques that combine EMG or E-stim with US may be efficacious in certain settings.
- Workplace ergonomics are important especially when performing US-guided procedures.

REFERENCES

1. Shaari CM, Sanders I. Quantifying how location and dose of botulinum toxin injections affect muscle paralysis. *Muscle Nerve*. 1993;16(9):964–969. https://doi.org.10.1002/mus.880160913

2. Childers MK, Kornegay JN, Aoki R, Otaviani L, Bogan DJ, Petroski G. Evaluating motor end-plate-targeted injections of botulinum toxin type a in a canine model. *Muscle Nerve*. 1998;21(5):653–655. https://doi.org.10.1002/(sici)1097-4598(199805)21:5<653::aid-mus15>3.0.co;2-w

3. Delagi EF. *Anatomic Guide for the Electromyographer: The Limbs*. C. C. Thomas; 1974:xiv, 207 p.

4. Perotto A, Delagi EF. *Anatomical Guide for the Electromyographer: The Limbs and Trunk*. 5th ed. Charles C. Thomas; 2011:xvii, 377.

5. Geiringer SR. *Anatomic Localization for Needle Electromyography*. 2nd ed. Hanley & Belfus; 1999.

6. Amirali A, Mu L, Gracies JM, Simpson DM. Anatomical localization of motor endplate bands in the human biceps brachii. *J Clin Neuromuscul Dis*. 2007;9(2):306–312. https://doi.org.10.1097/CND.0b013e31815c13a7

7. Harrison TP, Sadnicka A, Eastwood DM. Motor points for the neuromuscular blockade of the subscapularis muscle. *Arch Phys Med Rehabil*. 2007;88(3):295–297. https://doi.org.10.1016/j.apmr.2006.12.031

8. An XC, Lee JH, Im S, et al. Anatomic localization of motor entry points and intramuscular nerve endings in the hamstring muscles. *Surg Radiol Anat*. 2010;32(6):529–537. https://doi.org.10.1007/s00276-009-0609-5

9. Bickerton LE, Agur AM, Ashby P. Flexor digitorum superficialis: locations of individual muscle bellies for botulinum toxin injections. *Muscle Nerve*. 1997;20(8):1041–1043. https://doi.org.10.1002/(sici)1097-4598(199708)20:8<1041::aid-mus18>3.0.co;2-y

10. Munin MC, Navalgund BK, Levitt DA, Breisinger TP, Zafonte RD. Novel approach to the application of botulinum toxin to the flexor digitorum superficialis muscle in acquired brain injury. *Brain Inj*. 2004;18(4):403–407. https://doi.org.10.1080/02699050310001617334

11. Haig AJ, Goodmurphy CW, Harris AR, Ruiz AP, Etemad J. The accuracy of needle placement in lower-limb muscles: a blinded study. *Arch Phys Med Rehabil*. 2003;84(6):877–882. https://doi.org.10.1016/s0003-9993(03)00014-5

12. Schnitzler A, Roche N, Denormandie P, Lautridou C, Parratte B, Genet F. Manual needle placement: accuracy of botulinum toxin a injections. *Muscle Nerve*. 2012;46(4):531–534. https://doi.org.10.1002/mus.23410

13. Walker HW, Lee MY, Bahroo LB, Hedera P, Charles D. Botulinum toxin injection techniques for the management of adult spasticity. *PM R*. 2015;7(4):417–427. https://doi.org.10.1016/j.pmrj.2014.09.021

14. Lapatki BG, Van Dijk JP, Van de Warrenburg BP, Zwarts MJ. Botulinum toxin has an increased effect when targeted toward the muscle's endplate zone: a high-density surface EMG guided study (1872–8952 (Electronic)). *Clin Neurophysiol.* 2011;122(8):1611–1616. https://doi.org.10.1016/j.clinph.2010.11.018

15. Childers MK. Targeting the neuromuscular junction in skeletal muscles. (0894–9115 (Print)). *Am J Phys Med Rehabil.* 2004;83(10):S38–S44 httpoi//doi.org.10.1097/01. phm.0000141129.23219.42

16. Gracies JM, Lugassy M, Weisz DJ, Vecchio M, Flanagan S, Simpson DM. Botulinum toxin dilution and endplate targeting in spasticity: a double-blind controlled study. (1532–821X (Electronic)). *Arch Phys Med Rehabil.* 2009;90(1):9–16.

17. Matsumoto ME, Berry J, Yung H, Matsumoto M, Munin MC. Comparing electrical stimulation with and without ultrasound guidance for phenol neurolysis to the musculocutaneous nerve. *PM R.* 2018;10(4):357–364. https://doi.org.10.1016/j.pmrj.2017.09.006

18. Alter KE, Karp BI. Ultrasound guidance for botulinum neurotoxin chemodenervation procedures. *Toxins (Basel).* 2017;10(1). https://doi.org.10.3390/toxins10010018

19. Picelli A, Tamburin S, Cavazza S, et al. Relationship between ultrasonographic, electromyographic, and clinical parameters in adult stroke patients with spastic equinus: an observational study. *Arch Phys Med Rehabil.* 2014;95(8):1564–1570. https://doi.org.10.1016/j.apmr.2014.04.011

20. Moreta MC, Fleet A, Reebye R, et al. Reliability and validity of the modified Heckmatt scale in evaluating muscle changes with ultrasound in spasticity. *Arch Rehabil Res Clin Transl.* 2020;2(4):100071. https://doi.org.10.1016/j.arrct.2020.100071

21. Heckmatt JZ, Dubowitz V. Ultrasound imaging and directed needle biopsy in the diagnosis of selective involvement in muscle disease. *J Child Neurol.* 1987;2(3):205–213. https://doi.org.10.1177/088307388700200307

22. Picelli A, Bonetti P, Fontana C, et al. Is spastic muscle echo intensity related to the response to botulinum toxin type a in patients with stroke? a cohort study. *Arch Phys Med Rehabil.* 2012;93(7):1253–1258. https://doi.org.10.1016/j.apmr.2012.02.005

23. Boon AJ, Oney-Marlow TM, Murthy NS, Harper CM, McNamara TR, Smith J. Accuracy of electromyography needle placement in cadavers: non-guided vs. ultrasound guided. *Muscle & Nerve.* 2011;44(1):45–49.

24. Hong JS, Sathe GG, Niyonkuru C, Munin MC. Elimination of dysphagia using ultrasound guidance for botulinum toxin injections in cervical dystonia (1097–4598 (Electronic)). *Muscle & Nerve.* 2012;46(4):535–539.

25. Bayon-Mottu M, Gambart G, Deries X, Tessiot C, Richard I, Dinomais M. Pain during injections of botulinum toxin in children: influence of the localization technique. *Ann Phys Rehabil Med.* 2014;57(9–10):578–586. https://doi.org.10.1016/j. rehab.2014.09.010

26. Maneyapanda MB, Chang Chien GC, Mattie R, Amorapanth P, Reger C, McCormick ZL. Ultrasound guidance for technically challenging intrathecal baclofen pump refill: three cases and procedure description. *Am J Phys Med Rehabil.* 2016;95(9):692–697. https://doi.org.10.1097/PHM.0000000000000495

27. Grigoriu AI, Dinomais M, Rémy-Néris O, Brochard S. Impact of injection-guiding techniques on the effectiveness of botulinum toxin for the treatment of focal spasticity and dystonia: a systematic review. *Arch Phys Med Rehabil.* 2015;96(11):2067–2078.e1. https://doi.org.10.1016/j.apmr.2015.05.002

28. Chan AK, Finlayson H, Mills PB. Does the method of botulinum neurotoxin injection for limb spasticity affect outcomes? A systematic review. *Clin Rehabil.* 2017;31(6):713–721. https://doi.org.10.1177/0269215516655589

29. Picelli A, Lobba D, Midiri A, et al. Botulinum toxin injection into the forearm muscles for wrist and fingers spastic overactivity in adults with chronic stroke: a randomized controlled trial comparing three injection techniques. *Clin Rehabil.* 2014;28(3):232–242. https://doi.org.10.1177/0269215513497735

30. Francisco GE, Balbert A, Bavikatte G, et al. A practical guide to optimizing the benefits of post-stroke spasticity interventions with botulinum toxin a: an international group consensus. *J Rehabil Med.* 2021;53(1):jrm00134. https://doi.org.10.2340/16501977-2753

31. Kwon J-Y, Hwang JH, Kim J-S. Botulinum toxin A injection into calf muscles for treatment of spastic equinus in cerebral palsy: a controlled trial comparing sonography and electric stimulation-guided injection techniques: a preliminary report. *Am J Phys Med Rehabil.* 2010;89(4): 279–286.

32. Picelli A, Tamburin S, Bonetti P, et al. Botulinum toxin type A injection into the gastrocnemius muscle for spastic equinus in adults with stroke: a randomized controlled trial comparing manual needle placement, electrical stimulation and ultrasonography-guided injection techniques. *Am J Phys Med Rehabil.* 2012;91(11):957–964.

33. Karri J, Zhang B, Li S. Phenol neurolysis for management of focal spasticity in the distal upper extremity. *PM R.* 2020;12(3):246–250. https://doi.org.10.1002/pmrj.12217

34. Miracle AC, Fox MA, Ayyangar RN, Vyas A, Mukherji SK, Quint DJ. Imaging evaluation of intrathecal baclofen pump-catheter systems. *AJNR Am J Neuroradiol.* 2011;32(7):1158–1164. https://doi.org.10.3174/ajnr.A2211

35. Chiou-Tan F, Cianca J, Pandit S, John J, Furr-Stimming E, Taber KH. Procedure-oriented torsional anatomy of the proximal arm for spasticity injection. (1532–3145 (Electronic)) *J Comput Assisted Tomogr.* 2015;39(3):449–452.

36. Cianca J, Dy R, Chiou-Tan FY, John J, Taber KH. Torsional anatomy of the lower limb: the appearance of anatomy in hemispastic position. (1532–3145 (Electronic)) *J Comput Assisted Tomogr.* 2018;42(6):982–985.

37. Strakowski JA, Chiou-Tan FY. Musculoskeletal ultrasound for traumatic and torsional alterations. *Muscle Nerve.* 2020;62(6):654–663. https://doi.org.10.1002/mus.27025

38. Pike I, Russo A, Berkowitz J, Baker JP, Lessoway VA. The prevalence of musculoskeletal disorders among diagnostic medical sonographers. *J Diagn Med Sonogr.* 2022;13(5):219–227.

39. Lagnau P, Lo A, Sandarage R, et al. Ergonomic recommendations in ultrasound-guided botulinum neurotoxin chemodenervation for spasticity: an international expert group opinion. *Toxins (Basel).* 2021;13(4). https://doi.org.10.3390/toxins13040249

40. Scholl C, Salisbury H. Barriers to performing ergonomic scanning techniques for sonographers. *J Diagn Med Sonog.* 2022;33(5):406–411.

IV Disease Management: A Case-Based Approach

16 Cerebral Palsy Assessment: Nonsurgical and Surgical Treatments

Shatssa L. Wright

INTRODUCTION

Cerebral palsy (CP) describes disorders of movement control, tone, and posture resulting from a nonprogressive insult to an immature brain within the first few years of life.[1-6] Risk factors associated with the development of CP occur during the prenatal, perinatal, and postnatal periods of development.[1,2,7,8,6] CP is classified based on which limbs are affected, the type of motor deficit, and the location of the insult in the pediatric brain.[1,2,9] The motor disorders of CP are often accompanied by disturbances of sensation, cognition, behavior, language, hearing and vision, swallowing, epilepsy, and secondary musculoskeletal problems.[3,4,9]

Children with CP can develop head and truncal hypotonia, limb hypertonia, spasticity, dystonia, muscle weakness, and subsequent development of fixed and dynamic *contractures*.

Contracture: musculotendinous shortening resulting in difficult range of motion (ROM), pain, restricted functional activity, and musculoskeletal deformities of a limb. Contractures in children with CP are associated with spasticity resulting in abnormal joint positions, weakness of antagonistic muscles, impaired motor control, muscle imbalance, and fatigability.[10,11]

CP is the leading cause of childhood disability.[9] The most common type of CP is spastic CP in which the child will exhibit significant upper motor neuron (UMN) signs including but not limited to spasticity, stiffness, hyperreflexia, and clonus. The other types include hypotonia, dyskinetic ataxic, and mixed type.[1,7,9] Spastic CP is divided into subtypes that are named based on the body part involved. Spastic monoplegia is rare and involves one limb. Spastic diplegia is the most common overall type of CP, involves two limbs most commonly caused by prematurity, and affects lower limbs more than upper limbs. Spastic triplegia involves both legs and one arm, spastic hemiplegia involves one arm and leg on the same side, and spastic quadriplegia involves all extremities.[2,4,5,9]

It is important to understand the characteristics and anatomical associations as a result of CP. This is the foundation by which every clinical evaluation of a child is guided and every assessment and treatment plan is developed.

DIAGNOSTIC APPROACH

Spasticity can vary in severity from mild to moderate or severe in a child with CP.[3] In milder cases, it may not significantly impact or impair a child's function. In moderate cases, it may impact a child's function and can be treated conservatively with fewer therapeutic and medical interventions in order to improve ROM, achieve functional mobility, and ease caregiver burden.

Spasticity can also be functional for posture, positioning and transfers including assisting a child with weakened lower extremities by supporting them with standing and provide some stiffness and LE support with functional transfers.[1]

Severe spasticity can be very disabling and functionally limiting resulting in pain due to abnormal muscle positions and ROM restrictions that lead to muscle imbalanced forces on a tendon or bone. This can result in joint dislocations and long bone fractures that can lead to chronic pain. Spasticity can also lead to difficulty with activities of daily living (ADLs) due to restrictive joint motions with movements, positioning, and posture. Examples include severe spasticity of the hip adductors resulting in abnormal scissoring of the legs when standing upright or lying in bed, difficulty with diaper changes, difficulty straightening the knees during sitting at bath time, or difficulty standing during functional transfers. Spasticity can also result in skin breakdown and ulcerations due to abnormal postures of a limb leading to pressure injury from a brace or splint or a piece of equipment a child is placed in for prolonged periods of time, that is, wheelchair or stander. There is also the risk of impaired hygiene due to lack of ease of cleaning skin folds that can result in skin wounds and infections.

Spasticity in children with CP can also result in other systemic manifestations including disruption of sleep, slowing of the digestive system, delayed emptying of food contents, and chronic constipation that can then affect bladder compliance and lead to urinary retention.[2,3,9,12]

It is important to note that spasticity can acutely worsen in severity in a child with CP due to the impaired UMN system and abnormal stretch reflex. Several situations including acute medical illness or any noxious stimulation such as an ingrown toenail, wrinkled sheet, and prolonged position of discomfort can result in worsening spasticity. Gastrointestinal discomfort, formula intolerance, gas pain, worsening constipation, urinary retention, and UTI can also contribute to worsened spasticity, which is why evaluating a child with CP for overall health and wellness of their genitourinary and gastrointestinal systems is also of importance in order to optimize medical management and the spasticity treatment plan in a child with CP.

It is important that the treatment approach to spasticity is individualized in a child with CP.[2,12]

History

Pregnancy, Birth, Past Medical, and Family History

It is important to identify the risk factors for CP and identifying the inciting event that may have resulted in the nonprogressive injury to the child's brain prior to the age of 3. It is key to identify any prenatal care concerns, pregnancy complications or medical illness, and family history of any genetic conditions that would raise concern for an alternate neurodegenerative or neuromuscular disease. Prematurity, multiple gestation pregnancy, mother medical illness, placental abnormalities, breech birth, asphyxiation, infection, toxic exposures, blood incompatibility, and fetal distress are some of the etiologies during the prenatal, perinatal, and postnatal periods for a child who is later diagnosed with CP.[1,2,7,9.]A child with a history of feeding or swallowing difficulties, breathing and oxygenation difficulties, and hypotonia are also early presenting concerns.[9] It is important to ask the parent/caregiver age-appropriate developmental milestones and identify any concern for developmental delays by discussing not only the age in months of when a child achieved the milestones but also the characteristics.

Gross and Fine Motor Milestones

* Head control—Was there any torticollis or weakness noted with holding the head up? Was this achieved around 3 to 4 months of age?
* Movement of limbs—Did the child move their arms and limbs equally? Was there any concern for early hand dominance or neglect of using hand/limbs purposefully? Was there any difficulty with movement of one side compared to the other? Does the child hold items in both hands without difficulty? Does the child have a premature grasp or have fine motor skills such as pincer grasp?
* Muscle tone—Any differences in muscle tone of head and trunk in comparison to the limbs? Were they a floppy baby? Did the child develop any stiffness as they were getting older?
* Did the child roll around 4 to 6 months? Did the child roll to only one side or have difficulty rolling from back to front and vice versa?
* Did the child crawl around 6 to 9 months? Any difficulty with crawling and scooting, that is, commando crawl versus propping up on all fours?
* Pulling to stand and walking—Did the child stand earlier than expected? Did they have difficulty getting onto their legs or supporting their weight? Any scissoring noted?

Cognitive/Language/Vison/Hearing Milestones

* Social smile and tracking—Ask the caregiver or parent if the child tracks with their eyes or responds to sounds or lights appropriately.
* Speech/language—Ask if the child makes appropriate sounds or speaks words to assess for speech and cognitive delays that are also seen in children with CP.

Activities of Daily Living

From a functional standpoint, always include ADLs including but not limited to eating, drinking, and concerns for dysphagia or aspiration, sialorrhea, oral aversions, bathing, toileting or potty training, and bowel and bladder hygiene. Include gross and fine motor function in terms of mobility and transfers, that is, bed, bath, chair, and car. One should focus the discussion on the level of dependence or adaptation required and identifying areas for improved independence for a developing child.[2]

Social History

Home

A comprehensive evaluation should include the details of the child's primary residence.

It is imperative to avoid the assumption and perception that a family or caregiver of a child with CP is easily able to meet the positioning and mobility needs without barriers attributed to spasticity and disability. Included in the history should be key questions regarding a child's daily routine in terms of the type of bed and room they sleep in and whether or not it is meeting their needs for positioning and comfort. Reviewing transfer devices and equipment at home in terms of use, practicality, and safety to avoid harm to the caregiver and child is necessary. Further discussing ease of access into and within the home is also a helpful information. A parent or caregiver may experience a barrier from something designed to support a child with spasticity.

School/Day Care/Medical Day Program/Specialty Care Facilities
Having an understanding of the environment where a child spends a significant portion of their day is necessary to individualize the spasticity treatment plan. Involving school teams including nurses and therapist can be key to success. Equipment, orthotics, braces, and seating systems may be kept at school or a facility for various reasons, and it is often necessary to guide recommendations based on this information and involve those providers when developing ADLs, mobility and transfer goals, therapy goals (see section on Treatment Options), and targeted muscles for spasticity treatment plans, that is, botulinum toxin (BoNT; see section on Treatment Options).

Equipment/Braces/Orthotics/Splints
It is important to assess the current equipment and equipment needs as well as the condition and frequency of use of braces and orthotics.[1,2] Ill-fitting equipment, braces, and orthotics can contribute to pain, increased or lack of pressure support, and intolerance that may contribute to worsening of spasticity. For example, as a child grows or develops worsening contractures, they may no longer tolerate their stander, or braces, or splints due to pain. There may also be benefit to prescribing new equipment, braces, and splints to aide with spasticity management.

Overall as an examiner, the history is the key area where you can identify the barriers for a caregiver, a child, and their therapy teams that may be greatly improved by a spasticity management program.

Physical Examination
Observation
Initial examination of the child should include close observation of their behavior, any volitional or abnormal movements, as well as any functional tasks performed in the exam room such as sitting, reaching, grabbing, walking, etc. The examiner should pay close attention to see if the child is in any discomfort in addition to their cognitive abilities. This will provide key information regarding the child's neurologic awareness of their self and environment and help avoid an assumption that the child with CP and spasticity is too severely cognitively impaired to experience pain or discomfort or lacks functional goals for which spasticity treatment should be considered.

It is important to observe the child's posture, limb positioning, motor skills, and volitional movements of their limbs against gravity and resistance as well.

In the sitting and supine positions, a child with spasticity of the upper limbs will typically have their shoulders adducted and internally rotated and elbow and wrists flexed. The wrists may be pronated, plus or minus radial or ulnar deviation, and the fingers may be in flexion in a fist. One may observe a cortical or opposed and flexed thumb as well. For a child with dystonia, these postures may fluctuate[1] during sitting or lying position or with examination.

In the sitting and supine position, a child with spasticity of the lower limbs will commonly have some degree of hip flexion, hip adduction, knee flexion (or extension), and ankle plantar flexion that can be accompanied with equinovarus foot positioning. Depending on the active ROM the child has, the position of their limb can also reflect a posture in which gravity predominates resulting in windswept hips, extended knees, and varus ankles. For a child with dystonia, these postures may fluctuate as stated previously.[1]

Neuromuscular Exam

For young children, there are strategies to engage the child in play that helps the examiner with the assessment. A manual muscle test is typically not able to be performed in children younger than 5 years old; however, there are ways to test a child to see their strength against gravity and resistance. One strategy includes using a fun object such as a toy or sticker or light to engage the child with something familiar and comforting to them.

Spasticity

Assessing spasticity should be done in many ways with many considerations. A child may be fearful of the examiner or asleep and the exam may not reflect the predominant tone or posture. Strategies include examining a young child on a parents lap or in their wheelchair; however, whenever possible, examine a child on an exam table to get a better assessment of hip ROM, popliteal angles, leg lengths, and a spine exam (non-ambulatory children).

Use of an evaluation tool such as the Modified Ashworth Scale (MAS) or Modified Tardieu Scale (MTS) allows for consistent spasticity grading and is helpful when developing both a treatment plan and assessing response to treatment interventions.

Range of Motion and Strength

It is important to isolate each motion to the best of your ability and avoid causing pain to the child. If possible, have the child perform a functional movement such as reaching, grabbing, standing, or kicking their limbs as you observe active ROM. Next, passively range the joint and simultaneously perform your spasticity evaluation during this time. If the child can resist your movement during the full ROM movement, you can also evaluate their strength and perform the manual muscle test simultaneously. Restrictions in ROM, angles, and degrees of joint contractures can be assessed visually from experienced practitioners. Goniometry can be a useful assessment tool if done appropriately in the right setting.[1,7]

Reflexes

Testing for the presence of primitive and deep tendon reflexes provides information regarding central nervous system (CNS) injury in infants and small children. This is also useful to localize areas of the body affected.[1]

Gait

It is important to examine posture during stance and gait whenever possible as there may be components of the child's spasticity or dystonia that is more evident with gait. Examples of this include truncal weakness, flexion synergy of the upper limb, balance deficits, pelvic obliquity, severe hip flexion contracture, scissoring legs when advancing the limb, toe walking, etc. Pictures and videos from therapy or with use of equipment are also very helpful when provided by the parent, caregiver, and therapists.

Hips and Spine

Due to the mechanical muscle imbalances of pelvis, legs, and spine associated with trunk and limb weakness, impaired mobility, or decreased weightbearing, the child with CP is at risk of developing lower extremity contractures, developmental dysplasia of the hip (DDH),[10,11] windswept hip deformity, femoral neck anteversion, coxa valga, tibial torsion[11] subluxation, dislocation and fracture, and severe neuromuscular scoliosis. These conditions impair gait mechanics and increase joint instability and can result in pain.

Screening for DDH and neuromuscular scoliosis in children with CP is important as this can guide your early treatment plan for supportive orthotics, bracing, adaptive equipment and seating systems, imaging studies, antispasticity medications, etc. The risk and severity of hip dysplasia is directly correlated with the degree of neurologic impairment.[13,11] Concerning exam findings can include pain with palpation or restrictions in ROM, a positive Galeazzi sign, and unequal leg lengths.

A worsening positioning over time as it pertains to the hips and spine can result in pelvic obliquity, difficulty positioning upright or lying position,[13] difficulty with hygiene and caregiver burden, and poor cardiopulmonary health and may eventually require orthopedic surgical intervention (see section on Surgical Treatment Options).

Clinical Tools

There are many tools utilized for the assessment of spasticity, mobility, and function in a child with CP. These are briefly mentioned in the following.

Gross Motor Function Classification System (GMFCS) and GMFCS Expanded and Revised (E&R).

It is a five-level ordinal classification tool for children with CP that illustrates and predicts their gross motor function at age 2 to 18 years. GMFCS scores are useful indicators for treatment with BoNT for spasticity and for predicting procedural adverse events and surgical planning for orthopedic procedures.[1,7,5,11]

Functional Mobility Scale (FMS)

It is a scale that classifies the functional mobility in children taking into account the use of an assistive device.[14]

Manual Ability Classification System

It is a classification system that describes how children with CP age 4 to 18 years use their hands to handle objects during their ADLs.[15]

Three-Dimensional Gait Analysis

It is the gold standard for gait assessment that provides valid and accurate information regarding the child's gait pattern. It is useful to both recommendations and assessments in response to nonsurgical and surgical treatment plans, that is, intramuscular chemodenervation injections with BoNT and orthopedic and neurosurgical procedures[7] (see section on Treatment Options).

Diagnostic Imaging

Diagnostic imaging (DI) is useful for both diagnosing CP and medical management of spasticity. *Magnetic resonance imaging (MRI)* of the pediatric brain and spine and *newborn ultrasound (US)* studies help assess for areas of the brain involved, that is, periventricular leukomalacia, hypoxic ischemic encephalopathy, cerebral vascular injury, and other intracranial pathology.[9]

Radiographic imaging of the hips and spine provides useful surveillance of the stability of the hip affected by conditions such as DDH, coxa valga, hip subluxation and dislocation, leg length discrepancies, neuromuscular scoliosis, and pathologic fractures.[3,11] Radiographic studies are also useful to troubleshoot an improperly functioning intrathecal baclofen (ITB) pump to assessment of stool burden caused by chronic constipation related to antispasticity medications (see section on Treatment Options and Complications of Spasticity Treatment in Children with CP).

TREATMENT OPTIONS

Nonpharmacologic Treatment

Therapies and regular stretching and exercise are a key component to spasticity management and should always be goal directed and fun. Providers should have a conversation with each child and their families to determine measurable and achievable functional goals to guide the course of therapeutic intervention.[1,2,16,12]

Occupational therapy goals can include upper extremity strengthening, ROM and stretching programs, fine motor skills, and independence with ADLs. Key evaluation components include splinting, orthotics, adaptive utensils and instruments, adaptive seating and standing systems, and equipment for activities such as school work, feeding, play and leisure, bed, bath, and car.[1,2,16]

Physical therapy goals can include strengthening, stretching, and ROM programs, brace and gait training, and evaluation of transfer and mobility systems. Evaluation components include neuromuscular electrical stimulation (NMES), functional electrical stimulation (FES), vibrations systems, and US that have been helpful for spasticity treatment.[1,2,16] *Home Exercise Programs (HEP)* are key for consistency because a child will always need parental or caregiver support for motivation and assistance with their exercises and stretches in order to remain compliant.

Orthotics are extremely important for preserving ROM of a joint, preventing a contracture formation, and supporting a limb for a functional task including reaching, grabbing, sitting, standing, and walking. Orthotics should regularly be visualized, and the wearing programs should regularly be discussed during an evaluation to ensure proper fit and function.[1,2,16,6]

Adaptive equipment discussions are necessary to ensure the child is comfortable and tolerating their equipment. If they are experiencing difficulty, this can further be examined in terms of medications prescribed or spasticity treatments (see section on Pharmacologic Interventions).[1,2,16,6]

Serial casting is a beneficial treatment to improve ROM across a joint in a child with significant contracture. It is useful as an adjunct treatment with the use of oral antispasticity medications and intramuscular chemodenervation injections (see section on Pharmacologic Interventions).

It is a great option for younger children who do not tolerate their stretching orthotics or home exercise program or for children who have hit a plateau with therapies. It must be kept dry and monitored closely for fit and any pressure point of the limbs or toes disrupting circulation, causing pain or wounds.[1,2,7,16,6]

Inpatient rehabilitation provides a comprehensive spasticity rehabilitation program for a child with CP. This setting can provide goal-directed intensive therapies, equipment and orthotic evaluations, spasticity medication adjustments, and family and caregiver training due to functional decline following an acute illness, procedure, or prolonged hospitalization.

Pharmacologic Interventions

Oral medications: Several classes of medications indicated for the treatment of muscle spasms, spasticity, and pain related to spasticity can be safely utilized in children with CP. Medications are typically weight-based or age-based dosing and are started at low doses and slowly titrated up over several days to weeks. For discussion on adverse side effects, see section on Complications of Spasticity Treatment in Children with CP.[1,9,17,8] Table 16.1 is intended as a guide for medication consideration for treatment of spasticity in children with CP.

Valium
It is helpful for newborns and infants with spasticity and myoclonus.

Baclofen (Lioresal)
It is commonly used in infants >6 months old, >5 kg, and children for the treatment of spasticity, dystonia, and myoclonus.

Tizanidine (Zanaflex)
Useful in children >12 years old.

Clonidine
It is useful for pain and dysautonomia associated with worsening spasticity. Transdermal patch formulation should be considered to optimize steady state of medication release.

Dantrolene Sodium (Dantrium)
It is useful to avoid sedation and altered mental state.

Gabapentin
It is a GABA agonist, not typically a first- or second-line agent but can offer analgesic properties for neuropathic pain related to spasticity.[1,16,17]

Table 16.1 Oral Medications Used to Treat Spasticity in Children With Cerebral Palsy

Medication	Class	Oral Dosing	Adverse Side Effects
Valium	Benzodiazepine	Age >6 mo 0.01–0.3 mg/kg/d* q6–12 hrs Age >5 yrs 1–2 mg/dose q8	Altered mental state, respiratory depression
Baclofen	Skeletal muscle relaxant; GABA-B agonist	Age >4 mo–<2 yrs: 10–20 mg/day* q8 hrs** Age >2 yrs–7 yrs: 20–40 mg/day* q8 hrs Age >8 yrs: 30–40 mg/day* q8	Weakness, constipation, urinary retention, sedation ⇑
Tizanidine	Alpha-2 adrenergic agonist	Age 2–<10 yrs 1 mg qhs Age >10 yrs 2 mg qhs Age >12 yrs 0.3–0.5 mg/kg/day* q8–12 hrs	⇑ Sedation, dry mouth, dizziness

(continued)

Table 16.1 Oral Medications Used to Treat Spasticity in Children With Cerebral Palsy *(continued)*

Clonidine	Alpha-2 agonist	5–0 mcg/kg/day* q8–12 hrs	⇑ Sedation, dry mouth, hypotension
Dantrolene	Skeletal muscle relaxant; calcium inhibitor SR	<50 kg 0.5–1 mg/kg/dose q6–8 hrs >50 kg 25 mg–100 mg q6–9 hrs	Elevated LFTs, hepatitis, GI discomfort, dysphagia
Gabapentin	GABA agonist	5 mg/kg* q8–12 hrs	Vivid dreams, ⇑ sedation, fatigue

hrs, hours; kg, kilograms; LFT, liver function test; mg, milligrams; mcg, micrograms; q, every; yr/yrs, years old; <, less than.
*Divided doses. **Safety and efficacy not established in children <12 yrs. Sources: 4, 6, 8, 11, MedScape, UptoDate.

Minimally Invasive Procedures

BoNT injections is a useful agent for performing intramuscular chemodenervation of spastic and dystonic muscles in children with CP. A thorough history, examination, and functional assessment are needed to identify muscles to target for treatment. Discussion with the patient and family should include the dosing, risks, benefits, procedural aspects, and effectiveness of the medication, contraindications, and adverse side effects.

Prior to the procedure, a review of systems should include any contraindications to the procedure including acute illness, antibiotics, or recent vaccines and medications, that is, anticholinergics, anticoagulants, and antibiotics, due to risk of drug interaction, bleeding, and worsening side effects. Dosing of the medication should be based on the most current accurate weight, and one should ensure the patient has not had BoNT injections within a minimum of 3 months of the procedure and that the total dosing will not exceed a safe dosing regimen or be repeated in the same muscle groups. For example, a child may have had BoNT injections for salivary glands by another specialist.[1,7,16]

It is important to establish realistic goals and set expectations for an intended outcome. Discussion regarding sedation or in clinic procedures should be included prior to the injection appointment. Discussion regarding return to activity and treatment of pain or discomfort should be included as well as the benefits of resuming therapy programs, splinting and bracing regimens, and routine stretching and ROM of the joint/limb in order to improve expected outcomes. The procedure should be optimized by proper setup and preplanning of muscles and doses if possible to avoid delays during the procedure for the child.

Use of anatomic landmarks, anatomic maps, and textbooks are extremely useful. Studies also show that use of electromyography (EMG), electrical stimulation (e-stim), and ultrasonography are superior to anatomic landmarks alone.[2,7,17] Dosing regimens for BoNT are based on units/kg of body weight.

Alcohol/phenol injections: Neurolysis is another chemodenervation treatment involving protein denaturing and nerve signal inhibition contributing to the spasticity of a muscle. E-stim is utilized to localize a nerve. The procedure can be uncomfortable for children; however, the results are typically more sustained and lower in cost in comparison to BoNT injections.[1] This is dose dependent.[17]

Orthopedic Surgeries for Children With Spastic Cerebral Palsy

Due to progressive development of musculoskeletal imbalance, contractures, and deformities, orthopedic surgery plays a key role in the management of children with CP.[11] Goals for orthopedic surgery interventions include but are not limited to prevent medical complications, improve pain, reduce muscle imbalance, improve posture, joint protection, improve skin hygiene, and reduce caregiver burden.

The type of surgical intervention largely depends on the severity of the contracture, that is, dynamic versus fixed, previous failed therapeutic interventions as well as a child's Gross Motor Function Classification System (GMFCS) level. Common procedures performed on children with CP include musculotendinous lengthenings, tendon transfers, osteotomies, and arthrodesis for the correction of bony deformities and stabilization.[11]

It is important to note that for greater than 6 months after surgery, children are less functional and more dependent for cares by their caregivers. A physiatrist role is key in a comprehensive rehabilitation of a child in order to improve the goals of the procedure including an improved GMFCS level.[13]

Considerations for Timing of Surgery

One should include pediatric orthopedic surgeons into the therapeutic team as early as possible "to optimize motor development" and determine the best possible time of surgery to minimize the number of repeat surgeries the child may need during childhood.[13] The correct time for orthopedic surgery is determined by the following criteria: (1) the degree of maturation of the CNS, (2) the developmental rate of fixed contractures and skeletal deformities, (3) potential for independent gait and functional impact, (4) ineffectiveness of nonsurgical treatment modalities, and (5) inability of a child to make significant functional progress over the preceding 6 months. Age of consideration is key to avoid fixed contractures and decreased ambulatory function in children with GMFCS II and III as well as correction of fixed contractures and skeletal deformities or address functional decline.[10,13,11]

Indications for surgery include significant functional decline or pain related to fixed flexion or extension contractures and skeletal deformities of the hips, knees, ankles, and spine resulting in joint instability. Severe neuromuscular scoliosis caused compromised cardiopulmonary function, poor seating tolerance, pelvic obliquity, and unbalanced forces and pressure on the skin and muscles resulting in compromised skin integrity resulting in poor wound healing, pain, and infections.[10,13,11,14]

Orthopedic Surgeries

Multi-event single-level surgeries historically included yearly lower limb tendon lengthening surgeries that resulted in worsening gait mechanics until the final corrective surgery.[11] This ultimately impaired a child for many years due to a cycle of hospitalizations, immobility, rehabilitation, and deconditioning. In addition, due to psychosocial implications, costs, and caregiver burden, this is thought to be an unwise approach for children with CP.

Multilevel surgery previously referred to as single-event multilevel surgery (SEMLS) is the preferred approach for children with CP with the goal of reducing the period of hospitalization, rehabilitation, and recovery. Multilevel surgery is defined as two or more soft tissue or bony surgical procedures, performed at two or more anatomic levels, that is, hip, knee, and ankle.[8,13] Research shows when compared to multi-event surgeries, performing multiple levels of surgery at one interval improves the level of gross motor function in children with spastic CP.[11]

Scoliosis surgery is a surgical procedure for the treatment and stabilization of a child's spine due to neuromuscular imbalances that resulted in spinal deformities in children with CP. Several risk factors for severe neuromuscular scoliosis include but not limited to a spinal curvature of greater than 40 degrees before age 15, rapid growth, deteriorating neurologic function, progressive pelvic obliquity, neuromuscular disease, and shunt malfunction.[1,11,6]

Neurosurgical Procedures

Goals of neurosurgical procedures are individualized and largely focused on the reduction of spasticity in a child with CP. We will discuss two main procedures below.

ITB is a reservoir placed in a child's lower abdomen subcutaneously that is attached to a catheter that releases baclofen into the intrathecal space in order to reduce spasticity and diminish the hyperactive spinal reflex and subsequently relax the muscles.[1,7,16]

Indications and consideration for an ITB pump procedure include the advantage of route of administration, and smaller doses of baclofen is administered directly to the spinal cord, reducing the adverse side effect profile. This can result in improved arousal and cognition, improved functional abilities, decreased resistance of a child's muscles with ROM and purposeful tasks, and increased ease of caregiver burden.

Selective Dorsal Rhizotomy

Selective dorsal rhizotomy (SDR) is a surgical procedure in which selected sensory nerve rootlets are cut in order to disrupt the abnormal electrical impulses sent to the spinal cord and reduce spasticity in the lower extremities for children with CP.[9,12] This is a permanent procedure that is ideal for a child who has at least 3/5 motor strength in their lower extremities. This procedure may be considered if a child with CP experiences adverse side effects from antispasticity medications, is not a candidate for an ITB pump, and has failed conservative treatment with therapies, bracing, and orthotics in terms of having difficulty achieving their goal or improved gait and ambulation. The typical age is between 4 years and 7 years of age; however, the procedure may be considered at other stages in life including palliative care.[1,2,9]

COMPLICATIONS

Complications of antispasticity medications such as Valium, baclofen, and tizanidine may include decreased truncal head and neck control, worsening sialorrhea, drowsiness and sedation, constipation, urinary retention, and a lowered seizure threshold. Clonidine can result in hypotension and bradycardia. There is a risk of metabolic derangements including abnormal liver enzymes with the use of dantrolene. These medications should be slowly titrated up and carefully weaned to avoid withdrawal symptoms. Baclofen can lead to worsening of head and truncal control. Abrupt cessation can result in withdrawal symptoms that are life threatening in any form, that is, enteral or intrathecal. Symptoms include worsening agitation, altered mental status, worsening spasticity, hyperthermia, and seizures.[1,2,7,16,17]

Complications of BoNT injections include but are not limited to localized injection site reactions including pain, rash or allergic reaction, bleeding, and bruising. Systemic complications include flu-like illness, fever, headache, myalgias, nausea, vomiting, respiratory distress, dysphagia, sialorrhea, and facial weakness.[1,2,7,16]

Complications of alcohol/phenol injections include but are not limited to localized injection site reactions including pain, rash or allergic reaction, bleeding, bruising, and dyesthesias. Systemic complications include flu-like illness, fever, headache, myalgias, nausea, vomiting, respiratory distress, dysphagia, sialorrhea, and facial weakness.[1,2–7,16,17]

Complications of orthopedic surgeries include but are not limited to postoperative complications such as infections, pain, immobility, poor wound healing, and respiratory complications, adverse effects of anesthesia, weakness, impaired mobility, and decreased overall function. Consideration should be given to the great risks of complications with compounded multi-event surgeries as well as subsequent planned surgeries that are often required for removal of fixation plates and other implants.[10,13,11]

Complications of ITB pump include localized and systemic infections; catheter and pump malfunction; postoperative complications related to immobility, wound sites, pain, headache, drowsiness, nausea, constipation, CSF leak, and battery malfunction; and subsequent baclofen withdrawal that is life threatening[1,2,16,8] (see section on Complications of Antispasticity Medications).

Complications of SDR procedures includes postoperative complications as mentioned previously in this section. In addition, families should be counseled and informed regarding the intraoperative severe complications of significant lower extremity weakness and flaccid paralysis; bladder dysfunction; sensory impairment; CNS infections, that is, meningitis; and CSF leak. Additional hospitalizations and operations may be required.[9,12]

Caregiver Burden

Discussions prior to surgical and procedural interventions should be prioritized. Families and caregivers should have a clear understanding of indications for the procedures, goals of the interventions, aspects of the procedure itself, and post-procedural care and rehabilitation. Setting expectations improves outcomes. According to a study by Park et al., extracted from a 59-item questionnaire, the top five preoperative problems that concern the parents of children with CP are (a) postoperative rehabilitation, (b) duration and quality rehabilitation, (c) immediate postoperative pain, (d) general anesthesia, and (e) cost of medical expenses.[11]

CASE REPORT (◎ VIDEO 16.1)

 Video 16.1 can be accessed via the QR code or on Springer Publishing Connect™: https://connect.springerpub.com/content/book/978-0-8261 -3975-7/part/part04/chapter/ch16

A 2-year-old, left-hand dominant female presents due to concerns of delayed walking complicated by toe walking. Today, the mother would like to discuss spasticity treatment options.

Upon review of mother's *pregnancy history and birth history,* she had no apparent risk factors during the prenatal, perinatal, or postnatal period. Upon further review of her developmental milestones, the mom reports that at 3 months of age, the child had an early left-hand preference and at 18 months, she noticed toe walking on the right. MRI of the brain revealed encephalomalacia in the left frontotemporal lobe with ex vacuo dilatation of the left lateral ventricle confirming a left-sided neonatal stroke resulting in a static encephalopathy. She has no significant surgical and family history and has never taken antispasticity medications.

Neuromuscular exam is significant for spasticity of the distal right arm and leg. Pertinent findings on her right side include an MAS score of 1+ to 2 in her elbow flexor, MAS 1+ in her thumb held in adduction, MAS 1+ in her knee flexor, and an MAS 2 in her ankle plantar flexor. She has full PROM of her right and left shoulder, elbow, wrist, fingers, adductors, hamstrings, knee, and ankle. She does have dystonia of her right hand and fingers as well as difficulty isolating her thumb and dorsiflexing her right ankle. She has several beats of clonus on her right ankle as well.

Gait assessment is significant for a right lateral truncal lean, mildly flexed knee, and forefoot strike gait noted on the right leg. In stance, she can achieve a flat foot position. She does not demonstrate any pain, tripping, or falling with gait. She can run without difficulty.

Assessment and plan: A 2-year-old, left-hand dominant girl with spastic hemiplegic CP resulting in a right ankle contracture and subsequently altered gait that does not result in any significant pain, fatigue, or falls.

Recommendations include (a) stretching program, occupational and physical therapies for right fine motor control, stretching and strengthening of her right ankle, and gait training and (b) orthotic use of a nightly right ankle stretching splint, supportive shoe wear, and a daytime ankle foot orthotic as needed for fatigue, tripping, or falling and distances in the community. Lastly, we provided anticipatory guidance regarding brace wearing, spasticity and dystonia treatments, and potential challenges as she develops. We will serially re-evaluate her as she grows.

Table 16.1 is intended as a guide for medication consideration for treatment of spasticity in children with CP. All doses should be cross-referenced with a drug reference guide for accurate weight- or age-based dosing. Caution: Start at low suggested doses and titrate slowly as tolerated to minimize ASE. Consideration should be taken to any adverse side effects or cross-reactivity between the classes of medications.

REFERENCES

1. Braddom RL, Chan L, Harrast MA. *Physical Medicine and Rehabilitation*. 4th ed. Philadelphia, PA: Saunders/Elsevier. 2011. ISBN-13: 978-1437708844

2. Matthews DJM, Murphy KP. *Pediatric Rehabilitation: Principles and Practice*. Springer Publishing Company. 2015. https://doi.org/10.1891/9781617052255.0014

3. Novak I, Morgan C, Adde L, et al. Early, accurate diagnosis and early intervention in cerebral palsy: Advances in diagnosis and treatment. *JAMA Pediatr*. 2017;171(9): 897–907. https://doi.org/10.1001/jamapediatrics.2017.1689

4. Rosenbaum P, Paneth N, Leviton A, et al. A report: the definition and classification of cerebral palsy April 2006. *Dev Med Child Neurol Suppl*. 2007;109:8–14. PMID: 17370477. https://doi.org/10.1111/j.1469-8749.2007.tb12610.x

5. Rosenbaum PL, Palisano RJ, Bartlett DJ, et al. Development of the gross motor function classification system for cerebral palsy. *Dev Med Child Neurol*. 2008;50(4):249–253. https://doi.org/10.1111/j.1469-8749.2008.02045.x

6. Wimalasundera N, Stevenson VL. Cerebral palsy. *Pract Neurol*. 2016;16(3):184–194. https://doi.org/10.1136/practneurol-2015-001184

7. Multani I, Manji J, Hastings-Ison T, et al. Botulinum toxin in the management of children with cerebral palsy. *Paediatr Drugs*. 2019;21(4):261–281. https://doi.org/10.1007/s40272-019-00344-8

8. Shamsoddini A, Amirsalari S, Hollisaz MT, et al. Management of spasticity in children with cerebral palsy. *Iran J Pediatr*. 2014;24(4):345–351. https://doi.org/10.1007/978-3-319-74558-9_41

9. Sadowska M, Sarecka-Hujar B, Kopyta I. Cerebral palsy: current opinions on definition, epidemiology, risk factors, classification and treatment options. *Neuropsychiatr Dis Treat*. 2020;16:1505–1518. https://doi.org/10.2147/NDT.S235165

10. Park MS, Chung CY, Lee KM, et al. Issues of concern before single event multilevel surgery in patients with cerebral palsy. *J Pediatr Orthop*. 2010;30(5):489–495. https://doi.org/10.1097/BPO.0b013e3181e00c98

11. Skoutelis VC, Kanellopoulos AD, Kontogeorgakos VA, et al. The orthopaedic aspect of spastic cerebral palsy. *J Orthop*. 2020;22:553–558. https://doi.org/10.1016/j.jor.2020.11.002

12. Vitrikas K, Dalton H, Breish D. Cerebral palsy: an overview. *Am Fam Physician*. 2020;101(4):213–220. https://pubmed.ncbi.nlm.nih.gov/32053326/

13. Shrader MW, Wimberly L, Thompson R. Hip surveillance in children with cerebral palsy. *J Am Acad Orthop Surg*. 2019;27(20):760–768. https://doi.org/10.5435/JAAOS-D-18-00184

14. Yu S, Rethlefsen SA, Wren TA, et al. Long-term ambulatory change after lower extremity orthopaedic surgery in children with cerebral palsy: a retrospective review. *J Pediatr Orthop*. 2015;35(3):285–289. https://doi.org/10.1097/BPO.0000000000000251

15. Novak I, Morgan C, Fahey M, et al. State of the evidence traffic lights 2019: systematic review of interventions for preventing and treating children with cerebral palsy. *Curr Neurol Neurosci Rep*. 2020;20(2):3. https://doi.org/10.1007/s11910-020-1022-z

16. Reilly M, Liuzzo K, Blackmer AB. Pharmacological management of spasticity in children with cerebral palsy. *J Pediatr Health Care*. 2020;34(5):495–509. https://doi.org/10.1016/j.pedhc.2020.04.010

17. Davidson B, Schoen N, Sedighim S, et al. Intrathecal baclofen versus selective dorsal rhizotomy for children with cerebral palsy who are nonambulant: a systematic review. *J Neurosurg Pediatr*. 2020;25(1):69–77. Retrieved Mar 31, 2022 https://doi.org/10.3171/2019.8.peds19282

17 Spasticity in Spinal Cord Injury

Madeline A. Dicks and Heather W. Walker

INRODUCTION

Spasticity has been defined by Lance as "a motor disorder characterized by a velocity-dependent increase in tonic stretch reflexes (muscle tone) with exaggerated tendon jerks, resulting from hyperexcitability of the stretch reflex, as one component of the upper motor neuron syndrome (UMNS)."[1] Clinically positive and negative signs and symptoms are noted; the former includes clonus, hyperreflexia, and spasms, while the latter includes fatigue, incoordination, and weakness.[2] Spasticity commonly occurs after spinal cord injury (SCI) with an incidence of approximately 70%. Not all individuals require pharmacologic intervention, but at 1 year post discharge, 49% require pharmacologic treatment for management of spasticity.[3]

ASSESSMENT

Several outcome measures are available to objectively evaluate spasticity in the clinical setting including the Ashworth Scale (AS), Modified Ashworth Scale (MAS), Spasm Frequency Scale, and the Tardieu Scale. The AS and MAS are quite frequently used to measure muscle resistance to passive stretch throughout the entire range of motion (ROM) at the targeted joint. The AS is graded from 0 to 4, with a score of 0 indicating no increased tone, while a score of 4 indicates the affected joint is rigid in flexion and extension. The MAS added 1+ to the scale to characterize milder spasticity more specifically[4,5] (Table 17.1). The Penn Spasm Frequency Scale (PSFS) is used to quantify how often individuals are experiencing spasms, ranging from a score of 0 that correlates to no spasms within an hour to a score of 4, indicating 10 or more spasms per hour.[6] There is also a Modified PSFS that provides information regarding the severity of spasms being experienced as well as frequency of spasms[7] (Table 17.2). In addition to these scales that are commonly utilized for measurement of spasticity of various etiologies, there are tools available that were designed to evaluate spasticity specifically in individuals with SCI. The Spinal Cord Assessment Tool for Spastic Reflexes (SCATS) (Table 17.3) is a clinical tool measuring clonus and flexor/extensor spasms,[8] while the SCI-Spasticity Evaluation Tool (SCI-SET) is a self-reported scale measuring impact of SCI on a variety of activities of daily living (ADLs), mobility, and quality of life (QOL).[9]

Table 17.1 Clinical Measures of Spasticity

Ashworth Scale

0	No increased tone
1	Slight increase in tone, giving a "catch" when affected part is moved in flexion or extension
2	More marked increase in tone, but affected part easily flexed
3	Considerable increase in tone; passive movement difficult
4	Affected part rigid in flexion or extension

Modified Ashworth Scale

0	No increased tone
1	Slight increase in muscle tone, *manifested by a catch and release or by minimal resistance at the end of the ROM when the affected part(s) is moved in flexion or extension*
1 +	Slight increase in muscle tone, *manifested by a catch, followed by minimal resistance throughout the remainder (less than half) of the ROM*
2	More marked increase in tone, but affected part easily flexed
3	Considerable increase in tone; passive movement difficult
4	Affected part rigid in flexion or extension. (Changes compared to the standard AS are italicized.)

Table 17.2 Spasm Frequency Scales

Penn Spasm Frequency Score (Psfs)

0	No spasms
1	Mild spasms induced by stimulation
2	Infrequent spasms occurring less than once per hour
3	Spasms occurring more than once per hour
4	Spasms occurring more than 10 times per hour

Modified Psfs: 2 Parts

Part 1: spasm frequency score (as above)

Part 2: spasm severity scale

1	Mild
2	Moderate
3	Severe

Spasm Frequency Score

0	No spasms
1	1 or fewer spasms per day
2	Between 1 and 5 spasms per day
3	5 to >10 spasms per day
4	10 or more spasms per day, or continuous contraction

Table 17.3 Spinal Cord Assessment Tool for Spastic Reflexes

SCATS: Clonus

Clonus quantified in response to rapid dorsiflexion of the ankle

0	No reaction
1	Mild, clonus maintained less than 3 seconds
2	Moderate, clonus persists 3–10 seconds
3	Severe, clonus persists >10 seconds

SCATS: Flexor Spasms

Measurement of excursion of big toe into extension, ankle dorsiflexion, knee flexion, or hip flexion when pinprick stimulus is applied to plantar surface of the foot.

0	No reaction to stimulus
1	Mild, <10°
2	Moderate, 10°–30°
3	Severe, ≥30°

SCATS: Extensor Spasms

Starting position with hip and knee placed at 90°–110° of flexion with contralateral limb extended. Hip and knee joints then simultaneously extended and duration of quadriceps muscle contraction is measured

0	No reaction
1	Mild, contraction maintained <3 seconds
2	Moderate, contraction persists 3–10 seconds
3	Severe, contraction persists >10 seconds

Source: Adapted from Benz EN, Hornby TG, Bode RK, Scheidt RA, Schmit BD. A physiologically based clinical measure for spastic reflexes in spinal cord injury. *Arch Phys Med Rehabil*. 2005;86:52–59.

DIAGNOSTIC APPROACH

In order to diagnose spasticity in an individual with SCI, the clinician must gather information regarding the patient's objective complaints of spasms/spasticity, focusing on both negative and positive symptoms. Spasticity can negatively impact functional status; therefore, the clinician must elicit history regarding specific challenges that the patient is facing. In individuals with SCI, increased lower extremity spasticity can interfere with transfers and can make self-catheterization and perineal care/hygiene activities difficult to perform. It can affect positioning within the bed and wheelchair that may increase risk of pressure injury among other challenges. Frequent spasms may be painful and interfere with sleep, have a negative impact on QOL, and may lead to complications such as contractures; therefore, it is necessary to identify and treat problematic spasticity aggressively once identified. The outcome measures described above, including the SCI-specific measures, may be useful to elicit the desired history from the patient. It is also important to bear in mind that in individuals with SCI, spasticity can be exacerbated by other medical comorbidities including but not limited to urinary tract infection, bowel impaction, pressure injury, and syringomyelia. Before initiating treatment for spasticity, the clinician needs to inquire about potential concomitant medical issues that may be exacerbating the patient's baseline spasticity. Once the history is obtained, spasticity can objectively be measured using physical exam techniques as described above. Due to the COVID-19 pandemic, many in-person clinic visits have transitioned to telemedicine evaluations using telecommunication/video platforms. Gathering history from the patient relating to spasticity is easily accomplished in this setting; however, objective measurement of spasticity is more challenging. Verduzco-Gutierrez and colleagues suggest that a caregiver can demonstrate elements of the physical examination that would normally be conducted by the clinician; for example, the caregiver can demonstrate ROM at target joint and classify spasticity into three broad groups including severe tone/contracture, mild/moderate increase in tone, and no increase in tone/hypotonia.[10]

Once the history is obtained from the patient and physical examination is complete, whether in person or remote, the clinician and patient/caregiver need to determine goals of treatment. Goal Attainment Scaling (GAS) is a patient-reported outcome measure that allows patients to establish specific goals and track their response to treatment. Utilizing the SMART model, goals can be identified that are specific, measurable, achievable, realistic, and time bound. This method can be applied across multiple clinical domains within rehabilitation but has shown specific usefulness in setting goals with spasticity management and measuring response to treatment.[11–14]

TREATMENT OPTIONS

Nonpharmacologic Treatment Options
Identifying the type and severity of muscle tone and how it interferes with the patients' and families' QOL and functional goals enables providers to develop an appropriate treatment plan.[15] Initial treatment of spasticity typically starts with nonpharmacologic, noninvasive measures. This involves thorough evaluation of any precipitating factors that could be contributing to the patient's spasticity.[2,16] Some examples include complications related to the patient's neurogenic bladder and bowel, such as urinary tract infection and stool impaction, the development of pressure injuries, deep venous thromboses, and presence of heterotopic ossification. The avoidance of noxious stimuli is an important first step in the treatment and prevention of spasticity. It is important to maintain appropriate skin protocols to prevent pressure injury development as well as consistent bowel and bladder programs.

Muscle Stretching
Stretching is a common measure employed to decrease spasticity and maintain ROM at the affected joints. A regimen of both active and passive ROM coupled with strengthening exercises initiated by trained physical or occupational therapists and caregivers alike is the foundation for a successful spasticity management program.[15] Manually moving the joint through its ROM helps to normalize tone, maintain or increase soft tissue extensibility, and decrease stiffness.[17,18] Stretching may also improve motor function; however, evidence of clinical improvement in functional outcomes, such as walking, is limited.[19] It is also a useful adjunct to other treatment alternatives including oral antispasmodic medications, injections, and surgical intervention. Kunkel

et al. found that tilt-table standing not only reduces lower extremity spasticity via a prolonged stretch of the ankle plantar flexors but also improves passive ROM and psychological well-being in persons with SCI.[20]

Splinting and Casting
Splints and casts are often utilized to restore the proper biomechanics to the affected muscles and joints by reducing excitatory input from muscle spindles.[21] A splint is a noninvasive therapeutic tool that maintains the limb in a specific position, thus providing stability, maintaining ROM, and preventing contracture formation. A splint may be static, immobilizing the joint in a single position, or dynamic, allowing for a self-adjusting elastic component. It may be used in conjunction with chemodenervation; therefore, proper planning between the provider and therapist is paramount. Casting should occur at the time the toxin takes full effect, which is typically 2 to 3 weeks post injection.[15] Despite its common practice, practitioners should be aware of the possible complications that splints and casts carry including muscle atrophy, skin breakdown, and circulation impairment. Taping and bivalved casts are additional strategies to support the joint.

Positioning
Management of postural alignment to prevent or reduce muscle tone involves maintaining a balanced, symmetrical alignment when sitting, standing, and in bed.[22] Appropriate low back support to maintain lumbar lordosis with a firm, positive seat plane angle, with the knees and ankles at 90°, may reduce extensor tone.[2]

Physical Modalities
Several physical modalities are used to reduce spasticity, such as cryotherapy, thermotherapy, and functional electrical stimulation (FES). Cryotherapy refers to local muscle cooling that temporarily decreases spasticity by slowing nerve conduction velocity and reducing the sensitivity of muscle spindles to stretch.[18] Cold application includes ice packs, cold gel packs, ice massage, evaporative sprays, and cold whirlpool therapy. Lee et al. found that cold air therapy applied to spinally injured animal models optimally relieves spasticity for 30 to 60 minutes after treatment at an intramuscular temperature of 30°C.[23]

Thermotherapy refers to local muscle heating that temporarily decreases muscle tone by reducing the response of muscle spindles to stretch and inducing muscle and soft tissue relaxation.[18,23] Superficial heat application can penetrate soft tissue to a depth of 2 cm and includes hot packs, paraffin, fluidotherapy, and whirlpool therapy. Microwave diathermy and ultrasound (US) can penetrate deeper structures.[24]

Electrical Stimulation (E-Stim)
The application of electrotherapy has been shown to be beneficial in the treatment of spasticity of varying etiologies.[25-28] In addition, it has the potential to be less invasive, safer, and more user-friendly than various pharmacologic and other therapeutic options. There are a variety of different application techniques including:

- **FES:** An electrical current activates several muscles in a coordinated and sequenced fashion, thus creating purposeful movement. This system generates several action potentials in the intact peripheral nerve that activates the muscle.[29] It has been used to improve walking performance by stimulation of the common peroneal nerve, producing dorsiflexion and eversion of the foot when timed appropriately during the gait cycle.[28,30] It has also been shown to reduce spasticity, improve ROM, and facilitate stretching of spastic muscles.

- **Transcutaneous electrical nerve stimulation (TENS):** It is a modality commonly used in pain control that uses electrical current to stimulate large-diameter mechanosensitive afferent nerve fibers in the skin, which may reduce spinal spasticity through the modulation of abnormal spinal inhibitory circuits.[29] It has been reported that one TENS session is effective at reducing muscle tone and the results are prolonged with multiple sessions.[25,26]

Other Therapeutic Options

Other nonpharmacologic interventions include shock wave therapy, transcranial direct current stimulation, vibratory stimulation, electromyography (EMG) biofeedback, and acupuncture.[31] Zadnia et al. found the application of biofeedback techniques by providing visual and auditory signals can reduce spasticity.[32] Whole-body vibration has been shown to decrease lower extremity spasticity in the chronic SCI.[33] Hydrotherapy has also been studied in persons with SCI. Kesiktas et al. found that exercise in a 71°F pool, 3 times per week for 20 minutes, improved Functional Independence Measure (FIM) scores, decreased spasm severity, and decreased oral baclofen dose requirements.[34]

Oral Medications

There are several oral antispasmodic medications available for the treatment of generalized spasticity that function by altering neurotransmitters or neuromodulators in the central nervous system (CNS) or by working on peripheral neuromuscular sites. Only four agents are approved by the U.S. Food and Drug Administration (FDA) for treatment of spasticity related to the CNS that include baclofen (in adults), diazepam, dantrolene sodium, and tizanidine.[35]

- **Baclofen (Lioresal®)** is considered the first-line treatment in patients with spasticity of spinal origin that works pre- and postsynaptically as a gamma-aminobutyric acid (GABA) B agonist.[2,37,39] Upon binding to the GABA-B receptor, calcium influx into the presynaptic terminal is inhibited and the release of excitatory neurotransmitters is suppressed. Side effects include systemic muscle relaxation, sedation, and fatigue. Baclofen is primarily metabolized by the kidneys, although 15% is metabolized in the liver.[2,36] Liver function tests (LFTs) should be monitored due to risk of hepatotoxicity. Baclofen should be used with caution in patients with a history of seizure disorder, as the seizure threshold may be reduced.[37] The recommended initiating dose is 5 mg 3 times per day, and this can be titrated up every 2 to 3 days to a maximum dose of 80 mg per day.[2,36] Sudden withdrawal of baclofen therapy may lead to hyperthermia, seizures, worsening spasticity, and altered mental status.

- **Benzodiazepines**, including diazepam (Valium®) and clonazepam (Klonopin®), bind near GABA-A receptors and facilitate the postsynaptic effects of GABA, increasing presynaptic inhibition.[2,35] They are commonly used to decrease reflexes and treat painful spasms, rather than to treat increased tone related to spasticity. Diazepam is 98% protein-bound and it is metabolized by the liver; therefore, practitioners should maintain caution when using this medication to treat individuals with low serum albumin (i.e., acute SCI) or liver dysfunction. Diazepam has been shown to be effective in the management of spasticity compared to other drugs and placebo; however, there were more side effects in individuals treated with diazepam.[37,38] Common side effects include sedation, weakness, hypotension, reduced motor coordination, and impaired attention and memory (diazepam drug summary). Diazepam is typically dosed 2 to 10 mg 2 to 3 times a day. Clonazepam causes less sedation than diazepam and is often used to treat nighttime spasms at a dose of 0.5 mg to 1 mg.[2]

- **Dantrolene sodium (Dantrium®)** is the only antispasmodic medication that works directly on the skeletal muscle itself by inhibiting calcium ion release from the sarcoplasmic reticulum, thus preventing muscle contraction.[2,35,39] It is primarily metabolized by the liver that necessitates monitoring of LFTs due to the risk of hepatotoxicity and fatal hepatitis.[2] Due to its peripheral action, it is less likely to cause sedation or cognitive side effects compared to baclofen or benzodiazepines, making it a preferred agent for individuals with dual diagnosis, SCI, and cognitive dysfunction. Other common side effects include general muscle weakness, nausea, vomiting, diarrhea, malaise, and dizziness.[35] Dantrolene dosage is initiated at 25 mg per day and may be titrated up to a maximum dose of 400 mg per day divided into 3 or 4 times a day.

- **Tizanidine (Zanaflex®)** is a centrally acting alpha-2 agonist that decreases tone and spasm frequency in spastic muscles by preventing the presynaptic release of excitatory amino acids.[2,35] Common side effects include dry mouth, fatigue, dizziness, and hypotension. It is metabolized in the liver and should be used with caution in patients with known liver abnormality, necessitating monitoring of LFTs. Tizanidine is contraindicated in patients taking ciprofloxacin (Cipro®) and fluvoxamine (Luvox®) because the combination of tizanidine with CYP1A1 inhibitors can increase serum concentration of the drug, causing severe hypotension.[40] Tizanidine dosage is initiated at 2 to 4 mg dosages, typically at bedtime due to risk of sedation, with gradual increase to a maximum recommended dose of 36 mg per day.[35]

- **Clonidine (Catapres®)** is a centrally acting alpha-2 agonist antihypertensive medication that has been shown to decrease spasticity by inhibiting afferent sensory transmission below the level of injury.[2,39] Approximately half of the absorbed dose is metabolized by the liver and the other half is excreted in the urine.[35] Common side effects include orthostasis, dry mouth, bradycardia, and drowsiness.[2,39] The recommended initiation dose is 0.05 mg BID and can be increased to 0.1 mg per day after 3 days, titrating up to 0.1 mg per week to a maximum dose of 0.4 mg per day.[2] Caution should be taken while weaning off clonidine to prevent rebound hypertension.[41]

- **Gabapentin (Neurontin®)** is an anticonvulsant, which is renally cleared, that acts at the alpha-$2_{\delta 1}$ subunit of voltage-gated calcium channels, inhibiting the release of calcium ions.[39] Although it is rarely used as monotherapy for the treatment of spasticity, studies with gabapentin have shown a reduction in AS and spasticity Likert scores when compared with placebo.[42,43] Adverse effects include somnolence, tremor, and nystagmus.[39] Gabapentin is initiated at 300 mg 3 times a day and titrated up to a maximum dose of 3,600 mg per day.[44]

- **Cyproheptadine (Periactin®)** is a histamine and serotonin antagonist with mild anticholinergic activity that inhibits serotonergic excitatory input at the spinal and supraspinal levels.[2,35] It has been shown to reduce AS and increase amplitude of knee swing in the pendulum test in patient with SCI.[45] The most common side effects include CNS depression and dry mouth due to its anticholinergic properties.[35] It may be initiated at 4 mg at bedtime, increasing by 4 mg every 3 to 4 days to a maximum recommended dose of 36 mg per day.

- **Cannabinoids (Marinol®, Cesamet®)** are not FDA approved for the treatment of spasticity; however, the main active ingredient in cannabis, delta-9-tetrahydrocannabinol (THC), has been shown to reduce spasticity.[46,47] Hagenbach et al. found that a least 15 to 20 mg per day were needed to achieve a therapeutic effect in individuals with SCI.[47] THC is primarily hepatically metabolized and may cause cognitive and psychomotor impairment including sedation, anxiety, altered perception, and tachycardia.[48] Cannabinoid therapy is contraindicated in significant psychiatric, cardiovascular, and renal or hepatic disease.

Botulinum Toxin Injections

Botulinum toxin, produced by the bacteria *Clostridium botulinum*, was originally developed to treat blepharospasm and strabismus.[2] Treatment has since expanded to include various movement disorders such as torticollis, focal dystonias, overactive bladder, migraine, cosmetic injections, and upper and lower limb spasticity. Botulinum toxin is not recommended for the treatment of generalized spasticity; however, isolated muscle groups are often treated to facilitate functional activity, hygiene, and caregiving and improve patient comfort.

Botulinum toxin acts by inhibiting the release of acetylcholine (Ach) from the presynaptic motor axon, thereby blocking neuromuscular transmission and weakening the muscle.[2,49] There are seven neurotoxin subtypes (A through G). Each of the toxins prevent binding of Ach-containing vesicles to the nerve terminal; however, they do so in different ways. For instance, botulinum toxins A and E target the synaptosomal-associated protein (SNAP-25), while botulinum toxins B, D, F, and G target vesicle-associated protein (VAMP) and botulinum C targets both SNAP-25 and syntaxin.[49] Type A and B are the only formulations used clinically on the market today and include abobotulinumtoxinA (Dysport), incobotulinumtoxinA (Xeomin), onabotulinumtoxinA (Botox), and rimabotulinumtoxinB (Mybloc/Neurobloc).

There are several commonly practiced injection techniques, including the utilization of anatomic landmarks and guidance using EMG, e-stim, or US.[50] Anatomic localization is the easiest method and does not require equipment; however, it may not be accurate for small or deep muscles. Both EMG and e-stim require a hollow insulated monopolar needle electrode with an injection port that allows for attachment for a syringe. When using EMG guidance, the needle electrode is advanced into the spastic muscle until crisp, spontaneous motor units are heard, signifying appropriate localization at the motor end plate. When using e-stim, an electrical stimulus is delivered, producing contraction of the target muscle. US guidance allows for direct visualization of the anatomic structures, allowing the clinician to ensure injection into the target muscle while avoiding nerves and blood vessels.

The effect of botulinum toxin peaks at 2 to 6 weeks with local relief of spasticity lasting 3 to 5 months. Though the effect of botulinum toxin is irreversible, the response slowly diminishes, likely due to nerve terminal collateral sprouting.[2] If treatment is successful, the injections can be repeated at no shorter than 3-month intervals due to the risk of antibody formation that could render the treatment ineffective. Although botulinum toxin is typically well tolerated in therapeutic doses, it carries an FDA-mandated black box warning of the rare, but potentially life-threatening complications of systemic weakness, vision changes, dysarthria, dysphonia, dysphagia, and respiratory compromise.[51]

Intrathecal Baclofen

Intrathecal baclofen (ITB) is an effective treatment option for management of lower extremity spasticity and is FDA approved for the management of spasticity in SCI.[52–54] ITB is typically utilized in patients with SCI who have failed oral agents or do not tolerate side effects of the oral agents.[55] ITB is often preferable to oral medications as a means for lower extremity spasticity management as the medication is delivered directly to the cerebrospinal fluid (CSF). The dose that is delivered intrathecally is a fraction of the oral doses that would be required to produce similar results.[56] This allows for lower side effect profile and higher overall efficacy when compared to spasticity management using oral agents. In order to determine if the patient is an appropriate candidate for placement of an intrathecal pump, the patient must undergo an ITB trial. During the screening trial, a lumbar puncture is performed and 50 mcg is delivered intrathecally. In some cases, lower or higher doses are chosen, but 50 mcg is most frequently utilized. Peak efficacy is noted at 4 hours; therefore, assessment measures such as AS, MAS, and timed walking tests (if appropriate) are measured at baseline and again at the 4-hour mark. If the screening trial has a positive outcome, the patient can be referred to the appropriate surgeon for pump placement; however, if the trial is negative, it can be repeated at 24 hours with a higher dose of baclofen. The pump is surgically placed subcutaneously into the left or right lower quadrant of the abdomen, with catheter tunneled subcutaneously and inserted into the spinal canal in the lumbar region and tunneled to the subarachnoid space at the appropriate level. Typically, the catheter tip is placed in the low thoracic or high lumbar region; however, in some cases, the tip may be advanced to the midthoracic region or higher. ITB is most effective for managing lower extremity spasticity, but some report improvement in upper extremity spasticity if the catheter tip is placed in the upper thoracic region.[57–60] Once the pump is implanted, the patient is typically started on a continuous infusion of ITB, with dose increases of 10% to 20% no more frequently than every 24 hours.

Peripheral Nerve Blocks

Peripheral nerve blocks are an option for management of focal spasticity. Temporary diagnostic nerve blocks using anesthetic agents such as lidocaine or bupivacaine can be used to help differentiate severe spasticity from contracture and to identify appropriate targets for injection. Therapeutic nerve blocks using agents such as alcohol or phenol offer a more permanent and can last an average of 3 to 9 months.[61–63] The peripheral nerve is targeted using established anatomic landmarks and e-stim. The clinician attempts to obtain close proximity to the target nerve by eliciting desired muscular contraction while decreasing the current of e-stim. When an appropriate contraction is maintained with 1.0 mA or less of current being used, the clinician can be confident that the monopolar needle tip is near the nerve and the phenol or alcohol can be injected.[64] Typical concentrations of phenol are 5% to 7% in volumes up to 10 mL per nerve. Most common side effects from phenol injections are paresthesias and dysethesias that may occur in 10% to 32% of patients.[65–67] Common targets for peripheral nerve blocks include musculocutaneous nerve (elbow flexor spasticity), obturator nerve (hip adductor spasticity), and tibial nerve (plantar flexor spasticity).

Motor Point Blocks

Motor point injections use a similar approach to peripheral nerve blocks in that the clinician is attempting to sustain maximal contraction while delivering lower levels of current, with the goal as above to obtain maximal contraction at 1 mA or less. However, the motor point, rather than peripheral nerve, is being targeted in this technique and anatomic landmarks for the motor points of the target muscle are utilized. Results can last 3 to 8 months.[2]

Surgical Techniques

Surgical techniques can be delineated into those utilized to reduce spasticity and those that are necessary to manage complications of spasticity. The former includes neurosurgical options such as selective rhizotomy or neurotomy.[2] Anterior rhizotomy abolishes voluntary and involuntary activity in the targeted muscle, while dorsal rhizotomy disrupts the reflex arc thereby indirectly decreasing spasticity. Anterior rhizotomy will decrease the muscle bulk, in contrast to dorsal rhizotomy that does not have this effect; however, sensory function may be affected in the latter procedure. Neurotomy involves direct transection of the targeted peripheral nerve that will achieve results similar to a peripheral nerve; however, in contrast to the nerve block, the result is permanent. Spinal cord stimulation (SCS) has historically been used for management of pain; however, some studies have indicated that this therapy may decrease spasticity in individuals with SCI.[68,69] For individuals who develop complications from spasticity such as contracture, an orthopedic procedure may be necessary. These include tendon lengthening to decrease tension on the spastic muscle and improve positioning, tenotomy to release the tendon from the spastic muscle, and tendon transfer to improve joint positioning, such as the split anterior tendon transfer (SPLATT) that is used to improve an equinovarus deformity.[70]

COMPLICATIONS

Spasticity is not an inherently negative syndrome and, in some cases, can be beneficial. For example, some individuals with weakness in an extremity can use their spasticity to assist with weightbearing, transfers, and ambulation; if this spasticity is diminished with pharmacologic or other treatment interventions, the patient may suffer adverse functional impact. However, spasticity can be detrimental and lead to a variety of complications. There are physiological and histochemical changes that occur in spastic muscle that affect their contractile properties.[71] For muscles with spasticity that are held in a shortened position and are untreated, the muscle will lose sarcomeres and lead to loss of ROM and development of contracture.[72] Development of contractures can negatively impact positioning of the patient within a wheelchair or in bed, altering pressure distribution that will make the patient more susceptible to development of pressure injuries. Other complications of untreated spasticity include uncontrolled pain, negative impact on functional tasks including transfers, and self-consciousness due to abnormal limb positioning. Because these are complications that can be minimized or prevented with appropriate treatment, early identification and management of spasticity is necessary.

CASE REPORT

A 66-year-old male with T1 AIS B tetraplegia secondary to a ground-level fall in October 2018 complicated by neurogenic bowel (status post colostomy), neurogenic bladder (status post suprapubic tube), severe osteoarthritis of the right glenohumeral joint, and a chronic sacral pressure injury was transferred to the hospital from his long-term care facility for further evaluation and treatment of the pressure injury. He was admitted to the SCI unit for chronic wound care and medical optimization. The patient was found to have a stage IV sacral pressure injury with CT scan revealing cortical bone changes, concerning for osteomyelitis. He underwent wound debridement and bone biopsy with plastic surgery; pathology showed chronic osteomyelitis with negative cultures. Infectious disease was consulted and antibiotics were not recommended.

During the patient's admission, he was noted to have significant spasticity in the bilateral hip and knee flexors, measured as Ashworth score of 3. He reported that he had not been up in his wheelchair for several months due to declining function related to his lower limb spasticity. He could not perform independent slide board transfers or achieve appropriate ischial sitting in his power wheelchair. In addition, the patient's long-term care facility did not have a functioning Hoyer lift, so he had been essentially bedbound for several months and he suspects that is when his sacral pressure injury started to worsen. The patient was started on an aggressive stretching program and oral baclofen was initiated with some improvement. He was transferred back to his long-term care facility with follow-up appointment scheduled in the outpatient spasticity clinic for further evaluation and management. Upon reevaluation in spasticity clinic, he was noted to have continued significant hip and knee flexor spasticity despite initiation of oral baclofen and a stretching program. Decision was made to perform injections of botulinum toxin type A to bilateral hamstrings and iliopsoas muscles to assist with control of the flexor pattern of his lower extremities while facilitating wound healing and rehabilitation through proper positioning. Injections were performed with incobotulinumtoxinA using US guidance as seen in Table 17.4.

Table 17.4 Botulinum Toxin Type A Injections

Target Muscle	Units Injected
Left iliopsoas	100 units
Right iliopsoas	100 units
Left medial hamstrings	100 units
Right medial hamstrings	100 units

The patient was advised to continue with his daily stretching program at his long-term care facility and maintained on oral baclofen. He was seen in follow-up in spasticity clinic 6 weeks post injection and he reported some improvement in positioning in the bed and in his wheelchair. Examination revealed Ashworth score of 2 at the hip flexors and knee flexors. Plan was made to repeat injections at the 12-week point with a total dose of 600 units divided between bilateral medial hamstrings and iliopsoas muscles to gain improved control of spasticity. If higher doses are ineffective, consideration for baclofen pump implantation will be considered.

REFERENCES

1. Lance JW. The control of muscle tone, reflexes, and movement: Robert Wartenberg Lecture. *Neurology*. 1980;30(12):1303–1313. https://doi.org/10.1212/wnl.30.12.1303

2. Kirshblum S. Treatment alternatives for spinal cord injury related spasticity. *J Spinal Cord Med.* 1999;22(3):199–217. https://doi.org/10.1080/10790268.1999.11719570

3. Maynard FM, Karunas RS, Waring 3rd WP. Epidemiology of spasticity following traumatic spinal cord injury. *Arch Phys Med Rehabil.* 1990;71(8):566–569.

4. Bohannon RW, Smith MB. Interrater reliability of a modified Ashworth scale of muscle spasticity. *Phys Ther.* 1987;67(2):206–207. https://doi.org/10.1093/ptj/67.2.206

5. Ashworth B. Preliminary trial of carisoprodol in multiple sclerosis. *Practitioner.* 1964;192:540–2.

6. Penn RD, Savoy SM, Corcos D, et al. Intrathecal baclofen for severe spinal spasticity. *N Engl J Med.* 1989;320(23):1517–21. https://doi.org/10.1056/NEJM198906083202303

7. Priebe MM, Sherwood AM, Thornby JI, Kharas NF, Markowski J. Clinical assessment of spasticity in spinal cord injury: a multidimensional problem. *Arch Phys Med Rehabil.* 1996;77(7):713–716. https://doi.org/S0003-9993(96)90014-3

8. Benz EN, Hornby TG, Bode RK, Scheidt RA, Schmit BD. A physiologically based clinical measure for spastic reflexes in spinal cord injury. *Arch Phys Med Rehabil.* 2005;86(1):52–59. https://doi.org/S0003-9993(04)00297-7

9. Adams MM, Ginis KA, Hicks AL. The spinal cord injury spasticity evaluation tool: development and evaluation. *Arch Phys Med Rehabil.* 2007;88(9):1185–1192. https://doi.org/S0003-9993(07)00426-110.1016/j.apmr.2007.06.012

10. 1Verduzco-Gutierrez M, Romanoski NL, Capizzi AN, et al. Spasticity outpatient evaluation via telemedicine: a practical framework. *Am J Phys Med Rehabil.* 2020;99(12):1086–1091. https://doi.org/10.1097/PHM.0000000000001594

11. Turner-Stokes L. Goal Attainment Scaling (GAS) in rehabilitation: a practical guide. *Clin Rehabil.* 2009;23(4):362–370. https://doi.org/10.1177/0269215508101742

12. Hanlan A, Mills P, Lipson R, Finlayson H. Interdisciplinary spasticity management clinic outcomes using the goal Attainment scale: a retrospective chart review. *J Rehabil Med.* 2017;49(5):423–430. https://doi.org/10.2340/16501977-2228

13. Eftekhar P, Mochizuki G, Dutta T, Richardson D, Brooks D. Goal attainment scaling in individuals with upper limb spasticity post stroke. *Occup Ther Int.* 2016;23(4):379–389. https://doi.org/10.1002/oti.1440

14. Goldstine J, Knox K, Beekman J, et al. A patient-centric tool to facilitate goal attainment scaling in neurogenic bladder and bowel dysfunction: path to individualization. *Value Health.* 2021;24(3):413–420. https://doi.org/10.1016/j.jval.2020.10.023

15. Logan LR. Rehabilitation techniques to maximize spasticity management. *Top Stroke Rehabil.* 2011;18(3):203–11. https://doi.org/10.1310/tsr1803-203

16. Odeen I. Reduction of muscular hypertonus by long-term muscle stretch. *Scand J Rehabil Med.* 1981;13(2–3):93–99.

17. Page P. Current concepts in muscle stretching for exercise and rehabilitation. *Int J Sports Phys Ther.* 2012;7(1):109–119.

18. Smania N, Picelli A, Munari D, et al. Rehabilitation procedures in the management of spasticity. *Eur J Phys Rehabil Med.* 2010;46(3):423–438.

19. Bovend'Eerdt TJ, Newman M, Barker K, Dawes H, Minelli C, Wade DT. The effects of stretching in spasticity: a systematic review. *Arch Phys Med Rehabil.* 2008;89(7):1395–1406. https://doi.org/10.1016/j.apmr.2008.02.015

20. Kunkel CF, Scremin AM, Eisenberg B, Garcia JF, Roberts S, Martinez S. Effect of "standing" on spasticity, contracture, and osteoporosis in paralyzed males. *Arch Phys Med Rehabil.* 1993;74(1):73–78.

21. Lannin NA, Ada L. Neurorehabilitation splinting: theory and principles of clinical use. *NeuroRehabilitation*. 2011;28(1):21–28. https://doi.org/10.3233/NRE-2011-0628

22. Nair KP, Marsden J. The management of spasticity in adults. *BMJ*. 2014;349:g4737. https://doi.org/10.1136/bmj.g4737

23. Lee SU, Bang MS, Han TR. Effect of cold air therapy in relieving spasticity: applied to spinalized rabbits. *Spinal Cord*. 2002;40(4):167–173. https://doi.org/10.1038/sj.sc.3101279

24. Lehmann JF, deLateur BJ. Therapeutic heat. In: Lehmann JF, ed. *Therapeutic Heat and Cold*. 3rd ed. Williams and Wilkins; 1982.

25. Aydin G, Tomruk S, Keles I, Demir SO, Orkun S. Transcutaneous electrical nerve stimulation versus baclofen in spasticity: clinical and electrophysiologic comparison. *Am J Phys Med Rehabil*. 2005;84(8):584–592. https://doi.org/10.1097/01.phm.0000171173.86312.69

26. Ping Ho Chung B, Kam Kwan Cheng B. Immediate effect of transcutaneous electrical nerve stimulation on spasticity in patients with spinal cord injury. *Clin Rehabil*. 2010;24(3):202–210. https://doi.org/10.1177/0269215509343235

27. Granat MH, Ferguson AC, Andrews BJ, Delargy M. The role of functional electrical stimulation in the rehabilitation of patients with incomplete spinal cord injury--observed benefits during gait studies. *Paraplegia*. 1993;31(4):207–215. https://doi.org/10.1038/sc.1993.39

28. Krause P, Szecsi J, Straube A. Changes in spastic muscle tone increase in patients with spinal cord injury using functional electrical stimulation and passive leg movements. *Clin Rehabil*. 2008;22(7):627–634. https://doi.org/10.1177/0269215507084648

29. Sivaramakrishnan A, Solomon JM, Manikandan N. Comparison of Transcutaneous Electrical Nerve Stimulation (TENS) and Functional Electrical Stimulation (FES) for spasticity in spinal cord injury - A pilot randomized cross-over trial. *J Spinal Cord Med*. 2018;41(4):397–406. https://doi.org/10.1080/10790268.2017.1390930

30. Yan T, Hui-Chan CW, Li LS. Functional electrical stimulation improves motor recovery of the lower extremity and walking ability of subjects with first acute stroke: a randomized placebo-controlled trial. *Stroke*. 2005;36(1):80–85. https://doi.org/10.1161/01.STR.0000149623.24906.63

31. Khan F, Amatya B, Bensmail D, Yelnik A. Non-pharmacological interventions for spasticity in adults: an overview of systematic reviews. *Ann Phys Rehabil Med*. 2019;62(4):265–273. https://doi.org/10.1016/j.rehab.2017.10.001

32. Zadnia A, Kobravi HR, Sheikh M, Asghar Hosseini H. Generating the visual biofeedback signals applicable to reduction of wrist spasticity: a pilot study on stroke patients. *Basic Clin Neurosci*. 2018;9(1):15–26. https://doi.org/10.29252/nirp.bcn.9.1.15

33. Ness LL, Field-Fote EC. Effect of whole-body vibration on quadriceps spasticity in individuals with spastic hypertonia due to spinal cord injury. *Restor Neurol Neurosci*. 2009;27(6):621–631. https://doi.org/10.3233/RNN-2009-0487

34. Kesiktas N, Paker N, Erdogan N, Gulsen G, Bicki D, Yilmaz H. The use of hydrotherapy for the management of spasticity. *Neurorehabil Neural Repair*. 2004;18(4):268–273. https://doi.org/10.1177/1545968304270002

35. Gracies JM, Nance P, Elovic E, McGuire J, Simpson DM. Traditional pharmacological treatments for spasticity. Part II: general and regional treatments. *Muscle Nerve Suppl*. 1997;6:S92–120.

36. Baclofen--Drug Summary. 2022. https://www.pdr.net/drug-summary/Baclofen-baclofen-1058.3913

37. Stevenson VL. Rehabilitation in practice: spasticity management. *Clin Rehabil.* 2010;24(4): 293–304. https://doi.org/10.1177/0269215509353254

38. Corbett M, Frankel HL, Michaelis L. A double blind, cross-over trial of valium in the treatment of spasticity. *Paraplegia.* 1972;10(1):19–22. https://doi.org/10.1038/sc.1972.4

39. Chang E, Ghosh N, Yanni D, Lee S, Alexandru D, Mozaffar T. A review of spasticity treatments: pharmacological and interventional approaches. *Crit Rev Phys Rehabil Med.* 2013;25(1–2):11–22. https://doi.org/10.1615/CritRevPhysRehabilMed.2013007945

40. Tizanidine--Drug Summary. 2022. https://www.pdr.net/drug-summary/Tizanidine -tizanidine-3138

41. Clonidine hydrochloride--Drug Summary. Accessed 2022, https://www.pdr.net/ drug-summary/Catapres-clonidine-hydrochloride-1744

42. Gruenthal M, Mueller M, Olson WL, Priebe MM, Sherwood AM, Olson WH. Gabapentin for the treatment of spasticity in patients with spinal cord injury. *Spinal Cord.* 1997;35(10):686–9. https://doi.org/10.1038/sj.sc.3100481

43. Mueller ME, Gruenthal M, Olson WL, Olson WH. Gabapentin for relief of upper motor neuron symptoms in multiple sclerosis. *Arch Phys Med Rehabil.* 1997;78(5):521–4. https://doi.org/10.1016/s0003-9993(97)90168-4.

44. Gabapentin - Drug Summary. Prescribers' digital reference. http://www.pdr.net/ drug-summary/Neurontin-gabapentin-2477.4218 Accessed April 8, 2017.

45. Nance PW. A comparison of clonidine, cyproheptadine and baclofen in spastic spinal cord injured patients. *J Am Paraplegia Soc.* 1994;17(3):150–156. https://doi.org/10.108 0/01952307.1994.11735927

46. Petro DJ, Ellenberger C Jr. Treatment of human spasticity with delta 9-tet-rahydrocannabinol. *J Clin Pharmacol.* 1981;21(S1):413S-416S. https://doi. org/10.1002/j.1552-4604.1981.tb02621.x

47. Hagenbach U, Luz S, Ghafoor N, et al. The treatment of spasticity with delta9-tetra-hydrocannabinol in persons with spinal cord injury. *Spinal Cord.* 2007;45(8):551–62. https://doi.org/10.1038/sj.sc.3101982

48. Lucas CJ, Galettis P, Schneider J. The pharmacokinetics and the pharmacodynamics of cannabinoids. *Br J Clin Pharmacol.* 2018;84(11):2477–2482. https://doi.org/10.1111/ bcp.13710

49. Ozcakir S, Sivrioglu K. Botulinum toxin in poststroke spasticity. *Clin Med Res.* 2007;5(2): 132–138. https://doi.org/10.3121/cmr.2007.716

50. Walker HW, Lee MY, Bahroo LB, Hedera P, Charles D. Botulinum toxin injection tech-niques for the management of adult spasticity. *PM R.* 2015;7(4):417–427. https://doi. org/10.1016/j.pmrj.2014.09.021

51. Botox (onabotulinumtoxinA) package insert. AbbVie, Inc. 2022.

52. Lechner HE, Feldhaus S, Gudmundsen L, et al. The short-term effect of hippother-apy on spasticity in patients with spinal cord injury. *Spinal Cord.* 2003;41(9):502–505. https://doi.org/10.1038/sj.sc.3101492.

53. McIntyre A, Mays R, Mehta S, et al. Examining the effectiveness of intrathecal baclofen on spasticity in individuals with chronic spinal cord injury: a systematic review. *J Spinal Cord Med.* 2014;37(1):11–18. https://doi.org/10.1179/2045772313Y.0000000102

54. Khurana SR, Garg DS. Spasticity and the use of intrathecal baclofen in patients with spinal cord injury. *Phys Med Rehabil Clin N Am.* 2014;25(3):655–69. https://doi. org/10.1016/j.pmr.2014.04.008

55. Brennan PM, Whittle IR. Intrathecal baclofen therapy for neurological disorders: a sound knowledge base but many challenges remain. *Br J Neurosurg.* 2008;22(4): 508–519. https://doi.org/10.1080/02688690802233364

56. Penn RD, Kroin JS. Continuous intrathecal baclofen for severe spasticity. *Lancet.* 1985;2(8447):125–127. https://doi.org/10.1016/s0140-6736(85)90228-4

57. Heetla HW, Staal MJ, Proost JH, van Laar T. Clinical relevance of pharmacological and physiological data in intrathecal baclofen therapy. *Arch Phys Med Rehabil.* 2014;95(11):2199–206. https://doi.org/10.1016/j.apmr.2014.04.030

58. Grabb PA, Guin-Renfroe S, Meythaler JM. Midthoracic catheter tip placement for intrathecal baclofen administration in children with quadriparetic spasticity. *Neurosurgery.* 1999;45(4):833–836;discussion 836–837. https://doi.org/10.1097/00006123-199910000-00020

59. Vender JR, Hester S, Waller JL, Rekito A, Lee MR. Identification and management of intrathecal baclofen pump complications: a comparison of pediatric and adult patients. *J Neurosurg.* 2006;104(1 Suppl):9–15. https://doi.org/10.3171/ped.2006.104.1.9

60. Burns AS, Meythaler JM. Intrathecal baclofen in tetraplegia of spinal origin: efficacy for upper extremity hypertonia. *Spinal Cord.* 2001;39(8):413–419. https://doi.org/10.1038/sj.sc.3101178

61. Elovic E. Principles of pharmaceutical management of spastic hypertonia. *Phys Med Rehabil Clin N Am.* 2001;12(4):793–816, vii.

62. Botte MJ, Abrams RA, Bodine-Fowler SC. Treatment of acquired muscle spasticity using phenol peripheral nerve blocks. *Orthopedics.* 1995;18(2):151–159. https://doi.org/10.3928/0147-7447-19950201-14.

63. Chua KS, Kong KH. Alcohol neurolysis of the sciatic nerve in the treatment of hemiplegic knee flexor spasticity: clinical outcomes. *Arch Phys Med Rehabil.* 2000;81(10): 1432–1435. https://doi.org/10.1053/apmr.2000.9395

64. Zafonte RD, Munin MC. Phenol and alcohol blocks for the treatment of spasticity. *Phys Med Rehabil Clin N Am.* 2001;12(4):817–832, vii.

65. Khalili AA, Betts HB. Peripheral nerve block with phenol in the management of spasticity. Indications and complications. *JAMA.* 1967;200(13):1155–1157.

66. Spira R. Management of spasticity in cerebral palsied children by peripheral nerve block with phenol. *Dev Med Child Neurol.* r 1971;13(2):164–173. https://doi.org/10.1111/j.1469-8749.1971.tb03241.x

67. Moritz U. Phenol block of peripheral nerves. *Scand J Rehabil Med.* 1973;5(4):160–163.

68. Tapia Perez JH. Spinal cord stimulation: beyond pain management. *Neurologia (Engl Ed).* 2019;S0213–4853(19)30089–1. https://doi.org/10.1016/j.nrl.2019.05.009

69. Nagel SJ, Wilson S, Johnson MD, et al. Spinal cord stimulation for spasticity: historical approaches, current status, and future directions. *Neuromodulation.* 2017;20(4):307–321. https://doi.org/10.1111/ner.12591

70. Chambers HG. The surgical treatment of spasticity. *Muscle Nerve Suppl.* 1997;6:S121–S128.

71. Dietz V, Sinkjaer T. Spastic movement disorder: impaired reflex function and altered muscle mechanics. *Lancet Neurol.* 2007;6(8):725–733. https://doi.org/10.1016/S1474-4422(07)70193-X

72. Gracies JM. Pathophysiology of spastic paresis. I: Paresis and soft tissue changes. *Muscle Nerve.* 2005;31(5):535–551. https://doi.org/10.1002/mus.20284

18 Poststroke Spasticity

Jacob B. Jeffers, Harsha Ayyala, and Mary E. Russell

INTRODUCTION

The prevalence of spasticity following stroke is most frequently reported between 17% to 49%.[1-3] Varying prevalence reported in the literature may be due to different definitions or assessment measures utilized for evaluation. Given spasticity is a relatively common complication of stroke associated with functional deficits, pain, and decreased quality of life (QOL), it is very important for clinicians to identify and treat.

In addition to defining poststroke spasticity, it is important to consider recovery patterns. The Brunnstrom stages (Table 18.1) describe a typical recovery pattern following stroke, including the evolution of spasticity. The stages are a continuum from initial flaccid presentation, through emergence and increasing spasticity, to decreasing spasticity and resolution.[4] It is important to note that most patients will not return to "normal" function without spasticity and recovery may cease in any of the stages.

ASSESSMENT

Assessment of poststroke spasticity is multifaceted and multiple clinical tools have been developed to improve inter-rater reliability. Commonly, responses to passive movement are measured by ordinal scales such as Modified Ashworth Scale (MAS) and Tardieu Scale.[5-8] However, it has been noted that individual rater interpretation may affect objectivity of these scales; in addition, Ashworth Scale (AS) does not appear to measure neural components to spasticity that contributes to passive resistance.[9-15] Other assessment tools include combinations of electromyography (EMG) and torque; however, limitations such as equipment and specialized training are required for these procedures.[16,17]

A recent systematic review assessed 40 articles describing 15 different clinical tools for quality of study including reliability and validity.[5] In addition to AS, Tardieu Scales, force/torque, and EMG, electrophysiological testing explored the use of tonic stretch reflex threshold (TSRT) with the use of a wrist rig measuring muscle stretches at various speeds.[18,19] The knee pendulum test has also been used at elbow flexors with an accessory apparatus to assess stiffness, threshold angle, viscosity, and dampening ratio.[20] Multi-item scales such as Tone Assessment Scale (TAS) combined resting posture, ordinal measurements with MAS, and response to active efforts to identify associated reactions.[21] In addition, tone categorization (spastic, flaccid, normal) was used with Visual Analog Scale (VAS) as a 100-mm vertical mechanism to anchor points at highest and lowest muscle tone.[22] Lastly, this comprehensive review

Table 18.1 Brunnstrom Stages of Recovery

Stage	Description
1	Flaccid paralysis
2	Emergence of synergy patterns and spasticity
3	Voluntary synergy movements with movement across joints, increasing spasticity
4	Voluntary movements outside of synergy patterns, decreasing spasticity
5	Developing control of individual or isolated movements, decreasing spasticity
6	Return to near-normal motor control, spasticity nearly resolved

examined the Ankle Plantar Flexors Tone Scale (APTS), which assessed plantar flexor resistance of passive movement, middle range resistance, and final range of resistance on an ordinal scale.[23]

In examining the validity and quality of these studies, it was noted that the ability to discriminate between affected and unaffected sides was preserved; however, there was less clinically useful ability to discriminate between different levels of spasticity.[5] In addition, reliability was reported using intra-class correlation coefficient (ICC) for ordinal data such as MAS although more appropriate scales such as kappa statistic account for inherent heterogeneity.[24,25] Overall, while these clinical measures have been vital to poststroke spasticity assessment, further assessment tools should be considered to improve validity and reliability.

DIAGNOSTIC APPROACH

The diagnosis of spasticity following stroke is typically made during the physical examination utilizing the techniques discussed within the assessment section. Often, patients will have a medical history of stroke prior to the emergence of spasticity; however, it is possible that a patient did not receive medical care at the time of the stroke. In this case, additional workup would be necessary to establish etiology of spasticity. This would include a thorough history and physical examination. Depending on the information obtained, additional workup would likely include imaging of the brain and/or spinal cord. Other potential diagnostic tests include but may not be limited to EMG, EEG, serology (blood, CSF), and genetic testing. The focus for the remainder of this section will be on the diagnostic approach of spasticity in patients after stroke.

After suffering a stroke, the time to onset of spasticity is variable among patients. In a retrospective, observational study of patients with first-ever stroke complicated by poststroke spasticity (PSS), median time to emergence of poststroke spasticity defined as an MAS ≥1 was 34 days.[26] Approximately half of patients who developed spasticity were diagnosed in the first month after stroke; however, another quarter of patients were not diagnosed until after 2 months after stroke.[26] Several other studies suggest that spasticity onset occurs prior to this time, but the general consensus is that it occurs in most patients in the first month after stroke.[27–29] Close follow-up with serial physical examinations, especially in patients with paresis, may be necessary to aid in the diagnosis. Paresis is a precondition for spasticity, as it is seen in all patients with poststroke spasticity. Presence of paresis itself is not a predictor of spasticity; however, increasing severity of paresis correlates with increased poststroke spasticity incidence.[30,31] Reduced motor function and spasticity in the early phase (<4 weeks after stroke) is a predictor of severe spasticity.[32] In addition, worse functional impairment utilizing clinical assessments such as Barthel Index (BI), Modified Rankin Scale (mRS), and Mini Mental Status Examination is shown to be a significant predictor of PSS.[00]

Review of imaging obtained at the time of a stroke can also be of value. Lesions involving the motor network areas (precentral gyrus, parapyramidal tract, internal capsule, and basal ganglia) is also a precondition for PSS. Larger volume lesions in these areas are associated with increased risk of PSS, while pure cortical lesions do not appear to have a risk of PSS.[33] Another risk factor is hemorrhagic stroke; however, it remains unclear whether it is an independent risk factor.[31] Rather, this may be a result of the basal ganglia and internal capsule being commonly involved in hemorrhagic strokes.

Although the diagnosis is typically made at the bedside during physical examination, several have stated their concern regarding the validity of typically used scales such as the MAS and Tardieu Scale given its subjective nature.[34-36] Therefore, the argument can be made to supplement the physical examination with more objective measures. Utilization of ultrasound (US) is expanding given its increasing availability and cheaper cost compared to other advanced imaging techniques such as MRI. Some US techniques utilized to assess patients with after stroke spasticity include evaluation of pixel intensity of grayscale imaging and elastography (US strain imaging and shear wave elastography).[37] Spastic muscle appears more echogenic and have higher pixel intensity.[37,38] An added utility of the technique is the ability to evaluate for patients who will respond well to certain treatments. Patients with higher echogenicity tend to respond less favorably to botulinum toxin.[39]

EMG has also been used, largely in the laboratory setting and as a technique for injection guidance. Other techniques include advanced imaging with MRI and magnetic resonance elastography (MRE) of the extremities; however, these are not routinely used.

TREATMENT OPTIONS

The treatment of PSS often requires a multimodal approach with both pharmacologic and nonpharmacologic management. Nonpharmacologic management includes prevention and removal of noxious stimuli as well as rehabilitation techniques. It is common to see worsening of spasticity in the presence of noxious stimuli (i.e., infections, wounds, inadequate bowel and bladder management). It is important to address these issues directly, and patients may temporarily need additional pharmacologic treatment depending on severity of spasticity. There are also many rehabilitation techniques including but not limited to stretching, casting, orthoses, functional electrical stimulation (FES), US, vibration, and thermotherapy.[40]

The benefit of pharmacologic management for spasticity after stroke has been established although mechanisms of action are still being explored. While some medications act on neurotransmitters or neuromodulators within the central nervous system (CNS), other drugs appear to affect the peripheral neuromuscular sites.[41] In addition, these medications may reduce stretch reflexes but have not consistently demonstrated benefit in reducing after stroke disability.[42]

1) **Diazepam:** As a long-active benzodiazepine and originally developed for anxiety, it has been used for spasticity management although more commonly in spinal

cord injuries (SCIs) or cerebral palsy (CP) versus hemiplegia. It acts by increasing gamma-aminobutyric acid (GABA), an inhibitory neurotransmitter that acts at CNS synapses,[43] specifically at a system known as the GABA–benzodiazepine–chloride ion channel complex.[44] It is well absorbed through the gastrointestinal tract and binds to both the brainstem reticular formation (greater impact) and spinal polysynaptic pathways[45]; this results in inhibition at the GABA-B receptors by increasing potassium efflux from CNS neurons.[46] Dosage is initiated at 2 mg during the day or 5 mg at bedtime that can be increased to 10 mg with a maximum dosage of 60 mg/day.[41]

It has a half-life of 20 to 80 hours and effects can be seen within 15 to 45 minutes. Due to depressive CNS effects, it can produce fatigue and drowsiness at higher dosages to manage spasticity.[41] In two double-blind, placebo-controlled studies, the effects of diazepam were noted on spasticity.[47,48] In the first study, 6 to 15 mg/day of diazepam was administered and decreased grip force was noted, but no decrease in leg spasticity or range of motion (ROM) was noted.[47] In the second study, diazepam decreased spasticity specifically in the knee (measured by passive ROM) but reduced ambulation speed potentially due to improvement in motor control or quality of gait.[48]

2) **Dantrolene:** As a peripherally acting muscle relaxant, it alters the chemistry of muscle contraction by acting directly on skeletal muscle cells at the muscle fiber. Specifically, it interferes with the release of calcium from the sarcoplasmic reticulum and reduces muscle contractility.[49] It can cause generalized muscle weakness due to nonspecific action; however, it does not have active effects on the CNS. One of the main side effects is hepatotoxicity, requiring frequent liver function tests (LFTs).[50] For spasticity secondary to cerebral causes, dantrolene has shown reduction of resistance to passive ROM, clonus, and deep tendon reflexes in addition to activities of daily living (ADLs) in double-blinded, placebo-controlled trials.[51] However, it was noted to also produce weakness with a decline in gross motor performance by muscle force and stair climbing.[51] Dosage is usually started at 25 mg that can be increased to 100 mg 2 to 4 times per day with maximal dosage of 400 mg.[41,46,50]

3) **Baclofen:** As both an oral and implantable drug, baclofen acts on GABA-B receptors and increases inhibition both presynaptically and postsynaptically.[52] It causes hyperpolarization of the membrane and limits influx of calcium into the presynaptic terminal, therefore reducing release of excitatory endogenous transmitters.[40] It also decreases the activation of alpha motor neuron through either presynaptic inhibition of excitatory neurons or postsynaptic inhibition directly on the alpha motor neuron.[46] Oral administration can be limited due to systemic side effects including drowsiness, confusion, headache, and lethargy; there is also limited ability to cross the blood–brain barrier.[53] It is recommended to start dosing at 5 mg three times a day that can be increased by 15 mg/day increments at 3-day intervals with a maximum dosing of 80 mg/day.[46]

It has been used intrathecally by administering directly into the subarachnoid space of CNS via implantation of a programmable pump device. Therefore, a constant and continuous dosage can be administered in patients who do not benefit or tolerate baclofen in the oral dose form.[44] Fewer systemic side effects are noted although surgical complications such as wound healing, catheter dislocation, or pump malfunction may occur.[54] Overdose can result in respiratory depression, decreased cardiac function, or coma while withdrawal can be caused by abrupt cessation of drug administration.[55] Intrathecal baclofen pump (ITB) therapy in patients with after stroke spasticity has demonstrated functional improvement in 60% to 70% of studies.[56] A recent case series of 10 subjects showed that ITB administration improved walking speed, functional mobility ratings, and spasticity without significant impact on motor force in uninvolved extremities.[54] In another study, it was found that gait kinematics in patients with spastic hemiplegia improved with increased knee extension and ankle flexion 4 hours after initiating ITB therapy; in addition, MAS scores decreased in quadriceps femoris and triceps muscle with improved maximum walking speed.[57]

4) **Tizanidine:** As a centrally acting alpha-2 adrenergic agonist, tizanidine has both presynaptic and postsynaptic inhibition that are found in the brain and spinal cord. It increases presynaptic inhibition of excitatory spinal interneurons and decreases the amount of excitatory neurotransmitter release onto postsynaptic alpha motor neurons.[58] It has less cardiovascular side effects compared to clonidine (similarly acting) although it has been noted to cause dizziness, sedation, and dry mouth.[46] A double-blinded study of patients with after stroke spasticity found functional improvement in ambulation distance.[59] In addition, it has been shown to reduce spasticity measured by MAS, pain intensity, and QOL scores.[60] It has been noted that 13 out of 47 subjects in this study discontinued due to side effects although it has a more favorable side effect profile over oral baclofen and diazepam.[59,61] Dosage is initiated from 2 to 4 mg at bedtime and can be increased by 2 to 4 mg every 2 to 4 days with most efficacy at 4 to 8 mg three times a day. Maximum dosage is recommended at 36 mg/day.[41,62] Peak effect occurs approximately after 2 hours with a half-life of 2.5 hours.[63]

5) **Clonidine:** As a centrally acting medication that targets alpha-2 adrenergic receptors on the brainstem, it has been used mostly as an antihypertensive.[46] Similar to tizanidine, clonidine has been less used in spasticity due to its cardiovascular side effects.[46]

As previously discussed, oral medication use is often limited by adverse side effects. Therefore, focal treatment options such as botulinum neurotoxin and neurolysis should be considered. There have been several recent consensus articles and individual trials to support the use of botulinum toxin injections in the treatment of various diagnoses resulting in focal spasticity.[40] Botulinum toxin injections in the management of PSS has led to improvement in function[64] and prevention of complications of PSS such as contractures.[65] In addition, botulinum toxin use has been shown to be superior to tizanidine both in efficacy and safety.[66] Ultimately, an individualized approach for each patient should be utilized. A recent comprehensive overview of treatment with botulinum toxin within a multidisciplinary context utilizing adjunctive therapies was published.[67]

Phenol and ethanol neurolysis are additional effective interventions in the management of PSS. Compared to botulinum toxin, these options are less frequently utilized and studied.[68] This in part may be due to concern of side effects; however, these have been shown to be reduced with advanced guidance techniques such as US and electrical stimulation (e-stim). In one retrospective study with 293 procedures performed, reported sided effects included pain in 4.0%, swelling in 2.7%, and dysesthesia in 0.7%.[69] There have been limited studies to compare the efficacy of botulinum toxin versus phenol, but the results suggest similar or better results with phenol.[70,71]

Intrathecal baclofen is another option that some have considered underutilized in the treatment of PSS.[72] Some considerations into why that might be includes fear of surgical and device complications, weakness, worsening gait, and limited improvement in QOL.[72] Weighing the potential risks of a surgical procedure as well as device- and medication-related complications is important to consider. Several studies, however, provide evidence that would dispute some of these concerns. For instance, although it is not uncommon to see unmasking of weakness in the affected side during test doses, weakness was not seen in the unaffected sides of patients with spastic hemiparesis being treated with ITB.[73,74] This allows for a strengthening program to be implemented in the patient's therapy plan. In addition, improvements rather than worsening in gait have been seen in many patients.[53,73] It appears those with faster baseline walking speeds may benefit most, while those with slower baseline walking speeds may depend on increased tone for support and therefore have worsening of gait.[75] Lastly, the SISTERS trial has recently reported improvement in spasticity, pain, QOL, and patient satisfaction with ITB treatment for PSS.[76,77]

Alternatively, there are some newer treatment options emerging in the management of PSS that are reviewed as follows:

Repetitive Transcranial Magnetic Stimulation (rTMS)

This noninvasive technique has been commonly used after stroke by inducing cortical excitability at stimulation site and trans-synaptically at distant areas using either high-frequency or low-frequency modes.[78] High-frequency stimulation (>1 Hz) is applied to the affected hemisphere to increase excitability or low-frequency stimulation may be applied to the unaffected hemisphere to reduce excitability and decrease interhemispheric competition.[78] It has also been shown to modulate cortical excitability by affecting alpha motor neurons and changing descending corticospinal projections in both upper and lower limbs.[79,80] In one randomized clinical trial, five consecutive daily sessions of low-frequency rTMS over unaffected LE motor cortex can reduce LE spasticity and improve motor function poststroke for at least 1 week.[78] However, there were no electrophysiological changes on Hoffman reflex (H-reflex) measurements although LE motor performance improved possibly due to more isolated controlled movement with better speed.[78]

Hyaluronidase/Hyaluronan Hypothesis

Based on recent studies, spastic muscles have shown significantly lower tension than non-spastic muscles supporting the role of extracellular matrix (ECM) in spasticity.[81] The hyaluronan hypothesis proposed that muscle fiber atrophy after upper motor neuron (UMN) injury in the context of paresis leads to relative increase in proportion of ECM that could be occupied by hyaluronan. In addition, hyaluronan aggregate (high concentrations of hyaluronan and protein-crosslinked) increased viscoelasticity of ECM while reducing gliding movement and increasing muscle stiffness.[81] Addressing this complex intracellular signal transduction involved in nociception and inflammation may be a potential target for spasticity management by introducing the role of hyaluronidase.[82] A recent retrospective case series showed that injections of hyaluronidase into upper limb muscles not only decreased muscle stiffness and increased passive movement but also increased active movement.[81]

Hyperselective Neurectomy

Hyperselective neurectomy involves resection of part of nerve fascicles compared to neurotomy (complete section of nerve trunk). It has become a standard procedure in the lower limb, but not widely popular yet in the upper limb.[83] By following each motor ramus until its entry point into the target muscles, this procedure aims at improving selectivity and duration of results.[84] For patients with significant Poststroke spasticity, hyperselective neurectomy has been proposed to manage spastic muscles, reduce development of muscle or joint contracture, and reinforce paralyzed muscles.[85] A prospective study between 2012 and 2019 examined upper limb spasticity secondary to stroke as well as TBI, brain neoplasms, and congenital causes treated with hyperselective neurectomy.[83] It was found that there was significant improvement in resting position and AS and Tardieu Scale of elbow flexors, pronator teres, and wrist flexors. In addition, this study did not show any significant difference when comparing different joints apart from a significant increase in strength in antagonist muscles at the level of the forearm (WE).[83]

Selective Dorsal Rhizotomy

Selective dorsal rhizotomy (SDR) has been explored as a surgical procedure in refractory spasticity; it involves dissecting specific nerve rootlets and monitoring muscular responses to e-stim. Nerve rootlets that were considered "abnormal" with clonic or bilateral responses were then sectioned accordingly.[86] SDR has been performed for both upper and lower limbs, in particular in the cervical and lumbar levels. One study showed improvement in MAS scores from 3 to 1 in shoulder adduction, abduction, and extension and MAS scores from 2 to 1 in the elbow after cervical SDR at C5 to C7 levels.[86] In addition, two cases have been reported of unilateral selective posterior rhizotomy (SPR) to reduce spasticity and improve pain and ADLs. Both patients had unilateral lower extremity pain and spasticity secondary to cerebral infarctions; they underwent unilateral SPR on the spastic side with resulting improvement in pain and ADLs (one patient).[87]

Electro Shock Wave Therapy

Electro shock wave therapy (ESWT) therapy uses single, highly energetic, biphasic acoustic impulses directly into tissues without affecting global destruction.[88] It has been shown to promote activation of molecular and immunological reactions by improving blood microcirculation, stimulating angiogenesis, and increasing neurovascularization.[88] Two types of ESWT generators have been developed: focused ESWT (fESWT) and unfocused radial ESWT (rESWT). Studies have shown unambiguous and statistically significant improvement in both reduction of spasticity and relaxation of muscles studies, enhancement in ROM, and larger angle degrees in joints. However, no statistically significant differences between fESWT and rESWT was noted.[88]

COMPLICATIONS

If left untreated, PSS can lead to many complications. Increased spasticity alone can be a source of pain.[89] Untreated spasticity can lead to contracture of joints, skin breakdown, and pressure ulcers. Spasticity can lead to inability to perform ADLs, can interfere with mobility, and can cause an increased risk of fall. Caregiver burden can increase in the setting of untreated spasticity.[90]

CASE REPORT (◙VIDEO 18.1)

 Video 18.1 can be accessed via the QR code or on Springer Publishing Connect™: https://connect.springerpub.com/content/book/978-0-8261 -3975-7/part/part04/chapter/ch18

CT is a 42-year-old right hand dominant man with symptomatic severe calcific aortic stenosis who underwent percutaneous cutaneous intervention and was discharged home. At home, he started having headaches, left-sided facial droop, left-sided weakness, and confusion. EMS was called and he was brought to the hospital where a CT scan was consistent with large right intracranial hemorrhage and seizure activity prior to coming to the hospital. Neurosurgery was consulted and the patient underwent craniotomy with evacuation of intraparenchymal hematoma. Patient was premorbidly independent and working. He underwent acute inpatient rehabilitation, followed by intense outpatient rehabilitation. While in outpatient therapy, patient began to develop left-sided spasticity. He was referred to spasticity clinic for management where patient underwent phenol and botulinum toxin injections to the left upper and lower extremities. His tone was consistent with a flexor synergy pattern and injections were performed to the elbow flexors, wrist flexors, and gastrocsoleus complex. He is modified independent currently with walking stick and ankle foot orthosis.

REFERENCES

1. Sommerfeld DK, Gripenstedt U, Welmer AK. Spasticity after stroke: an overview of prevalence, test instruments, and treatments. *Am J Phys Med Rehabil.* 2012;91(9): 814–820. https://doi.org/10.1097/PHM.0b013e31825f13a3

2. Opheim A, Danielsson A, Alt Murphy M, et al. Upper-limb spasticity during the first year after stroke: stroke arm longitudinal study at the University of Gothenburg. *Am J Phys Med Rehabil.* 2014;93(10):884–886. https://doi.org/10.1097/PHM.0b013e31825f13a3

3. Dorňák T, Justanová M, Konvalinková R, et al. Prevalence and evolution of spasticity in patients suffering from first-ever stroke with carotid origin: a prospective, longitudinal study. *Eur J Neurol.* 2019;26(6):880–886. https://doi.org/10.1111/ene.13902

4. Brunnstrom S. Motor testing procedures in hemiplegia: based on sequential recovery stages. *Phys Ther.* 1966;46(4):357–75. https://doi.org/10.1093/ptj/46.4.357

5. Aloraini S, Gaverth J, Yeung E, et al. Assessment of spasticity after stroke using clinical measures: a systematic review. *Disabil Rehabil.* 2015;37(25):2313–2323. https://doi.org/10.3109/09638288.2015.1014933

6. Van Wijck FM, Pandyan AD, Johnson GR, et al. Assessing motor deficits in neurological rehabilitation: patterns of instrument usage. *Neurorehabil Neural Repair.* 2001;15(1):23–30. https://doi.org/10.1177/154596830101500104

7. Alhusaini AA, Dean CM, Crosbie J, et al. Evaluation of spasticity in children with cerebral palsy using Ashworth and Tardieu Scales compared with laboratory measures. *J Child Neurol.* 2010;25(10):1242–7. 13. https://doi.org/10.1177/0883073810362266

8. Thibaut A, Chatelle C, Ziegler E, et al. Spasticity after stroke: physiology, assessment and treatment. *Brain Inj.* 2013;27(10):1093–105. https://doi.org/10.3109/02699052.2013.804202

9. Ashworth B. Preliminary trial of carisoprodol in multiple sclerosis. *Practitioner.* 1964;192:540–2.

10. Bohannon RW, Smith MB. Interrater reliability of a modified Ashworth scale of muscle spasticity. *Phys Ther.* 1987;67(2):206–7. https://doi.org/10.1093/ptj/67.2.206

11. Boyd RN, Graham HK. Objective measurement of clinical findings in the use of botulinum toxin type A for the management of children with cerebral palsy. *Eur J Neurol.* 1999;6:S23–35.

12. Haugh AB, Pandyan AD, Johnson GR. A systematic review of the Tardieu scale for the measurement of spasticity. *Disabil Rehabil.* 2006;28(15):899–907. https://doi.org/10.1080/09638280500404305

13. Held JP, Pierrot-Deseilligny E. *Reeducation Mortrice Des Affections Neurologiques*. Paris: Baillie`re; 1969.

14. Pandyan AD, Johnson GR, Price CIM, et al. A review of the properties and limitations of the Ashworth and modified Ashworth Scales as measures of spasticity. *Clin Rehabil*. 1999;13(5):373–83. https://doi.org/10.1191/026921599677595404

15. Tardieu G, Shentoub S, Delarue R. A la recherche d'une technique de measure de la spasticite. *Rev Neurol (Paris)*. 1954;91:143–144.

16. Voerman GE, Gregoric M, Hermens HJ. Neurophysiological methods for the assessment of spasticity: the Hoffman reflex, the tendon reflex, and the stretch reflex. *Disabil Rehabil*. 2005;27(1-2):33–68. https://doi.org/10.1080/09638280400014600

17. Wood DE, Burridge JH, van Wijck FM, et al. Biomechanical approaches applied to the lower and upper limb for the measurement of spasticity: a systematic review of the literature. *Disabil Rehabil*. 2005;27(1-2):19–32. https://doi.org/10.1080/09638280400014683

18. Calota A, Feldman AG, Levin MF. Spasticity measurement based on tonic stretch reflex threshold in stroke using a portable device. *Clin Neurophysiol*. 2008;119(10):2329–37. https://doi.org/10.1016/j.clinph.2008.07.215

19. Kim KS, Seo JH, Song CG. Portable measurement system for the objective evaluation of the spasticity of hemiplegic patients based on the tonic stretch reflex threshold. *Med Eng Phys*. 2011;33(1):62–9. https://doi.org/10.1016/j.medengphy.2010.09.002

20. Lin CC, Ju MS, Lin CW. The pendulum test for evaluating spasticity of the elbow joint. *Arch Phys Med Rehubil*. 2003;84(1):69–74. https://doi.org/10.1053/apmr.2003.50066

21. Barnes S, Gregson J, Leathley M, et al. Development and inter-rater reliability of an assessment tool for measuring muscle tone in people with hemiplegia after a stroke. *Physiotherapy*. 1999;85(8):405–9.

22. Pomeroy VM, Dean D, Sykes L, et al. The unreliability of clinical measures of muscle tone: implications for stroke therapy. *Age Ageing*. 2000;29(3):229–33. https://doi.org/10.1093/ageing/29.3.229

23. Takeuchi N, Kuwabara T, Usuda S. Development and evaluation of a new measure for muscle tone of ankle plantar flexors: the ankle plantar flexors tone scale. *Arch Phys Med Rehabil*. 2009;90(12):2054–61. https://doi.org/10.1016/j.apmr.2009.08.141

24. Atkinson G, Nevill AM. Statistical methods for assessing measurement error (reliability) in variables relevant to sports medicine. *Sports Med*. 1998;26(4):217–38. https://doi.org/10.2165/00007256-199826040-00002

25. Brennan P, Silman A. Statistical methods for assessing observer variability in clinical measures. *BMJ*. 1992;304(6840):1491–4. https://doi.org/10.1136/bmj.304.6840.1491

26. Nam K, Lim S, Kim J, et al. When does spasticity in the upper limb develop after a first stroke? A nationwide observational study on 861 stroke patients. *J Clin Neurosci*.2019;66:144–8. https://doi.org/10.1016/j.jocn.2019.04.034

27. Opheim A, Danielsson A, Alt Murphy M, et al. Upper-limb spasticity during the first year after stroke: stroke arm longitudinal study at the University of Gothenburg. *Am J Phys Med Rehabil*. 2014;93(10):884–96. https://doi.org/10.1097/PHM.0000000000000157

28. Wissel J, Schelosky LD, Scott J, et al. Early development of spasticity following stroke: a prospective, observational trial. *J Neurol*. 2010;257(7):1067–72. https://doi.org/10.1007/s00415-010-5463-1

29. Sommerfeld DK, Eek EU, Svensson AK, et al. Spasticity after stroke: its occurrence and association with motor impairments and activity limitations. *Stroke*. 2004;35(1):134–9. https://doi.org/10.1161/01.STR.0000105386.05173.5E

30. Glaess-Leistner S, Ri SJ, Audebert HJ, et al. Early clinical predictors of post stroke spasticity. *Top Stroke Rehabil.* 2021;28(7):508–518. https://doi.org/10.1080/10749357.2 020.1843845.

31. Zeng H, Chen J, Guo Y, et al. Prevalence and risk factors for spasticity after stroke: a systematic review and meta-analysis. *Front Neurol.* 2021;11:616097. https://doi. org/10.3389/fneur.2020.616097

32. Sunnerhagen KS, Opheim A, Murphy MA. Onset, time course and prediction of spasticity after stroke or traumatic brain injury. *Ann Phys Rehabil Med.* 2019;62(6):431–434. https://doi.org/10.3389/fneur.2020.616097

33. Ri S, Glaess-Leistner S, Wissel J. Early brain imaging predictors of Poststroke spasticity. *J Rehabil Med.* 2021;53(3):jrm00169. https://doi.org/10.2340/16501977-2803

34. Balci BP. Spasticity measurement. *Noro Psikiyatr Ars.* 2018;55(suppl 1):S49–S53. https://doi.org/10.29399/npa.23339

35. Fleuren JFM, Voerman GE, Erren-Wolters CV, et al. Stop using the Ashworth Scale for the assessment of spasticity. *J Neurol Neurosurg Psychiatry.* 2010;81(1):46–53. https:// doi.org/10.1136/jnnp.2009.177071

36. Malhotra S, Pandyan AD, Day CR, et al. Spasticity, an impairment that is poorly defined and poorly measured. *Clin Rehabil.* 2009;23(7):651–658. https://doi. org/10.1177/0269215508101747

37. Tran A, Gao J. Quantitative ultrasound to assess skeletal muscles in post stroke spasticity. *J Cent Nerv Syst Dis.* 2021;13:1179573521996141. https://doi.org/10.1177/1179573521996141

38. Wu CH, Ho YC, Hsiao MY, et al. Evaluation of Poststroke spastic muscle stiffness using shear wave ultrasound elastography. *Ultrasound Med Biol.* 2017 ;43(6): 1105–1111. https://doi.org/10.1016/j.ultrasmedbio.2016.12.008. Epub 2017 Mar 9. PMID: 28285729.

39. Picelli A, Bonetti P, Fontana C, et al. Is spastic muscle echo intensity related to the response to botulinum toxin type A in patients with stroke? A cohort study. *Arch Phys Med Rehabil.* 932012;93(7):1253–1258. https://doi.org/10.1016/j.apmr.2012.02.005

40. Francisco GE, McGuire JR. Poststroke spasticity management. *Stroke.* 2012;43(11): 3132–3136. https://doi.org/10.1161/STROKEAHA.111.639831

41. Gracies JM, Nance P, Elovic E, et al. Traditional pharmacological treatments for spasticity, part II: general and regional treatments. *Muscle Nerve.* Suppl. 1997;6:S92–S120.

42. Davidoff RA. Antispasticity drugs: mechanisms of action. *Ann Neurol.* 1985;17(2): 107–116. https://doi.org/10.1002/ana.410170202

43. Tallman JF, Gallager DW. The GABA-ergic system: a locus of benzodiazepine action. *Annu Rev Neurosci.* 1985;8:21–44. https://doi.org/10.1146/annurev.ne.08.030185.000321

44. Gallichio JE. Pharmacologic management of spasticity following stroke. *Phys Ther.* 2004;84(10):973–981.

45. Tseng TC, Wang SC. Locus of action of centrally acting muscle relaxants, diazepam and tybamate. *J Pharmacol Exp Ther.* 1971;178(2):350–360.

46. Ciccone CD. *Pharmacology in Rehabilitation.* 3rd ed. Philadelphia, Pa: FA Davis Co; 2002.

47. Cocchiarella A, Downey JA, Darling RC. Evaluation of the effect of diazepam on spasticity. *Arch Phys Med Rehabil.* 1967;48(8):393–396.

48. Kendall H. The use of diazepam in hemiplegia. *Ann Phys Med.* 1964;7:225–228.

49. Young RR, Delwaide PJ. Drug therapy: spasticity (first of 2 parts). *N Engl J Med.* 1981;304:28–33. https://doi.org/10.1056/NEJM198101013040107.

50. Ward A, Chaffman MO, Sorkin EM. Dantrolene: a review of its pharmacodynamic and pharmacokinetic properties and therapeutic use in malignant hyperthermia, the neuroleptic malignant syndrome and an update of its use in muscle spasticity. *Drugs.* 1986;32(2):130–168. https://doi.org/10.2165/00003495-198632020-00003

51. Chyatte SB, Birdsong JH, Bergman BA. The effects of dantrolene sodium on spasticity and motor performance in hemiplegia. *South Med J.* 1971;64(2):180 185. https://doi. org/10.1097/00007611-197102000-00011

52. Al-Khodairy AT, Vuagnat H, Uebelhart D. Symptoms of recurrent intrathecal baclofen withdrawal resulting from drug delivery failure: a case report. *Am J Phys Med Rehabil.* 1999;78(3):272–277. https://doi.org/10.1097/00002060-199905000-00018

53. Francisco GE, Boake C. Improvement in walking speed in poststroke spastic hemiplegia after intrathecal baclofen therapy: a preliminary study. *Arch Phys Med Rehabil.* 2003;84(8):1194–1199. https://doi.org/10.1016/s0003-9993(03)00134-5

54. Levin AB, Sperling KB. Complications associated with infusion pumps implanted for spasticity. *Stereotact Funct Neurosurg.* 1995; 65(1–4):147–151. https://doi.org/10.1159/000098887

55. Peng CT, Ger J, Yang CC, et al. Prolonged severe withdrawal symptoms after acute-on-chronic baclofen overdose. *J Toxicol Clin Toxicol.* 1998;36(4):359–363. https://doi.org/10.3109/15563659809028033

56. Campbell SK, Almeida GL, Penn RD, et al. The effects of intrathecally administered baclofen on function in patients with spasticity. *Phys Ther.* 1995;75(5):352–362. https://doi.org/10.1093/ptj/75.5.352

57. Remy-Neris O, Tiffreau V, Bouilland S, et al. Intrathecal baclofen in subjects with spastic hemiplegia: assessment of the antispastic effect during gait. *Arch Phys Med Rehabil.* 2003;84(5):643–650. https://doi.org/10.1016/s0003-9993(02)04906-7

58. Milanov I, Georgiev D. Mechanisms of tizanidine action on spasticity. *Acta Neurol Scand.* 1994;89(4):274–279. https://doi.org/10.1111/j.1600-0404.1994.tb01680.x

59. Bes A, Eyssette M, Pierrot-Deseilligny E, et al. A multi-centre, double-blind trial of tizanidine, a new antispastic agent, in spasticity associated with hemiplegia. *Curr Med Res Opin.* 1988;10(10):709–718. https://doi.org/10.1185/03007998809111122

60. Gelber DA, Good DC, Dromerick A, et al. Open-label dose-titration safety and efficacy study of tizanidine hydrochloride in the treatment of spasticity associated with chronic stroke. *Stroke.* 2001;32(8):1841–1846. https://doi.org/10.1161/01.str.32.8.1841

61. Medici M, Pebet M, Ciblis D. A double-blind, long-term study of tizanidine ("Sirdalud") in spasticity due to cerebrovascular lesions. *Curr Med Res Opin.* 1989;11(6):398–407. https://doi.org/10.1185/03007998909110141

62. Emre M, Leslie GC, Muir C, et al. Correlations between dose, plasma concentrations, and antispastic action of tizanidine (Sirdalud). *J Neurol Neurosurg Psychiatry.* 1994;57(11):1355–1359. https://doi.org/10.1136/jnnp.57.11.1355

63. Shellenberger MK, Groves L, Shah J, et al. A controlled pharmacokinetic evaluation of tizanidine and baclofen at steady state. *Drug Metab Dispos.* 1999;27(2):201–204.

64. Cardoso E, Pedreira G, Prazeres A, et al. Does botulinum toxin improve the function of the patient with spasticity after stroke? *Arq Neuropsiquiatr.* 2007;65(3A):592–595. https://doi.org/10.1590/s0004-282x2007000400008

65. Lindsay C, Ispoglou S, Helliwell B, et al. Can the early use of botulinum toxin in post stroke spasticity reduce contracture development? A randomised controlled trial. *Clin. Rehabil.* 2021;35(3):399–409. https://doi.org/10.1177/0269215520963855

66. Simpson DM, Gracies JM, Yablon SA, et al. Botulinum neurotoxin versus tizanidine in upper limb spasticity: a placebo-controlled study. *J Neurol Neurosurg Psychiatry.* 2009;80(4):380–385. https://doi.org/10.1136/jnnp.2008.159657

67. Francisco GE, Balbert A, Bavikatte G, et al. A practical guide to optimizing the benefits of Poststroke spasticity interventions with botulinum toxin a: an international group consensus. *J Rehabil Med.* 2021;53(1):jrm00134. https://doi.org/10.2340/16501977-2753

68. Li S, Francisco GE. Current concepts in assessment and management of spasticity. In: Wilson R, Raghavan P, eds. *Stroke Rehabi.* St. Louis, MO: Elsevier. 2019; 133–54. http://doi.org/10.1016/B978-0-323-55381-0.00010-X

69. Karri J, Zhang B, Li S. Phenol neurolysis for management of focal spasticity in the distal upper extremity. *PM R.* 2020;12(3):246–50. https://doi.org/10.1002/pmrj.12217

70. Kirazli Y, On AY, Kismali B, et al. Comparison of phenol block and botulinus toxin type a in the treatment of spastic foot after stroke: a randomized, double-blind trial. *Am J Phys Med Rehabil.* 1998;77(6):510–5. https://doi.org/10.1097/00002060-199811000-00012

71. Manca M, Merlo A, Ferraresi G, et al. Botulinum toxin type a versus phenol. a clinical and neurophysiological study in the treatment of ankle clonus. *Eur J Phys Rehabil Med.* 2010;46(1):11–8.

72. Dvorak EM, Ketchum NC, McGuire JR. The underutilization of intrathecal baclofen in poststroke spasticity. *Top Stroke Rehabil.* 2011;18(3):195–202. https://doi.org/10.1310/tsr1803-195

73. Meythaler JM, Guin-Renfroe S, Brunner RC, et al. Intrathecal baclofen for spastic hypertonia from stroke. *Stroke.* 2001;32(9):2099–109. https://doi.org/10.1161/hs0901.095682

74. Ivanhoe CB, Francisco GE, McGuire JR, et al. Intrathecal baclofen management of poststroke spastic hypertonia: implications for function and quality of life. *Arch Phys Med Rehabil.* 2006;87(11):1509–15. https://doi.org/10.1016/j.apmr.2006.08.323

75. Horn TS, Yablon SA, Stokic DS. Effect of intrathecal baclofen bolus injection on temporospatial gait characteristics in patients with acquired brain injury. *Arch Phys Med Rehabil.* 2005;86(6):1127–1133. https://doi.org/10.1016/j.apmr.2004.11.013

76. Creamer M, Cloud G, Kossmehl P, et al. Intrathecal baclofen therapy versus conventional medical management for severe poststroke spasticity: results from a multicentre, randomised, controlled, open-label trial (SISTERS). *J Neurol Neurosurg Psychiatry.* 2018;89(6):642–650. https://doi.org/10.1136/jnnp-2017-317021

77. Creamer M, Cloud G, Kossmehl P, et al. Effect of intrathecal baclofen on pain and quality of life in poststroke spasticity. *Stroke.* 2018;49(9):2129-2137. https://doi.org/10.1161/STROKEAHA.118.022255

78. Rastgoo M, Naghdi S, Nakhostin Ansari N, et al. Effects of repetitive transcranial magnetic stimulation on lower extremity spasticity and motor function in stroke patients, *Disabil Rehabil,* 2016;38(19):1918–1926. https://doi.org/10.3109/09638288.2015.1107780

79. Valero-Cabre A, Oliveri M, Gangitano M, et al. Modulation of spinal cord excitability by subthreshold repetitive transcranial magnetic stimulation of the primary motor cortex in humans. *Neuro Rep.* 2001;12(17):3845–3848. https://doi.org/10.1097/00001756-200112040-00048

80. Perez MA, Lungholt BKS, Nielsen JB. Short-term adaptation in spinal cord circuits evoked by repetitive transcranial magnetic stimulation: possible underlying mechanisms. *Exp Brain Res.* 2005;162(2):202–212. https://doi.org/10.1007/s00221-004-2144-2

81. Adam A, Kim S, Stecco A, et al. "Hyaluronan Homeostasis and its Role in Pain and Muscle Stiffness". *PM R*. 2022:14(12):1490–1496. https://doi.org /10.1002/pmrj.12771

82. Raghavan P. "Emerging Therapies for Spastic Movement Disorders". *Phys Med Rehabil Clin N Am*.2018;29(3):633–644. https://doi.org/10.1016/j.pmr.2018.04.004

83. Leclercq C, Perruisseau-Carrier A, Gras M, et al. "Hyperselective neurectomy for the treatment of upper limb spasticity in adults and children. a prospective study". *J Hand Surg Eur Vol*. 2021;46(7):708–716. https://doi.org/10.1177/17531934211027499

84. Leclercq C, Gras M. "Hyperselective neurectomy in the treatment of the spastic upper limb". *Phys Med Rehabil Int*. 2016; 3(1): 1075.

85. Sitthinamsuwan B, Chanvanitkulchai K, Ploypetch L et al. "Surgical outcomes of microsurgical selective peripheral neurotomy for intractable limb spasticity". *StereotactFunct Neurosurg*. 2013;91(4):248–57. https://doi.org/10.1159/000345504

86. Duan Y, Luo X, Gao X, et al. "Cervical selective dorsal rhizotomy for treating spasticity in upper limb neurosurgical way to neurosurgical technique." *Interdisciplinary Neurosurgery*. 2015;2(1):57–60.

87. Fukuhara T, Kamata I. "Selective posterior rhizotomy for painful spasticity in the lower limbs of hemiplegic patients after stroke: report of two cases." *Neurosurgery,* 2004;54(5):1268–1273. https://doi.org/10.1227/01.neu.0000119605.32216.2e

88. Dymarek R, Ptaszkowski K, Ptaszkowska L, et al. Shock waves as a treatment modality for spasticity reduction and recovery improvement in Poststroke adults - current evidence and qualitative systematic review. *Clin Interv Aging*. 2020;15:9–28. https://doi.org/10.2147/CIA.S221032

89. Paolucci S, Iosa M, Toni D, et al. Prevalence and time course of Poststroke pain: a multicenter prospective hospital-based study. *Pain Medicine*. 2016;17(5),924–930. https://doi.org/10.1093/pm/pnv019

90. Zorowitz RD, Gillard PJ, Brainin M. Poststroke spasticity: sequelae and burden on stroke survivors and caregivers. *Neurology*.2013;80(3 Suppl 2):S45-S52. https://doi.org/10.1212/WNL.0b013e3182764c86

19 Brain Injury-Related Spasticity: A Case-Based Approach

Blaise Langan and Katherine Lin

INTRODUCTION

Prevalence of spasticity in traumatic brain injury (TBI) has wide interstudy variance. Prevalence data can be seen as low as 18%[1] and as high as 89%.[2,3] However, sources agree that an increase in severity of TBI is associated with increased likelihood of spasticity.[4]

As is true in all cases of spasticity, in the setting of TBI, treatment goals should be individualized to each patient. Goals should include pain management, improvement in patients' functional goals, and reduction of caregiver burden, among many others. It is important to consider that a complete absence of spasticity can be harmful to some patients. Spasticity can facilitate improved function and accomplishment of tasks. Each treatment modality considered by the clinician should first be seen through the lens of each patient's specific goal. These goals should be thoroughly discussed with the patient (if able), caregivers, and the treatment team prior to treatment initiation and should continue to evolve throughout the disease course. Given that functional prognosis after TBI is often difficult to predict, close observation and follow-up are needed to clarify goals and optimize treatment throughout a patient's life. To demonstrate these principles and best practices in managing patients with TBI, the following case will be utilized throughout this chapter.

ACUTE INPATIENT SETTING

Diagnostic Approach

In the acute phase after brain injury, spasticity is often not seen. However, evaluation prior to the onset of spasticity can give a provider invaluable information as a patient case progresses. The provider should regularly assess for the development of spasticity in order to effectively track symptoms as they arise.

A good assessment of spasticity in any patient, including patients with TBI, starts with a thorough history. In addition to obtaining a good understanding of the initial injury and any subsequent injuries, it is important to understand what muscle groups are most affected by spasticity. One should inquire if there are certain positions or movements that trigger tone and if there are certain times of the day that are more problematic. However, in brain injury, patients often have impaired cognition, arousal, or other communication challenges. This can make obtaining a thorough history from the patient difficult or impossible. In these circumstances, thorough chart review and obtaining history from collateral historians is vital. Without a true sense of the patient's social situation, one cannot fully form adequate goals for spasticity management.

Initial assessment in TBI spasticity can vary widely based on patient presentation and should incorporate a cognitive assessment. The widely accepted cornerstone of the physical examination is the Glasgow Coma Scale (GCS). Other important areas of emphasis include pupillary size, symmetry, and responsiveness; motor examination, including the evaluation of possible posturing; cranial nerve function; and deep tendon reflexes. Serial physical examinations throughout a patient's acute inpatient stay are of critical importance. Any decline in the patient's mental status or changes in physical exam should be assumed to indicate a worsening in the patient's brain injury and should produce an immediate response for further assessment and therapeutic interventions. Additionally, factors such as new fractures, heterotopic ossification, and hydrocephalus must be considered and ruled out as possible sources of increased spasticity if it arises.

Often in the initial stages after injury, patients are receiving numerous procedures or medication changes that could affect their tone.

It is important in these early stages and beyond to view the patient in a wholistic manner. The practitioner should consider all possible sources of pain, including the spasticity itself, that could be contributing to an acute increase in tone. In disorders of consciousness, pain assessments can be very difficult; however, the Nociceptive Coma Scale (NCS)[5] can be used in order to provide objective data about pain perception. This scale showed good inter-rater reliability and good concurrent validity compared to NIPS, FLACC, CNPI, and PAINAD scales. Given many patients with TBIs cannot effectively communicate, painful stimuli may present as agitation, sleep cycle disruptions, dysautonomia, increased tone, and slowed recovery from disorders of consciousness.

As is true for most facets of TBI, the effect of anesthetics and other medications on spasticity has not been well studied and can vary widely from patient to patient. Overall, it can be said that general anesthesia has the effect of slightly reducing tone; however, the added nociceptive stimulus of surgical intervention of any kind can increase spasticity. Likewise, one should consider possible sources of tone reduction such as oral medications. Many patients after TBI are receiving one if not multiple medications that could unintentionally mask the development of spasticity, and these include but are not limited to neuroparalytics, opioids, and benzodiazepines. A thorough medication review must be performed prior to each examination in order to determine what factors might be influencing the practitioner's physical exam findings.

In addition to the factors listed above, patients may also have concomitant polytrauma injuries or mobility precautions that could impair the physical exam. For example, foot and ankle fractures may preclude full evaluation of the lower extremity. Nevertheless, serial joint-by-joint assessments of range of motion (ROM) should be performed with preservation of ROM being a primary goal of treatment at this critical stage.

For a further discussion on physical exam maneuvers and techniques involved in spasticity evaluation, please refer to Chapter 4, Measurements and Scales.

Treatment Options

After a thorough history and physical exam, treatment options can be considered. In determining treatment options for spasticity in TBI, it can be difficult to obtain sufficient, high-quality evidence to support individual treatment options over others. The vast majority of evidence regarding this topic is limited secondary to small sample sizes and patients with TBI often representing only a small portion of the total study participants. However, it is clear that spasticity management is of vital importance both in the acute and chronic phases of TBI. As in all forms of spasticity management, a functional approach to treatment is necessary in order to achieve individualized patient goals. Reduction in spasticity can allow for a fuller ROM resulting in a decreased need for physical assistance from others and assistive devices. Effective spasticity management can also decrease caregiver burden by allowing patients to be more easily positioned for dressing, bathing, and grooming.

Optimizing patient function to participate in daily activities and reducing allostatic load via pain management are of vital importance. However, this must also be balanced with the preservation of cognitive function and progression given spasticity treatment methods can negatively impact cognition. It is also vital that the practitioner considers individual-specific functions that are desired by the patient and family.

Nonpharmacologic Treatment Modalities
In this acute inpatient rehab setting, providers are allotted a wide range of treatment options as many resources are available and follow-up is close. Let us first consider nonpharmacologic modalities.

Splinting
In the acute setting, providers should involve occupational therapists and prosthetists early in a patient's course to obtain or create effective orthoses to aid in prevention of contractures and maintenance of neutral joint positioning. This can be accomplished through a variety of techniques including active and/or passive ranging of joints multiple times a day, splinting, and casting. All three of these techniques aim to provide a period stretch whether transient or prolonged. There is limited evidence to support the benefit of active and passive ROM stretching[6]; however, casting has been shown to increase joint ROM and reduce spasticity.[7] Attention must be given to monitoring for pain, skin breakdown, and other adverse side effects when implementing these techniques.

Physiotherapy
The Bobath,[8,9] Brunnstrom,[10] and Car and Shepherd[11] methods have been shown to effectively treat spasticity. Cryotherapy to spastic muscles has been shown to provide a 35° improvement in ROM.[12] Electrical stimulation (E-stim) has been shown to reduce spasticity in patients recovering from a stroke, and this could be extrapolated to patients with brain injury.[13] A myriad of other modalities including ultrasound have been used to treat spasticity; however, there is very limited evidence for their use.[14] Physiotherapy is the standard of care for all patients in the acute inpatient rehab setting, but close monitoring is still necessary given patients with brain injury may have limited ability to communicate and/or sense when a certain modality is causing harm.

Pharmacologic Treatment Modalities
Oral Medications
If an oral medication is needed, baclofen is the most widely used. However, there are no comparative studies of oral medications in the TBI population. Below is a

description of four of the most common medications used to treat spasticity.[15] Although there are many other medications that could be used, they will not be discussed in this chapter.

Baclofen: A GABA-B receptor agonist that inhibits the release of excitatory neurotransmitters at the presynaptic neuromuscular junction. Dosing should start with 5 mg 3 times per day and increase by 5 mg every 3 to 5 days with a maximum dose of 80 mg per day.

Tizanidine: An alpha-2 adrenergic receptor agonist that indiscriminately targets supraspinal and intraspinal regions. Dosing should start with 2 to 4 mg per day and can be increased to a maximum dose of 36 mg per day, usually separated over three doses.

Diazepam: A GABA-A agonist that results in presynaptic inhibition of stretch reflexes. Dosing should start with 2 mg BID and can be titrated to a maximum dose of 60 mg per day if needed. It is important to note that diazepam has a half-life of approximately 30 hours.

Dantrolene: An inhibitor on calcium ion release from the sarcoplasmic reticulum. Dosing should start at 25 mg per day and titration can progress to a maximum dose of 400 mg per day. Of note, dantrolene is peripherally acting and thus avoids the cognitive effects of other antispasmodics.

CHRONIC OUTPATIENT SETTING

Diagnostic Approach

Many challenges that are seen in the acute inpatient setting continue into the outpatient setting. Impaired cognition and communication continue to prove significant throughout outpatient follow-up; however, through utilization of caregiver and family reports, the impact of these challenges can be lessened. In addition, through routine follow-up, practitioners can observe long-term changes not appreciated during acute hospitalization. The importance of practitioners maintaining thorough, accurate, and objective documentation cannot be understated. In order to make direct comparisons across time periods of months between follow-ups, one cannot rely on memory alone to make clinical observations.

During the physical exam, the examiner should thoroughly assess ROM paying special attention to velocity-dependent changes in tone. Physical exam findings can be interpreted using scales such as the Ashworth Scale (AS), the Modified Ashworth Scale (MAS), and/or Tardieu Scale. The principal limitation of clinical scales such as MAS and Tardieu is reliability and inter-examiner reproducibility.[16] Despite their limitations, the MAS and Tardieu Scale can provide a practical and inexpensive way to measure spasticity that requires little to no equipment. These scales can give the examiner a rough idea of how effective treatments have been in reducing spasticity. Ultimately, spasticity treatment should focus on the patient's ability to regain function and improve quality of life (QOL), which may not always correlate with objective findings.

There are settings, however, in which having a more precise method to measure spasticity would be important, with research and development of new treatments being a prime example. In order to demonstrate the superiority of one treatment over another, the developer will need to be able to collect reliable data and use that data to demonstrate clinical significance. Single-channel surface electromyography (sEMG) is one such method that is widely used in the research setting. It has proven to be effective in measuring muscle activity intensity and activity pattern in patients with spasticity. This method is noninvasive, convenient, and low cost, which has led to it being widely used in the clinical setting as well.[17]

Another method of objectively quantifying spasticity is using the pendulum test to measure and calculate the resistance of passive joint movement. The swing of the limb can be evaluated using an isokinetic dynamometer. One limitation to this method is it does not differentiate between the neural component and nonneural components of spasticity such as changes in viscoelastic properties of the muscle. However, this limitation can be mitigated if the examiner incorporates a measurement of the resistance to passive movement as slow passive movement is primarily affected by the nonneural component.[16]

Treatment Options

Although all treatment options discussed in this chapter can be applied to both inpatient and outpatient settings, the methods below are most often seen in an outpatient setting given delayed onset of action or having failed prior therapy as a prerequisite for initiation.

Botulinum Toxin Injection

Botulinum toxin injection is discussed in detail in several other chapters in this text. Specifically in the brain injury population, botulinum toxin injection can be very effective given its lack of systemic effects that could impair cognition and long-lasting effects in many patients. However, limitations include delayed onset of action, need for repeated injections throughout a patient's life, and high cost.

Intrathecal Baclofen Pump Management

Intrathecal baclofen (ITB) can be effective in managing spasticity, especially lower extremity spasticity when oral agents have produced undesired effects or have been discontinued secondary to intolerable side effects. For more information regarding baclofen pump management, please see Chapter 12; however, there are specific considerations to make for individuals with TBI. There has been limited evidence suggesting an increased risk of complications occurring in those with concurrent implantation of both an ITB pump and a ventriculoperitoneal shunt.[18] ITB has been used in several studies to treat dysautonomia, and as such, one must be cautious when decreasing intrathecal dosing that symptoms of dysautonomia do not increase or reappear.[19] In addition, the importance of caregiver education surrounding baclofen withdrawal and overdose is paramount when patient cognition has been impaired by their injury.

Nerve Blocks

Nerve blocks can provide temporary or sustained spasticity management by reducing or eliminating the neural input responsible for the spasticity. Practitioners should target motor-only branches of nerves using a variable intensity stimulator as targeting combined sensory and motor nerves can result in dysesthesias. Lidocaine or bupivacaine can result in blocks lasting 1 to 6 hours. Phenol or ethanol can result in blocks lasting 3 to 9 months.[15]

Surgical Treatment

If spasticity is refractory to the above treatments, orthopedic and neurosurgical procedures can be considered. Tendon lengthening, muscle transposition, neurotomy, and rhizotomy, among many others, could be considered by a surgical team. As in all treatment modalities, surgical intervention should always be aimed at accomplishing functional goals specific to the individual patient.

COMPLICATIONS

Oral Medications

Baclofen: Side effects include sedation, hallucinations, convulsions, rigidity, lowered seizure threshold, and severe withdrawal symptoms if medication is discontinued abruptly.

Tizanidine: Side effects include sedation, asthenia, hallucinations, convulsions, and rigidity. There is a low incidence of hepatic dysfunction and rare cases of hepatic failure.[20]

Diazepam: Side effects include dampened cognition, sedation, drowsiness, memory impairment, and weakness.

Dantrolene: Side effects include gastrointestinal intolerance, sedation, and hepatotoxicity that necessitates monitoring of liver function tests (LFTs) at a regular interval.

Botulinum Toxin Injections

Side effects include muscular weakness, distant spread of effect, and dysphagia.

Intrathecal Baclofen Pump

Complications include risk of surgery, device malfunction, catheter malfunction, baclofen overdose, and baclofen withdrawal.

Nerve Blocks

Side effects include weakness, injection site pain, phlebitis, central nervous system (CNS) and cardiovascular compromise, phenol nerve fibrosis, and dysesthesias.

CASE REPORT

Ms. J is a 58-year-old female with a past medical history of hypertension, diabetes mellitus type 2, and chronic kidney disease stage 2 who was the only passenger in a single-car motor vehicle collision. She was unresponsive at the scene of the incident and was airlifted to the closest hospital. Patient was found to have a depressed skull fracture over the left frontal bone, diffuse axonal injury, kidney laceration, right humerus and scaphoid fractures, and many fractures in the left foot and ankle. The patient is stabilized in the trauma bay and admitted to the intensive care unit for further evaluation.

She has been through multiple early surgical interventions and a revision at the end of her second week of hospitalization. Craniectomy was performed on day 1 of hospitalization with open reduction and internal fixation of the right scaphoid and left foot and ankle the following day. Revision of the right scaphoid fixation was performed on day 13 after injury. On initial examination, the patient was found to have no increased tone, but by day 11, she had begun to develop mild tone in all four extremities with symptoms subtly worse on the left than right. However, spasticity was considerably worse following fixation revision.

At the time of evaluation, she is minimally conscious and is actively developing increased spasticity in her left greater than right extremities. At this time, the goals of treatment should be aimed at preserving ROM, reducing pain, and removing barriers to increased arousal. Complicating factors include right scaphoid fracture that has been internally fixed and placed in a fixed splint and exacerbation of chronic kidney disease due to kidney trauma.

Ms. J has been stabilized in the acute hospital and has been transitioned to an acute rehabilitation unit. She is minimally conscious and has developed profound left-sided spasticity with generalized flexor tone of the upper extremity (MAS 2 in finger, wrist, and elbow flexors and shoulder adductors) and milder tone in the left lower extremity (MAS 1 in knee flexors and hip flexors). Her only family support remains her elderly mother who has been at bedside throughout her admission. Ms. J has flexion withdrawal with facial expression startle response to painful stimuli, but no eye movement or vocal response.

For Ms. J, physiotherapy was initiated while in the acute hospital but was furthered in the acute rehab setting. This included an emphasis on Bobath method-directed physical and occupational therapy. In addition, she received a customized resting hand splint from in-house orthotists. Patient remained in a CAM boot for much of her inpatient stay, but custom AFO was fitted to prevent ankle contracture upon its removal.

Ms. J was initiated on baclofen 5 mg three times daily during her acute inpatient hospitalization. This was subsequently titrated to 10 mg three times daily. During her acute rehabilitation stay, she emerged from her minimally conscious state. At that time, it was determined that she would be weaned off baclofen in order to judge the effect, if any, it could be having on her cognition. Ms. J showed a marked improvement in her cognition over the next week, but spasticity also slightly increased. At that time, a discussion was had with the patient's family in order to determine whether baclofen should be resumed. For this patient, the goal of improved cognition outweighed the goal of decreased spasticity. Patient remained off oral spasticity medications and treatment of her tone shifted to more localized treatment in order to preserve cognitive function. These treatment modalities began during her inpatient stay and continued throughout her outpatient course.

Ms. J was discharged from acute rehabilitation 6 weeks after her admission and 2 months after the initial injury. Follow-up was scheduled for the patient to be seen in a neurologic rehabilitation clinic 2 weeks after her discharge and she was subsequently seen every 3 months. On initial presentation to the clinic, patient was able to interact with the treatment team through yes/no answers to simple questions. The patient's mother and cousin functioned as the sole caregivers to the patient. Ms. J's spasticity had diminished slightly in the left upper and lower extremities since her inpatient stay.

For Ms. J, botulinum toxin injections began in the last week of her inpatient stay with mild improvement in spasticity seen at her first follow-up visit. However, her spasticity continued to make caretaking challenging, especially in hygiene tasks. Ms. J also stated that hygiene tasks caused her pain. After discussion with the patient, family members, and treatment team, the decision was made to trial increased dosing of botulinum toxin at her next clinic visit. Over the course of several treatments at 3-month intervals, optimal dosing was found to manage spasticity.

Over 1 year after her injury, Ms. J underwent surgical tendon lengthening in her left upper extremity in order to relieve pain and aid in ease of bathing, grooming, and dressing. She continues to be seen in the neurologic rehabilitation clinic on a regular basis for botulinum toxin injections and continues to be satisfied with her spasticity care.

REFERENCES

1. Nakase-Richardson R, McNamee S, Howe LL, et al. Descriptive characteristics and rehabilitation outcomes in active duty military personnel and veterans with disorders of consciousness with combat- and noncombat-related brain injury. *Arch Phys Med Rehabil.* 2013 ;94(10):1861–9. https://doi.org/10.1016/j.apmr.2013.05.027. Epub 2013 Jun 26. PMID: 23810353.

2. Thibaut FA, Chatelle C, Wannez S, et al. Spasticity in disorders of consciousness: a behavioral study. *Eur J Phys Rehabil Med.* 2015;51(4):389–97. Epub 2014 Nov 6. PMID: 25375186.

3. Martens G, Laureys S, Thibaut A. Spasticity management in disorders of consciousness. *Brain Sci.* 2017;7(12):162. https://doi.org/10.3390/brainsci7120162

4. Ganesh S, Guernon A, Chalcraft L, et al. Medical comorbidities in disorders of consciousness patients and their association with functional outcomes. *Arch Phys Med Rehabil.* 2013;94(10):1899–907. https://doi.org/10.1016/j.apmr.2012.12.026. Epub 2013 Jun 2. PMID: 23735521.

5. Caroline Schnakers, Camille Chatelle, Audrey Vanhaudenhuyse, Steve Majerus, Didier Ledoux, Melanie Boly, Marie-Aurélie Bruno, Pierre Boveroux, Athena Demertzi, Gustave Moonen, Steven Laureys, The Nociception Coma Scale: A new tool to assess nociception in disorders of consciousness, PAIN, Volume 148, Issue 2, 2010, Pages 215–219, ISSN 0304-3959, https://doi.org/10.1016/j.pain.2009.09.028.

6. Thibaut A, Deltombe T, Wannez S, et al. Impact of soft splints on upper limb spasticity in chronic patients with disorders of consciousness: a randomized, single-blind, controlled trial. *Brain Inj.* 2015;29(7–8):830–6. https://doi.org/10.3109/02699052.2015.100 5132. Epub 2015 Apr 27. PMID: 25915721.

7. Leung J, King C, Fereday S. Effectiveness of a programme comprising serial casting, botulinum toxin, splinting and motor training for contracture management: a randomized controlled trial. *Clin Rehabil.* 2019;33(6):1035–1044. https://doi.org/10.1177/0269215519831337. Epub 2019 Feb 27. PMID: 30813776.

8. Abradimene. *Bobath Evolutionary Treatment. Brazilian Association for the Development and Dissemination of the Bobath Concept 2017.* (Online). http://www.abradimene.org.br/bobath.asp. Accessed March 23, 2022.

9. Alcântara CB, Costa CMB, Lacerda HS. *Neuroevolutionary Treatment-Bobath Concept.* 2014. (Online). http://www.bobath.com.br/wpcontent/uploads/2014/08/Curycap-20.pdf. Accessed March 23, 2022.

10. Freitas E. *Practical Manual for Upper Limb Motor Re-Education in Hemiplegia: Based on the Brunnstrom Method.* São Paulo: Memnon; 2000:20.

11. Carr J, Shepherd, R. The changing face of neurological rehabilitation. *Brazilian J Physiother.* 2006;10(2):147–156.

12. Kaplan M. Upper motor neuron syndrome and spasticity. In: Nesathurai S, ed. *The Rehabilitation of People with Spinal Cord Injury.* Whitinsville, MA: AAP; 2003:75–80.

13. Oo W. Efficacy of addition of transcutaneous electrical nerve stimulation to standardized physical therapy in subacute spinal spasticity: a randomized controlled trail. *Arch Phys Med Rehabil.* 2014;95(11):2013–2020. https://doi.org/10.1016/j.apmr.2014.06.001

14. dos Santos Silva Borges C, Rodrigues Neto G. Therapeutic exercise protocols in patients with traumatic brain injury: a systematic review. *J Exerc Physiol*. 2020;23(2):71–82. https://www.asep.org/asep/asep/JEPonlineAPRIL2020_Borges.pdf

15. Zollman FS, Iaccarino MA, Bhatnagar S, Zafonte R. Spasticity in traumatic brain injury. In: *Manual of Traumatic Brain Injury: Assessment and Management* (pp. 400–407). essay, Demos Medical Publishing; 2016.

16. Aloraini SM, Gäverth J, Yeung E, MacKay-Lyons M. Assessment of spasticity after stroke using clinical measures: a systematic review. *Disabil Rehabil*. 2015;37(25):2313–23. https://doi.org/10.3109/09638288.2015.1014933. Epub 2015 Feb 18. PMID: 25690684.

17. Luo Z, Lo WLA, Bian R, Wong S, Li L. Advanced quantitative estimation methods for spasticity: a literature review. *J Int Med Res*. 2020;48(3):300060519888425. https://doi.org/10.1177/0300060519888425. Epub 2019 Dec 4. PMID: 31801402; PMCID: PMC7607521.

18. Pucks-Faes E, Dobesberger J, Halbmayer LM, Hitzenberger G, Matzak H, Saltuari L. Complications after dual placement of a baclofen pump and ventricular shunt in individuals with severe brain injury. *Arch Rehabil Res Clin Transl*. 2020;2(4):100082. https://doi.org/10.1016/j.arrct.2020.100082. ISSN 2590-1095

19. Cuny E, Richer E, Castel JP. (2001) Dysautonomia syndrome in the acute recovery phase after traumatic brain injury: relief with intrathecal Baclofen therapy, *Brain Inj*. 2001;15(10):917–925. https://doi.org/10.1080/02699050110065277

20. *LiverTox: Clinical and Research Information on Drug-Induced Liver Injury* [Internet]. Bethesda (MD): National Institute of Diabetes and Digestive and Kidney Diseases; 2012-. Tizanidine. Updated January 30, 2017. https://www.ncbi.nlm.nih.gov/books/NBK548048

20 Upper Limb Spasticity With Botulinum Neurotoxin

Matthew David Wilhelm, Faiza Khan Humayun, and Marissa McCarthy

INTRODUCTION

In the upper limb, chemodenervation is primarily used to decrease muscle tone in elbow flexors, wrist flexors, finger flexors, and thumb flexors. Understanding the etiology of spasticity is essential for patient evaluation in the context of their larger disease process. Upper extremity hypertonicity is commonly encountered following stroke. Upper limb spasticity may also affect patients with multiple sclerosis (MS), chronic childhood encephalopathy, adult cerebral palsy (CP), amyotrophic lateral sclerosis, spinal cord injury (SCI), traumatic brain injury (TBI), anoxic encephalopathy, and basal ganglia disease.[1] The upper limb is most frequently in a position of adduction and internal rotation at the shoulder, elbow flexion, wrist flexion, wrist pronation, and finger flexion. Thus, the muscles most frequently targeted for chemodenervation include the biceps brachii, brachioradialis, brachialis, pronator teres, flexor carpi radialis (FCR), flexor carpi ulnaris (FCU), flexor digitorum superficialis (FDS), flexor digitorum profundus (FDP), flexor pollicis longus (FPL), and adductor pollicis.

Spasticity in the upper extremity can have wide ranging negative impact on a person's quality of life (QOL). The clinical assessment of spasticity is based on quantifying the degree of increased muscle tone and its effect on pain, function, hygiene, or positioning. Physical exam is necessary to differentiate spasticity from contracture as a fixed deformity cannot be treated with botulinum toxin (BoNT). The skin should be inspected for pressure wounds and intertriginous breakdown. Functional limitations are measured using the Barthel Index (BI) for activities of daily living (ADLs) performance and the Functional Independence Measure (FIM) for severity of overall disability. Additionally, there are several clinical tests for the upper limbs: nine-hole peg test, Frenchay Arm Test, Fugl–Meyer Assessment, Action Research Arm Test, and robotic evaluation devices. These methods are often utilized by occupational therapists for further documentation of functional impairments. A thorough patient assessment must include identification of spasticity-related barriers to social participation, employment, fulfilment of family roles, and performance of daily tasks.

The Modified Ashworth Scale (MAS) is the most widely used instrument for grading spasticity with high inter-rater reliability and reproducibility, which is described elsewhere. Other evaluation methods include the Tardieu Scale, Spasm Frequency Scale, electromyography (EMG) testing with H-reflex, and biomechanical measurements with goniometry, also described elsewhere.

DIAGNOSTIC APPROACH

Diagnosis of spasticity begins with a thorough history and physical examination. Medical history should identify the primary etiology of upper motor neuron (UMN) pathology as well as the chronicity of increased muscle tone. The five most common causes of spasticity are stroke, MS, TBI, SCI, and adult CP.[2] Patients and caregivers should be questioned on current symptoms, functional limitations, pain level, care needs, and treatment goals. Response to prior treatments with oral antispasticity medications, rehabilitation techniques, physical modalities, or nerve blocks should also be documented.

Physical Examination

Physical exam is focused on quantifying the severity of spasticity in involved muscles while also identifying possible complications and coexisting impairments. Physical exam should be performed with full exposure of the involved limb. The MAS is the most utilized clinical tool for measurement of spasticity. While examining the patient, spasticity should be differentiated from weakness, soft tissue contractures, dystonia, and synergistic limb patterns that may be associated with upper motor neuron syndromes (UMNSs). Skin should be inspected for breakdown or decubitus ulcers. Figure 20.1 illustrates seven common patterns seen in patients with upper limb spasticity as described by Simpson et al.[3]

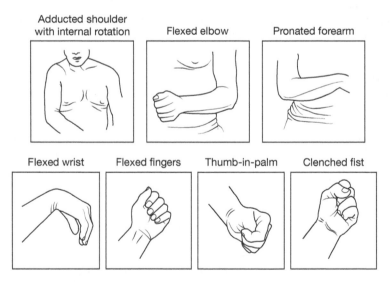

Figure 20.1 Common postures of upper limb spasticity.

Source: From Simpson DM, Patel AT, Alfaro A, et al. Onabotulinumtoxina injection for poststroke upper-limb spasticity; guidance for early injectors from a delphi panel process. PM & R. 2017;9(2):136-148. https://doi.org/10.1016/j.pmrj.2016.06.016

Goal Setting

Realistic treatment goals must be established prior to initiation of rehabilitation therapies, interventional procedures, or prescription of oral medications. In treating upper extremity spasticity, both passive and active goals may be identified.

Table 20.1 Treatment Goals for Upper Limb Spasticity
Improved positioning and orthotic fit
Decreased pain and spasms
Decreased nursing or caregiver burden
Improved axillary and palmar hygiene
Contracture prevention
Improved grasp and release
Improved overhead activities
Reduced time and effort to perform activities of daily living

Use of oral antispasticity medications is often limited by systemic complications of cognitive decline, hypotension, drug–drug interactions, or end organ toxicity. Rehabilitation techniques are valuable in augmenting function but do not alter underlying pathologic muscle contraction. Chemical neurolysis with phenol or alcohol denatures proteins in nerve axons and membranes leading to denervation of muscle fibers.[4] Nerve blocks are best used in pure motor nerves due to potential for postinjection dysesthesias in mixed motor sensory nerves. Botulinum neurotoxins are advantageous in their localized and targeted treatment of muscles affected by spasticity.

Therapeutic benefit from chemodenervation is optimized when BoNT is injected at the muscle motor points. There are several methods utilized to increase the accuracy of toxin delivery. The most common localization techniques include anatomic palpation, EMG guidance, sonographic guidance, and electrical stimulation (e-stim). Surface anatomic guidance is least precise and reliable. Anatomic landmarks may be obscured by adipose tissue, contractures, or muscle atrophy. Deeper muscles are particularly difficult to isolate through this method. EMG guidance allows the practitioner to visualize or auscultate motor unit action potentials (MUAPs) and thus better target the motor end plate. Unfortunately, this method is not specific to individual muscles and is limited by the patient's ability to activate muscle contractions. Ultrasound (US) guidance is a painless method to isolate both superficial and deep muscles but is dependent on practitioner skill and experience. E-stim is performed by advancing the needle tip into the desired muscle and injecting BoNT once contraction is observed in the selected muscle. This is often a painful and time-consuming process that also requires adequate training. Ultimately, anatomic localization for BoNT delivery will depend on practitioner training, available equipment, and patient-specific factors.

Response to chemodenervation will vary based on specific formulation, muscle selection, dosage, and individual patient factors. Postinjection rehabilitation techniques can assist with maximizing gains through restoration of biomechanics, improved motor control, and facilitation of augmented function. Patients should return for a 4- to 6-week follow-up evaluation to assess for changes in spasticity and achievement of goals. Muscle selection and dosage for subsequent treatment sessions may be adjusted based on the patient's clinical response.

TREATMENT OPTIONS

As upper extremity spasticity varies in degree and severity, treatment options additionally vary in both modality and invasiveness. **Nonpharmacologic, pharmacologic,** and **interventional/surgical options** are available and can be utilized on a case-by-case basis to best suit each patient and their unique, individual needs.

Nonpharmacologic treatments remain within the primary scope of upper extremity spasticity management given their varying efficacies, relatively benign adverse effect profiles, and wide range of modalities.

Physical and/or occupational therapy with a focus on mobilization of the spastic upper extremity remains as first-line management; the cornerstone of which includes passive stretching and limb positioning maneuvers or braces to regulate muscle tone and prevent contractures.[5] Along similar lines, splinting or casting of the upper extremities may benefit passive range of motion (ROM) and stretching, when utilized appropriately and given breaks.

Hydrotherapy, cryotherapy, heat therapy, and electrotherapy may be used in adjuvant therapies on an as-needed basis to provide additional support. These therapies may prove more cumbersome or ineffective if utilized in true contractures.

Novel research has cast light on extracorporeal shock wave therapy (ESWT) as an upcoming, promising, safe modality to reduce spasticity and improve motor function via muscle rheological changes and increasing nitric oxide production, causing neuromuscular dysfunction and decreasing motor neuron excitability.[6,7]

Lastly, reintegration into a daily routine (work, school, extracurriculars, hobbies) are paramount to maintaining function and improving daily QOL.

Pharmacologic options for spasticity treatment are comprised of oral, intrathecal, or intramuscular administrations of systemic or localized medications acting on a number of neuroreceptors and ion channels to reduce muscle tone. Careful titration of medications is advised in order to minimize a myriad of possible adverse effects, including alterations of consciousness, respiratory drive, and changes to intracranial pressure of cerebral oxygenation. These are discussed in detail elsewhere. A table of on-label dosing of BoNTs available to treat upper limb spasticity is included here in Table 20.2.

Interventional or surgical options have been well documented in historical medical text and are increasingly studied and utilized as modern surgical techniques are applied and perfected.

One of the most studied pharmacologic interventions for spasticity, botulinum toxin A (BoNTA), has been proven to be a primary option for focal upper extremity spasticity across many patient populations. BoNTA acts upon the neuromuscular junction by cleaving soluble N-ethylmaleimide-sensitive attachment protein receptor (SNARE) proteins, specifically SNAP-25, at the synaptic cleft, preventing acetylcholine vesicles binding to the intracellular cell membrane leading to an inability of acetylcholine to release. BoNTA is injected directly into the target spastic muscle group, typically utilizing EMG or US guidance.

The classic spastic upper extremity posturing of the flexed elbow, flexed wrist, and clenched hand can be seen in the imbalance of spastic upper extremity flexor muscles unhindered by the weakness of unused upper extremity extensor muscles. Canonically, BoNTA injections into spastic muscles may aid in "rebalancing" the muscular imbalances around the joint, augmenting the rehabilitation process. After injecting upper extremity flexors, strengthening and stretching therapies aimed at upper extremity extensors are more effective and greatly aid in rehabilitation efforts.

Effects of BoNTA injection may take upward to 1 to 4 weeks to take full effect, with effects lasting on average 3 to 6 months in duration. Maintaining a strict regimen with reevaluations prior to injections is recommended to adequately dose patients' and their individual needs and requirements. Keeping considerations for patient

Table 20.2 Principal Patterns of Upper Limb Spasticity, Key Muscles, and Suggested Dosage of OnabotulinumtoxinA, IncobotulinumtoxinA, and AbobotulinumtoxinA

Principal Patterns	Key Muscle Involved	Suggested Dosage of OnabotulinumtoxinA	Suggested Dosage of IncobotulinumtoxinA	Suggested Dosage of AbobotulinumtoxinA
Flexed elbow	Biceps	60–200 units	50–200 units	200–400 units
	Brachialis	30–50 units	25–100 units	200–400 units
	Brachioradialis	45–75 units	25–100 units	100–200 units
Pronated forearm	Pronator teres	15–25 units	25–75 units	100–200 units
	Pronator quadratus	10–50 units	10–50 units	
Wrist flexion	Flexor carpi radialis	12.5–50 units	25–100 units	100–200 units
	Flexor carpi ulnaris	12.5–50 units	25–100 units	100–200 units
Finger flexion/ clenched fist	Flexor digitorum sublimis/ superficialis	30–50 units	25–100 units	100–200 units
	Flexor digitorum profundus	30–50 units	25–100 units	100–200 units
	Lumbricals/interossei	5–10 units each		
Thumb in palm	Flexor pollicis longus	20 units	10–50 units	
	Adductor pollicis	20 units	5–30 units	
	Flexor pollicis brevis/ opponens pollicis	5–25 units	5–30 units	

independence, or for caregivers and their responsibilities for patients' care, is best practice given the far-reaching utility of BoNTA beyond rehabilitation into ADLs.

Selective peripheral neurotomies remain an additional treatment option for severe focal spasticity, refractory to BoNTA injections. Prior to the procedure, preoperative motor blocks that mimic the post-surgical outcome are performed. In the upper extremity, neurotomies of the median and ulnar nerves are indicated for spasticity in the pronators and wrist and finger flexor musculature, while neurotomies of the musculocutaneous nerve is indicated for elbow flexor spasticity.

Dorsal rhizotomies remain nearly entirely limited to patients with CP with spastic diplegia, or global bilateral lower extremity spasticity.

Lastly, as mentioned above, intrathecal baclofen (ITB) therapy remains a routine, valid treatment option for lower extremity spasticity, with limited efficaciousness for upper extremity involvement.

COMPLICATIONS

A myriad of adverse reactions and unwanted side effects exist for the pharmacologic agents previously mentioned. In this section, we focus on intramuscular BoNTA and its inherent complications with administration for spasticity.

Prior to performing an injection of BoNTA for spasticity, an informed consent must be provided and completed between the provider(s) and patient. A general informed consent includes all of the following information regarding the possible reactions and adverse effects of BoNTA injections:

First, the introduction of a needle into the skin and subcutaneous tissues, including fat and muscle, provides opportunities for any number of possible skin or soft tissue infections. The use of "best-as-possible" sterile practices, utilizing antiseptic techniques such as prepping the injection site with alcohol and wearing gloves, is both recommended and expected.

In addition to infection, the risk of bleeding from the injection site can be expected with the puncturing of the skin and advancing of the needle into deeper structures, including the risk of vascular penetration. Pain at the injection site may additionally accompany a routine BoNTA injection. Generally, BoNTA produces strictly local changes to the targeted musculature. However, a black box warning revolving

---

Box 20.1 U.S. Food and Drug Administration

Postmarketing reports indicate that the effects of all BoNT products may spread from the area of injection to produce symptoms consistent with BoNT effects. These may include asthenia, generalized muscle weakness, diplopia, ptosis, dysphagia, dysphonia, dysarthria, urinary incontinence, and breathing difficulties. These symptoms have been reported hours to weeks after injection. Swallowing and breathing difficulties can be life threatening, and there have been reports of death. The risk of symptoms is probably greatest in children treated for spasticity, but symptoms can also occur in adults treated for spasticity and other conditions, particularly in those patients who have an underlying condition that would predispose them to these symptoms. In unapproved uses and in approved indications, cases of spread of effect have been reported at doses comparable to those used to treat cervical dystonia and spasticity and at lower doses.

around BoNTA was released in 2009 under the direction of the US Food and Drug Administration (FDA) following several rare, fatal adverse reactions directly linked to BoNTA injection:

CASE REPORT (◉VIDEO 20.1)

 Video 20.1 can be accessed via the QR code or on Springer Publishing Connect™: https://connect.springerpub.com/content/book/978-0-8261 -3975-7/part/part04/chapter/ch20

A 42-year-old male presents to your clinic with right hemiparesis and spasticity following a left thalamic infarct sustained during a right frontal craniotomy for a large intraventricular tumor concerning for malignancy. The patient underwent extensive inpatient rehabilitation following the injury at his previous home and relocated to your area to establish care. The patient additionally suffers from significant expressive aphasia (Broca's), of which he is receiving outpatient speech therapy on a regular basis.

The patient ambulates to your room independently without use of an assistive device and sits comfortably on the examination table. The patient utilized oral pharmacologics

Table 20.3 Modified Ashworth Scale Ratings for Patient's Associated Musculature in His Right Upper Extremity

Muscle(s)	Modified Ashworth Scale Rating
Right flexor carpi ulnaris	0
Right flexor carpi radialis	0
Right flexor digitorum profundis	0
Right flexor digitorum superficialis	2
Right triceps	0
Right biceps brachii	1
Right lumbricals (four)	2
Right adductor pollicis	2
Right flexor pollicis longus	0

for his upper extremity spasticity in the past; however, he has required BoNTA injections recently for effective management. He endorses past tightness in his wrist flexion and elbow extension, but during this visit, he endorses tightness in his biceps and fingers. The patient's most recent injection was 3 months ago, and he notes that 2 to 3 weeks after a series of injections, he received roughly 8 to 12 weeks of therapeutic benefit. On examination, you determine the following muscle groups and their respective ratings on the MAS:[8]

The patient was subsequently consented for chemodenervation of the right upper extremity using BoNTA; the risks and benefits of the procedure were explained to the patient with a time-out, performed immediately prior to the start of the procedure.

Benefits discussed included, but were not limited to, decreased muscle tightness, increased ROM, and decreased pain. Risks discussed included, but were not limited to, pain and discomfort, bleeding, bruising, excessive weakness, venous thrombosis, and muscle atrophy.

Table 20.4 AbobotulinumtoxinA Treatment Doses for Patient's Targeted Musculature in His Right Upper Extremity

Target Muscle	Units Injected
Right flexor digitorum superficialis	300 units
Right biceps brachii	200 units
Right lumbricals (four)	200 units
Right adductor pollicis	100 units

Muscles to be treated were identified using anatomic landmarks described by Perotto et al. (2005).[9] Skin was cleaned and prepared with alcohol. A 27-gauge hollow monopolar needle was introduced into the target muscles. Limited EMG confirmed needle location within the muscle. There was increased activity in the muscle even at rest. In some muscle, e-stim was utilized to localize the muscle. Prior to injection, the needled plunger was aspirated to make sure the needle was not within a surrounding blood vessel. With negative aspiration, the muscles were injected with the appropriate amount of BoNTA product (abobotulinumtoxinA):

The patient tolerated the procedure well with no complications. The patient was educated to resume his normal activities and utilize acetaminophen and ice packs for pain at the injection sites as needed. Education regarding expectations and time frames of treatment were provided.

REFERENCES

1. McGuire JR. Epidemiology of spasticity. In: Brasher A, Elovic E, eds. *Spasticity: Diagnosis and Management*. New York: Demos Medical Publishing, LLC; 2011:5–15.

2. Lyle RC. A performance test for assessment of upper limb function in physical rehabilitation treatment and research. *Int J Rehabil Res*.1981;4(4):483–492. https://doi.org/10.1097/00004356-198112000-00001

3. Simpson DM, Patel AT, Alfaro A, et al. OnabotulinumtoxinA injection for poststroke upper-limb spasticity: guidance for early injectors from a Delphi panel process. *PM & R*. 2017;9(2):136–148. https://doi.org/10.1016/j.pmrj.2016.06.016

4. Romanoski N, Moser K, Cherin N. Chemodenervation and Neurolysis. In: *PM&R Knowledge Know*. American Academy of Physical Medicine and Rehabilitation; 2019.

5. Enslin JMN, Rohlwink UK, Figaji A. Management of spasticity after traumatic brain injury in children. *Front Neurol*. 2020;11:126. https://doi.org/10.3389/fneur.2020.00126

6. Dymarek R, Ptaszkowski K, Ptaszkowska L, et al. Shock waves as a treatment modality for spasticity reduction and recovery improvement in post-stroke adults - current evidence and qualitative systematic review. *Clin Interv Aging*. 2020;15:9–28. https://doi.org/10.2147/CIA.S221032

7. Yang E, Lew HL, Özçakar L, et al. Recent advances in the treatment of spasticity: extracorporeal shock wave therapy. *J Clin Med*. 2021;10(20):4723. https://doi.org/10.3390/jcm10204723

8. Cha Y, Arami A. Quantitative modeling of spasticity for clinical assessment, treatment and rehabilitation. *Sensors (Basel)*. 2020;20(18):5046. https://doi.org/10.3390/s20185046

9. Delagi EF, Perotto A. *Anatomical Guide for the Electromyographer: The Limbs and Trunk.* Springfield, IL: Thomas; 2005.

FURTHER READING

Bose P, Hou I, Thompson FJ. Traumatic Brain Injury (TBI)-induced spasticity: neurobiology, treatment, and rehabilitation. In: Kobeissy FH, ed. *Brain Neurotrauma.* Boca Raton, FL: CRC Press; 2015:182–193. https://doi.org/10.1201/b18126-17

Farag SM, Mohammed MO, El-Sobky TA, et al. Botulinum toxin A injection in treatment of upper limb spasticity in children with cerebral palsy: a systematic review of randomized controlled trials. *JBJS* Rev. 2020;8(3):e0119. https://doi.org/10.2106/JBJS. RVW.19.00119. PMID: 32224633; PMCID: PMC7161716.

Francisco GE, McGuire JR. Poststroke spasticity management. *Stroke.* 2012;43(11):3132–6. https://doi.org/10.1161/STROKEAHA.111.639831. Epub 2012 Sep 13. PMID: 22984012.

Hughes C, Howard IM. Spasticity management in multiple sclerosis. *Phys Med Rehabil Clin N Am.* 2013;24(4):593–604. https://doi.org/10.1016/j.pmr.2013.07.003. PMID: 24314678.

Lui J, Sarai M, Mills PB. Chemodenervation for treatment of limb spasticity following spinal cord injury: a systematic review. *Spinal Cord.* 2015;53(4):25264. https://doi. org/10.1038/sc.2014.241. Epub 2015 Jan 13. PMID: 25582713.

Orsini M, Leite MAA, Chung TM, et al. Botulinum neurotoxin type a in neurology: update. *Neurol Int.* 2015;7(2):5886. https://doi.org/10.4081/ni.2015.5886

21 Lower Limb Spasticity Management With Botulinum Neurotoxin

Eve Boissonnault, Heather Finlayson, Farris Kassam, and Rajiv Reebye

INTRODUCTION

Lower limb spasticity (LLS) is a motor disorder that affects muscles from the hip girdle to the toes. It results from central nervous system (CNS) dysfunction and is an element of the upper motor neuron (UMN) syndrome (UMNS), which includes both positive and negative features as outlined in Table 21.1.[1]

Table 21.1 Features of the Upper Motor Neuron Syndrome	
Negative Features	Positive Features
Muscle weakness	Increased tendon reflexes with radiation
Loss of dexterity	Clonus
Fatigability	Babinski sign
	Spasticity
	Extensor spasms
	Flexor spasms
	Mass reflex
	Dyssynergic patterns of co-contraction during movement
	Associated reactions and other dyssynergic and stereotypical spastic dystonias
Source: Barnes MP. An overview of the clinical management of spasticity. In Johnson GR and Barnes MP, (Eds.), Upper Motor Neurone Syndrome and Spasticity: Clinical Management and Neurophysiology (2nd ed, pp. 1-8). Cambridge University Press. http://doi.org/10.1017/CBO9780511544866.002	

Botulinum neurotoxin (BoNT) injections are a form of chemodenervation that cause a temporary blockade of neurotransmitter release at the neuromuscular junction, leading to reduced muscle contraction. The mechanism of action of BoNT has been reviewed extensively elsewhere in this book. BoNT is an important management option for focal spasticity (spasticity that is confined to one joint or functional body area) or multifocal spasticity (affecting two or more joints or areas) as part of a multimodal approach to the management of LLS.

When compared to the upper limb, there is a knowledge gap for LLS as more studies focus on after stroke upper limb spasticity.[2] In this chapter, we discuss the assessment, diagnostic approach, and treatment options for LLS with a focus on the use of BoNT. Our case study illustrates a patient-centered approach to BoNT therapy in the management of LLS.

DIAGNOSTIC APPROACH

When assessing a patient with LLS for possible BoNT treatment, the following elements are essential: (a) a focused spasticity history, (b) a physical examination including the identification of the key muscles involved in problematic LLS, and (c) goal setting.

Spasticity History

The assessment of LLS begins with a focused but thorough history to identify the location, onset, severity, timing, alleviating factors, and potential noxious triggers for spasticity. We recommend the use of a structured and systematic approach when taking the history regarding LLS. The mnemonic "ILOSTWAR" can be helpful to ensure that the key spasticity issues are addressed:

I: Impact on function
L: Location
O: Onset
S: Severity
T: Timing
W: Worsening/noxious stimuli
A: Alleviating factors
R: Radiation/pain

Physical Examination

The LLS-focused physical examination builds upon data gathered from the history. It consists of neurologic and relevant musculoskeletal examinations of the affected body parts.

The examination begins with inspection. This includes the identification of common postural patterns of LLS, which is discussed in the next section. Muscle tone, power, sensation, reflexes, and gait (if feasible) are assessed. When considering BoNT treatment, it is important to evaluate the presence and strength of voluntary activation within a) the spastic muscles and b) their antagonists. For example, when assessing spastic equinovarus, it is important to know whether there is potential for active ankle dorsiflexion and eversion that is being overpowered by the spastic plantar flexors and inverters. For ambulatory patients, gait assessment helps to identify muscles that are contributing to an abnormal pattern and impairing function.

Observing the patient as they transfer to the bed/examining table provides valuable information about the ways in which their spasticity affects their transfers, both negatively and positively. Some patients may experience an exacerbation of spasms in the process of transferring that sheds light on treatment targets, while other patients may demonstrate dependence on lower limb tone to act as a support. In the latter case, there is a significant risk that interventions to reduce spasticity would unmask underlying weakness and reduce their ability to transfer safely. For patients who use wheelchairs, their position in the wheelchair should be closely observed to evaluate the impact of spasticity on their positioning, for example, head position on a head support, truncal lean, upper limb position on an armrest, foot position on footplates, etc. If these patients cannot be safely transferred, they can be examined in their wheelchair, but this needs to be documented for consistency of future examinations.

Quantifiable and reproducible measures should be used in the LLS assessment. The most commonly used spasticity scales were described in the chapter on upper limb spasticity. These are the Modified Ashworth Scale (MAS)[3] and the Tardieu Scale.[4]

Specific to the lower limb, the Wartenberg pendulum test is a simple, objective, and repeatable biomechanical method of spasticity assessment. The affected limb is extended and then let to swing freely against gravity.[5-7] Although it can be used for different muscle groups, it is classically used to assess spasticity of the quadriceps muscles. To perform the test, the patient should sit in a relaxed position with their legs hanging freely over the edge of a seat or a table. The examiner then lifts the affected leg to a horizontal position and lets it swing freely. This induced pendulum-like movement of the lower limb allows different measures to be taken with instrumentation such as a goniometer, potentiometer, electro-goniometer, accelerometer, gyro sensor, computerized video motion analysis, and electromyography (EMG) to quantify the spasticity.[5-7] It is a sensitive test to detect subtle changes in spasticity, it requires a simple setup, and it correlates well with clinical measures of spasticity.[5-7] It also has some limitations including its lack of reliability when testing the same patient multiple times, the need for equipment, and the fact that it cannot be used to assess all muscle groups. Variables that have the potential to alter the reliability of the pendulum test include positioning of the limb, muscle length, and the level of muscle relaxation.[5-7]

Gait speed measurement is a simple and effective way to monitor the functional effects of LLS treatment. As noted above, when resources are available, instrumented gait analysis is optimal. If this is not possible, we recommend pre- and posttreatment video capture of the patient's gait in the frontal and sagittal planes. These tools provide an objective record of the patient's treatment response and progression over time. Sharing the videos with patients can also enhance their engagement in their care and strengthen the therapeutic relationship.

The focus of this chapter is not on upper limb spasticity, but it is important to consider the effects of upper limb spasticity and posturing on balance and gait. Thus, an upper limb assessment should always be a part of the evaluation for LLS.[8]

Goal Setting

The decision about whether and where to inject BoNT for LLS requires patient-centered goal setting. A key element in the art of setting goals is devising goals that are in accordance with the SMART principle (specific, measurable, attainable, realistic, timely).[9,10] Goal setting should be a multidisciplinary or interdisciplinary process and must involve the patient and/or their caregivers.

All LLS treatment goals should relate to specific active or passive functions and consider the impact on activity and participation.[11-13] Examples of passive functions impaired by LLS are adductor spasticity that makes peri-care challenging for caregivers; knee flexor spasticity that leads to uncomfortable wheelchair seating and contributes to wound development; knee extensor tone that prevents proper positioning on wheelchair footplates; or painful spasms that interfere with sleep. Active functions that may be affected by LLS include equinovarus posturing at the foot and ankle that slows gait and leads to an unstable base of support and knee extensor clonus that causes falls while attempting to stand or transfer.

It is crucial to set goals with realistic expectations. When formulating their goals, patients may focus on the recovery of negative symptoms of the UMNS (e.g., they expect to regain active motor function in a plegic limb). If it is true that spasticity and motor recovery are interrelated, then treating the first will not necessarily improve the second [14,15] and the patient may be disappointed with the treatment outcome, despite a decrease in their LLS.

If BoNT treatment is deemed appropriate, goals should be reviewed after each round of BoNT. If treatment goals are not achieved, this stimulates reevaluation of the BoNT dosage, muscle selection, injection technique, and adjunctive therapies. Follow-up assessments should ideally be scheduled 4 to 6 weeks after injections when the BoNT is at its peak effect.[16]

LOWER LIMB SPASTICITY PATTERNS

Once the assessment is complete and goals are set, the diagnostic impression can be refined and the treatment approach planned. BoNT is often the optimal management option for focal LLS. Mastering and refining the injection technique is an art to develop with specific training and experience.

Each patient is unique, and different pathologies of the UMN system are associated with different patterns. Therefore, there is a high degree of variability in how LLS presents, making it difficult for clinicians with limited experience to identify a common posture and target the appropriate muscle for injection of BoNT. Figure 21.1 shows the seven patterns of after stroke LLS identified by Esquenazi et al.[17]

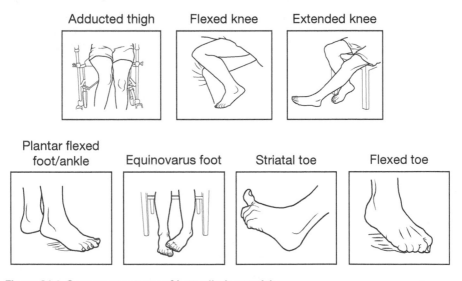

Figure 21.1 Common postures of lower limb spasticity.

Source: Esquenazi A, Alfaro A, Ayyoub Z et al. OnabotulinumtoxinA for lower limb spasticity: guidance from a delphi panel approach. *PM & R*, 2017;9(10):960-968. https://doi.org/10.1016/j.pmrj.2017.02.014

Based on the work of Esquenazi et al.,[17] we focus on three common patterns of LLS that can be seen independently or as an aggregate. For each pattern, we indicate the three key muscles to inject with BoNT and provide a suggested dosage range for onabotulinumtoxinA and abobotulinumtoxinA. As incobotulinumtoxinA is not currently approved for injection of the lower extremity, we did not include it in the table (Table 21.2).[17,18]

Table 21.2 Principal Patterns of LLS, Key Muscles, and Suggested Dosage of OnabotulinumtoxinA and AbobotulinumtoxinA

Principal Patterns	Key Muscle Involved	Suggested Dosage of OnabotulinumtoxinA	Suggested Dosage of AbobotulinumtoxinA
Plantar flexed foot/ankle	Gastrocnemius	50–250 units	300–800 units
	Soleus	50–200 units	250–500 units
Equinovarus foot	Tibialis posterior	50–100 units	100–350 units
	Gastrocnemius	50–250 units	300–800 units
	Soleus	50–200 units	250–500 units
Flexed toe	Flexor digitorum longus	25–125 units	150–300 units
	Flexor digitorum brevis	20–80 units	40–200 Units
	Flexor hallucis longus	15–95 units	100–200 units

Source: Esquenazi A, Alfaro A, Ayyoub Z et al. OnabotulinumtoxinA for lower limb spasticity: guidance from a delphi panel approach. *PM & R*, 2017;9(10):960-968. https://doi.org/10.1016/j.pmrj.2017.02.014; Alter KE, Wilson NA. *Botulinum neurotoxin injection manual*. 2015 Demos Medical Publishing, LLC. http://site.ebrary.com/id/10998335

With respect to the flexed toe pattern, a clinical pearl is to remember that the flexor hallucis longus (FHL) has a tendinous slip with a variable number of branches to the flexor digitorum longus (FDL) in the plantar aspect of the foot.[19-21] This means that when addressing a classic flexed toe pattern with BoNT injections, omission of FHL injections may lead to a suboptimal treatment outcome.

Variation of LLS is further increased when considering patient active patterns. This is highlighted in Armand et al.'s and Rodda et al.'s analysis of gait patterns in children with cerebral palsy. When examining spastic hemiplegia alone, six classic gait patterns can be identified.[22,23] With guidelines still to be developed, physicians must rely on patient feedback and an understanding of how treatment of a stationary pattern will impact a patient's activities of daily living (ADLs). Physicians must be especially diligent when treating pediatric patients, as a child's growth rate is estimated at 6 to 7 cm and 3 to 3.5 kg per year.[24] These findings emphasize the complexity of the diagnostic approach and how a solid understanding of the patterns observed will lead to optimal patient outcomes in pediatric and adult populations.[22,17,23]

NERVE BLOCKS

Once the problematic LLS pattern is identified, diagnostic motor nerve blocks with an anesthetic such as lidocaine can be helpful, especially for complex cases or those who do not respond as expected to focal treatment with BoNT. Nerve blocks can help to differentiate between a reducible deformity due to spasticity that should respond to conservative treatment including BoNT injections, and a non-reducible contracture requiring a surgical approach. With respect to LLS, Picelli et al. recently confirmed that a diagnostic nerve block is a valuable tool in deciding whether to treat spastic equinovarus with BoNT.[25]

TREATMENT OPTIONS

Other chapters in this book reviewed the range of nonpharmacologic, pharmacologic, and interventional/surgical options for the treatment of spasticity. We therefore focus on clinical pearls specific to the treatment of LLS with BoNT injections. Chemodenervation with BoNT can be used to reduce spasticity, increase range of motion (ROM), and improve gait for patients with focal symptomatically distressing LLS.[26,27] It can also reduce spasticity-associated pain and improve passive functions such as positioning and peri-care.

A multimodal approach to LLS management can include nonpharmacologic therapies and modalities, oral medication, as well as nonsurgical and surgical interventions. This approach is a cornerstone of a dynamic, goal-specific, and patient-centered rehabilitation program. More specifically, this is essential to optimize the outcomes of BoNT injections for spasticity management.[28,13,8,29]

Localization Techniques

Once it has been established that intervention with BoNT is needed, the clinician should consult and collaborate with the patient's healthcare team prior to administering BoNT for LLS. Localization techniques can be used to correctly locate and place injections. These localization techniques include EMG, electrostimulation, and ultrasound (US) guidance[30] and are described in detail elsewhere in this text.

It is important to consider the optimization of ergonomics while injecting BoNT. This consists of analyzing the physical relationships between the physician, their patient, and their work environment. A proper ergonomic arrangement for the injector and for the patient is essential, not only to decrease injuries and improve safety but also to increase efficiency, reduce discomfort, and optimize treatment outcomes by improving the accuracy of muscle identification under US. If the patient is non-ambulatory, they can often be injected while sitting in their wheelchair to maximize their comfort.[31]

Timing and Management

The timing of initial intervention and long-term management with BoNT is important. In order to optimize patient outcomes and minimize the negative effects of spasticity, BoNT should be administered as soon as a patient's function is affected, regardless of the duration of time from the initial stroke.[16] Early intervention with BoNT may reduce the progression of prior spinal cord injury (SCI) and poststroke spasticity (PSS), prevent the development of contractures and deformities, and modify the long-term course of overall muscle overactivity.[32,33] Thus, we recommend initiating BoNT treatment when spasticity develops, even within the first 12 weeks after stroke.

Multimodal Therapy

While BoNT is often a key treatment for LLS, patients should be prescribed adjuvant therapies as part of a multimodal approach.[28] Physiotherapy, splinting, casting,[8] extracorporeal shock wave therapy (ESWT),[34] and transcutaneous electrical nerve stimulation (TENS)[35] have been shown to decrease spasticity and should be considered as part of the management strategy to maximize outcomes. For example, patients with LLS who can ambulate indoors and/or outdoors will benefit from self-rehabilitation or physiotherapy-focused gait training in order to improve motor control, leading to increased walking speed and walking distance.[36]

COMPLICATIONS

Risk of Falls

BoNT injections generally have an excellent safety profile in adults and children with LLS. Muscle weakness and pain are the most commonly reported complications.[37,17,38] In the context of LLS, practitioners must pay special attention to the potential for unmasked weakness leading to an increased risk of falls.[39] This risk is particularly great for patients with knee extensor spasticity who have BoNT injections to the quadriceps muscles. For patients with toe flexor spasticity, tone in the FDL and FHL muscles may be a dynamic reaction that helps to compensate for proprioceptive deficits. In this case, BoNT injections to the FDL and FHL could decompensate a patient with precarious balance and also increase their risk of falls. In these scenarios, diagnostic nerve blocks can be helpful to assess the risk of impairing balance before performing BoNT injections.

Poor Response to Treatment

A poor response to treatment can be thought of as a possible complication if patient and healthcare practitioner goals are not achieved. When this occurs, the team should reevaluate and try to understand the reasons for the lack of effectiveness. There are multiple factors that may contribute to this, including factors related to the patient, the injector, or the BoNT, as outlined in Table 21.3.

Table 21.3 Potential Reasons for Poor Outcome of BoNT Therapy

Patient-Related	Injector-Related	BoNT-Related
Unrealistic expectations	Incorrect diagnosis	Incorrect dose (over- or underdose)
Disease conditions	Incorrect muscle selection	Incorrect preparation
Concurrent medications that interact with spasmolytic drugs or alter muscle tone	Improper injection technique	Inactive medication
Immunoresistance		
Secondary muscle changes, fibrosis, etc.		

Source: Li S, Francisco GE. The use of botulinum toxin for treatment of spasticity. *Handb Exp Pharmacol*, 2021;263:127-146. https://doi.org/10.1007/164_2019_315

Unrealistic expectations from patients and/or caregivers is probably the most common reason for treatment failure with BoNT, which highlights the importance of the goal-setting conversation. With respect to immune resistance, the latest literature reveals that it is rarely a cause for non-response to treatment with BoNT.[40,41] Finally, as discussed in the diagnostic approach section, the assessment of the muscle echo intensity[42] or a pre-BoNT diagnostic nerve block[25] may help to predict a poor outcome to BoNT, such that the treatment plan should be adjusted before injecting.

CASE REPORT

To illustrate our assessment and treatment approach, we present a case of PSS. This is the most frequent, studied, and predictable form of spasticity, and it usually presents with the classic patterns previously described. However, we must be aware that other UMN pathologies such as multiple sclerosis (MS) and SCI present with different LLS patterns, including stiff knee gait and bilateral hip flexion and adductor spasticity.

Mr. S. is a 50-year-old right-handed man who works in the construction industry. He has been referred to your care after suffering a left middle cerebral artery occlusion 4 weeks ago, leading to right-sided spastic hemiplegia.

He was recently diagnosed with hypertension, hypercholesterolemia, and type 2 diabetes. His medications are perindopril 4 mg, rosuvastatin 20 mg, and aspirin 80 mg, all once a day, and metformin 1 g twice a day.

Prior to his stroke, he was not very active and did not exercise. His work has mostly been office-based for the last few years. He used to smoke 20 cigarettes per day but tried to cut down due to his high blood pressure.

Since he returned home after his stroke, his wife has been the main caregiver. He currently has minimal use of his upper limb and has some active function of his lower limb. He requires assistance from one person for ADLs including dressing, eating, and bathing. He is independent for transferring and is able to walk 30 meters with a cane and close supervision. Mr. S. feels afraid about his future and has a low mood—his wife has seen him tearful at times. His wife says they are both concerned about him losing more function. They both noticed that his right side has been stiffer lately, especially in the morning after waking up. The stiffness seems to improve as he stretches and activates, but since it is a new phenomenon for him, he has a hard time giving more details. He does feel that it is getting worse overall and that it is impairing his ability to transfer, which concerns him significantly.

Your first physical exam reveals weakness on the right side, with a Medical Research Council (MRC) scale of muscle strength 1/5 to 2/5 for the upper limb and 2/5 to 3/5 for the lower limb. Right elbow flexor and ankle plantar flexor spasticity is a grade 2 on the MAS. The Modified Tardieu Scale (MTS) results are illustrated in Table 21.4.

The pendulum test for the right rectus femoris reveals a catch at 60° from the horizontal. Sustained clonus is noted in both soleus and gastrocnemius (though greater in gastrocnemius) in the right lower limb. The sensory examination reveals deficiency only on the right side, but this is difficult to assess due to aphasia. There is no significant pain elicited by our assessment.

You have a goal-setting conversation with Mr. S. and his wife about what improvements and goals they would like to work toward as part of a management program.

Table 21.4 Modified Tardieu Scale, Initial Visit			
Muscle Group	V1	V2	V3
Elbow flexors	80°	120°	125°
Ankle plantar flexors	−15°	−30°	−35°

It is explained that, ideally, two to three goals should be agreed upon for now. They are asked to provide a list of all possible goals they would like to discuss.

They provide a list of the following possible goals:

- Improvement in hand function
- Improvement in gait
- Improvement in independence when doing daily activities

After discussing this with them, you suggest focusing on these two goals for now as they seem to be the most realistic and attainable in a reasonable time frame:

- Improvement in hand function
- Improvement in gait

Mr. S. and his wife agree with the recommendations and ask what the next steps will be.

In accordance with a multidisciplinary and multimodal approach, you write a referral for a physiotherapist to work on improving the function of his upper limb and for gait training, and you also refer him to a speech and language pathologist to work on his communication. For spasticity management, you encourage regular stretching and utilization of a TENS machine.[35]

You decide to start by injecting, under US guidance, a total of 50 units of onabotulinumtoxinA to the right upper extremity: 25 units to the brachialis and 25 units to the brachioradialis. Because you are only 4 weeks after the stroke, you consider it an early intervention and you decide to start with half of the dose you would normally use.[43] You also cast the right elbow in extension 2 weeks after the injection, for 1 week, based on the protocol suggested by Kotteduwa Jayawarden et al.[8]

At your follow-up appointment, 6 weeks after the first BoNT injections, the MAS is reduced to 1 for elbow flexors and the MTS reveals increased ranges of motion compared to your first assessment (Table 21.5). He is also using his right upper extremity more and more, notably to stabilize a piece of paper and to carry light objects. He is now able to feed himself independently with adapted utensils if his food is prepared. In the right lower extremity, the MAS is still a 2 for ankle plantar flexors, and the MTS is only slightly improved (Table 21.5). The sustained clonus is still present at the ankle, and still stronger at the gastrocnemius, with the knee extended, compared to the soleus, with the knee bent. Interestingly, despite the fact that you did not directly address the LLS and that relative to the upper limb, the objective improvement is more subtle in the lower limb, Mr. S.'s ability to transfer and his gait are better. He feels that he has better balance and movement fluidity. These results please you but do not surprise you as you know that literature suggests that improvement in elbow flexor spasticity may improve gait without directly treating the lower limbs.[44,8]

Table 21.5 Modified Tardieu Scale, Second Visit, After BoNT Injection to Right Brachialis and Brachioradialis

Muscle Group	V1	V2	V3
Elbow flexors	70°	90°	100°
Ankle plantar flexors	−10°	−25°	−30°

Mr. S. and his wife are also pleased with the overall result. The GAS is +1 for the goal of improvement to hand function and GAS of 0 for improvement of gait. This time, they would like to focus on the latter goal. According to your assessment, you agree with them. You feel that you do not need to repeat the BoNT injections to the upper extremity at the moment, but you decide to inject a total of 150 units of onabotulinumtoxinA to the right lower extremity: 50 units to the medial head of the gastrocnemius, 40 units to the lateral head of the gastrocnemius, and 60 units to the soleus using US guidance for localization. You also refer to an orthotist for a right ankle foot orthosis (AFO).

On your follow-up appointment 6 weeks later, Mr. S. and his wife are extremely satisfied with the outcome. The GAS is +1 for both goals (improvement of hand function and improvement of gait). They do not feel that the spasticity has come back to the upper extremity. You can now focus on their third goal of improving Mr. S.'s independence with daily activities. They also want to discuss a new goal with you today. They noticed that since you treated the equinus foot by injecting the gastrocnemius and soleus with BoNT, he does not drag his foot anymore, but he noticed a new tendency to curl the toes, causing discomfort and limiting his progress with gait training. They also give you a report written by the community physiotherapist highlighting Mr. S.'s good progress with gait training and wondering if he would be a candidate for BoNT to the toe flexors.

The physical exam today **(see also PowerPoint Audio/Video 21.1 via Springer Connect™)*** reveals steady gains in the upper extremity. In the lower extremity, the MAS is now at 0 for gastrocnemius and soleus. The MTS is also significantly improved (Table 21.6). There is no residual clonus at the ankle. The pendulum test for the right rectus femoris is still positive at 60° from the horizontal. The gait assessment with his articulated AFO and a cane reveals improved gait balance, symmetry, and fluidity. The right arm still has spasticity with associated reaction, but the arm swing amplitude is greater. The equinus deformity is resolved, leading to increased tibial progression during stance phase and improved clearance of the foot during swing phase. When assessing gait with bare feet and a cane, you notice toe flexion during the stance phase and the swing phase, associated with abduction of the forefoot and pronation of the midfoot. However, the hindfoot remains well aligned.

You are hesitant to inject the FDL and FHL with BoNT, because of the risk of impairing his gait and increasing his risk of falls. However, because of the pain component, you agree to consider a trial of focal BoNT injections to FDL and FHL, as he currently has an AFO to help compensate for any post-toxin weakness and proprioceptive deficit. You review the different options as well as the pros and cons of each option with Mr. S. and his wife. You also clarify the new goals with them, which are to reduce toe pain to improve his walking tolerance and walking distance and to improve shoe wear. After the discussion, you inject, under US guidance, small

Table 21.6 Modified Tardieu Scale, Third Visit, After BoNT Injection to Right Gastrocnemius and oleus

Muscle Group	V1	V2	V3
Elbow flexors	70°	90°	100°
Ankle plantar flexors	+5°	0°	−5°

---

*Access to the PowerPoint Audio/Video 21.1 presentation related to the physical exam can be found via Springer Connect™ (http://connect.springerpub.com/content/book/978-0-8261-3975-7) by clicking onto the supplementary tab via Student Materials.

doses of onabotulinumtoxinA: 25 units to his right FDL and 15 units to his right FHL. You also optimize the conservative approach with stretching, TENS, and ESWT, and you ask the orthotist to reassess the AFO to make sure it provides adequate arch support and does not contribute to the discomfort. You will review him in 6 weeks to monitor the response to the latest injection.

REFERENCES

1. Barnes MP. An overview of the clinical management of spasticity. In Johnson GR and Barnes MP, (Eds.), *Upper Motor Neurone Syndrome and Spasticity: Clinical Management and Neurophysiology* (2nd ed, pp. 1–8). Cambridge University Press. https://doi.org/10.1017/CBO9780511544866.002

2. Sun LC, Chen R, Fu C, et al. Efficacy and safety of botulinum toxin type a for limb spasticity after stroke: a meta-analysis of randomized controlled trials. *Biomed Res Int*, 2019;8329306. https://doi.org/10.1155/2019/832930657. Turner-Stokes L. Goal attainment scaling (GAS) in rehabilitation: a practical guide. *Clin Rehabil*. 2009;23(4):362–370. https://doi.org/10.1177/0269215508101742

3. Bohannon RW, Smith MB. Interrater reliability of a modified Ashworth scale of muscle spasticity. *Phys Ther*. 1987;67(2):206–207. https://doi.org/10.1093/ptj/67.2.206

4. Tardieu G, Shentoub S, Delarue R. Research on a technic for measurement of spasticity. *Rev Neurol (Paris)*. 1954;91(2):143–144. https://www.ncbi.nlm.nih.gov/pubmed/14358132 (A la recherche d'une technique de mesure de la spasticite.

5. Bethoux F. Spasticity management after stroke. *Phys Med Rehabil Clin N Am*. 2015;26(4):625–639. https://doi.org/10.1016/j.pmr.2015.07.003

6. Hsieh JT, Wolfe DL, Miller WC, et al. Spasticity outcome measures in spinal cord injury: psychometric properties and clinical utility. *Spinal Cord*. 2008;46(2):86–95. https://doi.org/10.1038/sj.sc.3102125

7. Rahimi F, Eyvazpour R, Salahshour N, et al. Objective assessment of spasticity by pendulum test: a systematic review on methods of implementation and outcome measures. *Biomed Eng Online*. 2020;19(1):82. https://doi.org/10.1186/s12938-020-00826-8

8. Kotteduwa Jayawarden S, Sandarage R, Farag J, et al. Effect of treating elbow flexor spasticity with botulinum toxin injection and adjunctive casting on hemiparetic gait parameters: a prospective case series. *Journal of Rehabilitation Medicine*. 2020;52(10): jrm00110. Retrieved 2020/10//, from http://europepmc.org/abstract/MED/32939558 https://doi.org/10.2340/16501977-2743

9. Bovend'Eerdt TJ, Botell RE, Wade DT. Writing SMART rehabilitation goals and achieving goal attainment scaling: a practical guide. *Clin Rehabil*. 2009;23(4):352–361. https://doi.org/10.1177/0269215508101741

10. Hanlan A, Mills P, Lipson R, et al. Interdisciplinary spasticity management clinic outcomes using the Goal Attainment Scale: a retrospective chart review. *J Rehabil Med*. 2017;49(5):423–430. https://doi.org/10.2340/16501977-2228

11. Ashford S, Fheodoroff K, Jacinto J, et al. Common goal areas in the treatment of upper limb spasticity: a multicentre analysis. *Clin Rehabil*. 2016;30(6): 617–622. https://doi.org/10.1177/0269215515593391

12. Choudhry S, Patritti BL, Woodman R, et al. Goal attainment: a clinically meaningful measure of success of botulinum toxin-a treatment for lower limb spasticity in ambulatory patients. *Arch Rehabil Res Clin Transl*. 2021;3(2):100129. https://doi.org/10.1016/j.arrct.2021.100129

13. Francisco GE, Balbert A, Bavikatte G, et al. A practical guide to optimizing the benefits of post-stroke spasticity interventions with botulinum toxin a: an international group consensus. *J Rehabil Med*. 2021;53(1): jrm00134. https://doi.org/10.2340/16501977-2753

14. Li S. Spasticity, motor recovery, and neural plasticity after stroke. *Front Neurol*. 2017; 8:120. https://doi.org/10.3389/fneur.2017.00120

15. Li S, Francisco GE. The use of botulinum toxin for treatment of spasticity. *Handb Exp Pharmacol*. 2021;263:127–146. https://doi.org/10.1007/164_2019_315

16. Baricich A, Wein T, Cinone N, et al. BoNT-a for post-stroke spasticity: guidance on unmet clinical needs from a Delphi panel approach. *Toxins (Basel)*. 2021;13(4):236.

17. Esquenazi A, Alfaro A, Ayyoub Z, et al. OnabotulinumtoxinA for lower limb spasticity: guidance from a Delphi panel approach. *PM R*. 2017;9(10):960–968. https://doi.org/10.1016/j.pmrj.2017.02.014

18. Alter KE, Wilson NA. *Botulinum neurotoxin injection manual*.2015 Demos Medical Publishing, LLC. http://site.ebrary.com/id/10998335

19. Edama M, Kubo M, Onishi H, et al. Anatomical study of toe flexion by flexor hallucis longus. *Ann Anat*. 2016;204:80–85.

20. Hirota K, Watanabe K, Teramoto A, et al. Flexor hallucis longus tendinous slips and the relationship to toe flexor strength. *Foot Ankle Surg*. 2021; 27(8):851–854. https://doi.org/10.1016/j.fas.2020.11.002.

21. Plaass C, Abuharbid G, Waizy H, et al. Anatomical variations of the flexor hallucis longus and flexor digitorum longus in the chiasma plantare. *Foot Ankle Int*. 2013;34(11):1580–1587. https://doi.org/10.1177/1071100713494780

22. Armand S, Decoulon G, Bonnefoy-Mazure A. Gait analysis in children with cerebral palsy. *EFORT Open Rev*. 2016;1(12):448–460. https://doi.org/10.1302/2058-5241.1.000052

23. Rodda J, Graham HK. Classification of gait patterns in spastic hemiplegia and spastic diplegia: a basis for a management algorithm. *Eur J Neurol*. 2001;8(5):98–108. https://doi.org/10.1046/j.1468-1331.2001.00042.x

24. Kliegman RM, Stanton BF, St. Geme, et al. *Nelson Textbook of Pediatrics E-Book*. 2015; 1. Elsevier.

25. Picelli A, Battistuzzi E, Filippetti M, et al. Diagnostic nerve block in prediction of outcome of botulinum toxin treatment for spastic equinovarus foot after stroke: a retrospective observational study. *J Rehabil Med*. 2020;52(6): jrm00069. https://doi.org/10.2340/16501977-2693

26. Canada Ha. S. F. o. (2018a, 2019). *5.2. Range of Motion and Spasticity in the Shoulder, Arm and Hand*. Heart & Stroke. Retrieved May 18, 2022 from https://www.strokebestpractices.ca/recommendations/stroke-rehabilitation/range-of-motion-and-spasticity-in-the-shoulder-arm-and-hand

27. Canada, H. a. S. F. o. (2018b, 2019). *6.2. Lower Limb Spasticity following Stroke*. Stroke Best Practices Retrieved May 18, 2022 from https://www.strokebestpractices.ca/recommendations/stroke-rehabilitation/lower-limb-spasticity-following-stroke

28. Bussmann JBJ, Pangalila RF, Stam HJ, et al. The role of botulinum toxin in multimodal treatment of spasticity in ambulatory children with spastic Cerebral Palsy: extensive evaluation of a cost-effectiveness trial. *J Rehabil Med*. 2020; 52(5):jrm00059. https://doi.org/10.2340/16501977-2680

29. Moore EJ, Olver J, Bryant AL, et al. Therapy influences goal attainment following botulinum neurotoxin injection for focal spasticity in adults with neurological conditions. *Brain Inj*. 2018;32(7): 948–956. https://doi.org/10.1080/02699052.2018.1469044

30. Chan AK, Finlayson H, and Mills PB. Does the method of botulinum neurotoxin injection for limb spasticity affect outcomes? a systematic review. *Clin Rehabil.* 2017; 31(6):713–721. https://doi.org/10.1177/0269215516655589.

31. Lagnau P, Lo A, Sandarage R, et al. Ergonomic recommendations in ultrasound-guided botulinum neurotoxin chemodenervation for spasticity: an international expert group opinion. *Toxins (Basel).* 2021;13(4):249 https://doi.org/10.3390/toxins13040249

32. Stampas A, Hook M, Korupolu R, et al. Evidence of treating spasticity before it develops: a systematic review of spasticity outcomes in acute spinal cord injury interventional trials. *Ther Adv Neurol Disord.* 2022;15:17562864211070657.

33. Wissel J, Bavikatte G, Sposito M, et al. Development of an early identification tool in post-stroke spasticity (PSS): the PSS risk classification system. *Arch Phys Med Rehabil.* 2020;101: e35. https://doi.org/10.1016/j.apmr.2020.09.101

34. Picelli A, La Marchina E, Gajofatto F, et al. Sonographic and clinical effects of botulinum toxin Type a combined with extracorporeal shock wave therapy on spastic muscles of children with cerebral palsy. *Dev Neurorehabil.* 2017;20(3):160–164.

35. Mahmood A., Veluswamy, S. K., Hombali, A., Mullick, A., N, M., Solomon, J. M. Effect of Transcutaneous Electrical Nerve Stimulation on Spasticity in Adults With Stroke: A Systematic Review and Meta-analysis. *Arch Phys Med Rehabil.* 2019;100(4), 751–768. https://doi.org/10.1016/j.apmr.2018.10.016

36. Gupta AD, Chu WH, Howell S, et al. A systematic review: efficacy of botulinum toxin in walking and quality of life in post-stroke lower limb spasticity. *Syst Rev.* 2018;7(1):1. https://doi.org/10.1186/s13643-017-0670-9.

37. Camargo CH, Teive HA, Zonta M, et al. Botulinum toxin type a in the treatment of lower-limb spasticity in children with cerebral palsy. *Arq Neuropsiquiatr.* 2009;67(1):62–68. https://doi.org/10.1590/s0004-282x2009000100016

38. Esquenazi A, Stoquart G, Hedera P, et al. Efficacy and safety of abobotulinumtoxinA for the treatment of hemiparesis in adults with lower limb spasticity previously treated with other botulinum toxins: a secondary analysis of a randomized controlled trial. *PM R,.*2020;12(9):853–860. https://doi.org/10.1002/pmrj.12348.

39. Yoshizaki S, Yokota K, Kubota K, et al. The beneficial aspects of spasticity in relation to ambulatory ability in mice with spinal cord injury. *Spinal Cord.* 2020;58(5):537–543. https://doi.org/10.1038/s41393-019-0395-9.

40. Jankovic J, Truong D, Patel AT, et al. Injectable daxibotulinumtoxinA in cervical dystonia: a phase 2 dose-escalation multicenter study. *Mov Disord Clin Pract.* 2018;5(3): 273–282. https://doi.org/10.1002/mdc3.12613

41. Mathevon L, Declemy A, Laffont I, et al. Immunogenicity induced by botulinum toxin injections for limb spasticity: a systematic review. *Ann Phys Rehabil Med.* 2019;62(4): 241–251. https://doi.org/10.1016/j.rehab.2019.03.004.

42. Picelli A, Bonetti P, Fontana C, et al. Is spastic muscle echo intensity related to the response to botulinum toxin type a in patients with stroke? a cohort study. *Arch Phys Med Rehabil.* 2012;93(7):1253–1258. https://doi.org/10.1016/j.apmr.2012.02.005

43. Rosales RL, Efendy F, Teleg ES, et al. Botulinum toxin as early intervention for spasticity after stroke or non-progressive brain lesion: a meta-analysis. *J Neurol Sci.* 2016;371: 6–14. https://doi.org/10.1016/j.jns.2016.10.005

44. Esquenazi A, Mayer N, Garreta R. Influence of botulinum toxin type a treatment of elbow flexor spasticity on hemiparetic gait. *Am J Phys Med Rehabil.* 2008; 87(4):305–310; quiz 311, 329.

FURTHER READING

Alter KE, and Karp BI. Ultrasound Guidance for Botulinum Neurotoxin Chemodenervation Procedures. *Toxins (Basel).* 2017;10(1):18. https://doi.org/10.3390/toxins10010018 https://search.ebscohost.com/login.aspx?direct=true&scope=site&db=nlebk&db=nlabk&AN=924883 https://public.ebookcentral.proquest.com/choice/publicfullrecord.aspx?p=1887328 http://www.vlebooks.com/vleweb/product/openreader?id=none&isbn=9781617052095

Ashford S, Turner-Stokes L. Goal attainment for spasticity management using botulinum toxin. *Physiother Res Int.* 2006;11(1):24–34. https://doi.org/10.1002/pri.36 https://doi.org/10.3390/toxins13040236

Bavikatte G, Subramanian G, Ashford S, et al. Early identification, intervention and management of post-stroke spasticity: expert consensus recommendations. *J Cent Nerv Syst Dis.* 2021;13:11795735211036576. https://doi.org/10.1177/11795735211036576

Cosenza L, Picelli A, Azzolina D, et al. Rectus femoris characteristics in post stroke spasticity: clinical implications from ultrasonographic evaluation. *Toxins (Basel).* 2020; 12(8):490 https://doi.org/10.3390/toxins12080490 https://doi.org/10.1016/j.aanat.2015.11.008 https://doi.org/10.1097/phm.0b013e318168d36c

Filippetti M, Di Censo R, Varalta V, et al. Is the outcome of diagnostic nerve block related to spastic muscle echo intensity? a retrospective observational study on patients with spastic equinovarus foot. *J Rehabil Med.* 2022;54, jrm00275. https://doi.org/10.2340/jrm.v54.85

Grigoriu AI, Dinomais M, Remy-Neris O, et al. Impact of injection-guiding techniques on the effectiveness of botulinum toxin for the treatment of focal spasticity and dystonia: a systematic review. *Arch Phys Med Rehabil.* 2015;96(11): 2067–2078 e2061. https://doi.org/10.1016/j.apmr.2015.05.002

Hara T, Abo M, Hara H, Effects of botulinum toxin A therapy and multidisciplinary rehabilitation on lower limb spasticity classified by spastic muscle echo intensity in post-stroke patients. *Int J Neurosci.* 2018;128(5):412–420. https://doi.org/10.1080/00207454.2017.1389927 http://ebookcentral.proquest.com/lib/umontreal-ebooks/detail.action?docID=2036219

Moreta MC, Fleet A, Reebye R, et al. Reliability and validity of the modified Heckmatt scale in evaluating muscle changes with ultrasound in spasticity. *Arch Rehabil Res Clin Transl.* 2020:2(4), 100071. https://doi.org/10.1016/j.arrct.2020.100071 https://doi.org/10.1016/j.apmr.2014.08.025

Pereira S, Richardson M, Mehta S, et al. Toning it down: selecting outcome measures for spasticity management using a modified Delphi approach. *Arch Phys Med Rehabil.* 2015;96(3):518–523 e518.

Picelli A, Baricich A, Chemello E, et al. Ultrasonographic evaluation of botulinum toxin injection site for the medial approach to tibialis posterior muscle in chronic stroke patients with spastic equinovarus foot: an observational study. *Toxins (Basel).* 2017; 9(11):375. https://doi.org/10.3390/toxins9110375

Picelli A, Bonetti P, Fontana C, et al. Accuracy of botulinum toxin type A injection into the gastrocnemius muscle of adults with spastic equinus: manual needle placement and electrical stimulation guidance compared using ultrasonography. *J Rehabil Med.* 2012;44(5); 450–452. https://doi.org/10.2340/16501977-0970 https://doi.org/10.3109/17518423.2015.1105320

Picelli A, Tamburin S, Bonetti P, et al. Botulinum toxin type A injection into the gastrocnemius muscle for spastic equinus in adults with stroke: a randomized controlled trial comparing manual needle placement, electrical stimulation and ultrasonography-guided injection techniques. *Am J Phys Med Rehabil.* 2012;91(11):957–964. https://doi.org/10.1097/PHM.0b013e318269d7f3

Pill J. The Delphi method: substance, context, a critique and an annotated bibliography. *Socio-Economic Planning Sciences.* 1971;5(1):57–71. https://doi.org/https://doi.org/10.1016/0038-0121(71)90041-3

Schroeder AS, Berweck S, Lee SH, et al. Botulinum toxin treatment of children with cerebral palsy - a short review of different injection techniques. *Neurotox Res.* 2006;9(2–3):189–196. https://doi.org/10.1007/BF03033938 https://doi.org/10.1177/17562864211070657

Wissel J, Ward AB, Erztgaard P, et al. European consensus table on the use of botulinum toxin type a in adult spasticity. *J Rehabil Med.* 2009;41(1):13–25. https://doi.org/10.2340/16501977-0303

Yang EJ, Rha DW, Yoo JK, et al. Accuracy of manual needle placement for gastrocnemius muscle in children with cerebral palsy checked against ultrasonography. *Arch Phys Med Rehabil.* 2009;90(5):741–744. https://doi.org/10.1016/j.apmr.2008.10.025

22 Chemoneurolysis

Andrea Paulson and Mark Gormley Jr.

INTRODUCTION

Patients who have had injury or abnormalities to their central nervous system (CNS) can have varying degrees of neurologic impairment that can include cognitive impairment, sensory deficits, weakness, incoordination, loss of selective motor control, as well as movement disorders including hypertonia. In general, movement disorders are classified as hyperkinetic movements, hypokinetic movements, disorders of tone, and negative symptoms. Hypokinetic disorders are more common in adults than children. One example is Parkinson's disease. In children, hyperkinetic disorders are more common and you are more likely to see mixed tone movement disorders including spasticity and dystonia. A single patient may demonstrate one, or more commonly many, movement disorder patterns. Spasticity and dystonia are the two most common forms of hypertonia. Spasticity is the velocity-dependent muscle resistance in response to stretch. Dystonia is the sustained or intermittent muscle contraction that result in twisting or posturing. In dystonia, there often is co-contracture of the agonist and antagonist muscles and the muscle contraction can be secondary to any stimulus. In dystonia, the muscle contraction is not velocity dependent.[1,2,3]

Common etiologies of hypertonia include cerebral palsy (CP), spinal cord injury (SCI), or traumatic or acquired brain injury, for example, a stroke or brain tumor, inborn errors of metabolism, autoimmune disorders, neurodegenerative disorders, and other genetic disorders.[2] Hypertonia includes spasticity, dystonia, chorea, athetosis, and ballismus and can result in functional challenges or musculoskeletal concerns, contractures, and pain.[1]

Common Causes of Movement Disorders[4]

- CP
- Traumatic brain injury (TBI)
- Acquired brain injury
- Stroke
- SCI
- Inborn errors of metabolism (Glut-1 deficiency syndrome)
- Autoimmune disorders (Sydenham chorea)

- Neurodegenerative disorders (pantothenate kinase-associated neurodegeneration, PKAN)
- Genetic disorders (hereditary spastic paraplegia, HSP)

Table 22.1 The Five Types of Hypertonia and Their Definitions

Type of Hypertonia	Definition
Spasticity	Resistance to muscle stretch that is velocity dependent
Dystonia	Abnormal, intermittent, or sustained muscle contraction that results in twisting or posturing; can be truncal or in a limb
Chorea	Continuous, random-appearing movements; seen during active movement; made up of identifiable discrete movements
Athetosis	Involuntary, slow, writhing movements
Ballismus	Sudden, high-amplitude movement of a limb

Source: Murphy KP, McMahon MA, Houtrow AJ. (eds.). *Pediatric Rehabilitation: Principles and Practice*. Springer Publishing Company; 2020:100–123.

ASSESSMENT AND DIAGNOSTIC APPROACH

There are four commonly used hypertonia measurement tools: the Modified Ashworth Scale (MAS), the Tardieu Scale, the Barry–Albright Dystonia Scale (BADS), and the Hypertonia Assessment Tool (HAT). Both the MAS and the Tardieu scale measure spasticity, but not dystonia.[5,6] The BADS only measures dystonia and the HAT identifies both spasticity and dystonia.[1,3]

The BADS was published in 1999 and is based on a 5-point ordinal severity score.[18] The body is divided into eight regions and each is assessed on a 0 to 4 point, with a total of five choices. Each of the eight body region scores are then added together for a total score of 0 to 32. The eight body regions include eyes, mouth, neck, trunk, upper extremities (right and left), and lower extremities (right and left). For all the body regions except eyes, the following scores apply: A score of 0 represents the absence of dystonia and score of 1 indicates slight, which is defined as less than 10% of the time and no effect on function; a score of 2 indicates mild, which is less than 50% of the time and does not interfere with function; 3 indicates moderate, which is more than 50% of the time and interferes with function or positioning; and 4 indicates severe, which is more than 50% of the time or dystonia that prevents normal positioning or function. The scoring for eyes are as follows: 0 is the absence of dystonia, 1 is slight and less than 10% of the time, 2 is mild with frequent blinking without prolonged spasms and less than 50% of the time, 3 is moderate with prolonged spasms of eyelid closure but eyes open most of the time, and 4 is severe with prolonged spasms of eyelid closure and eyes closed more than 30% of the time.[7]

The Barry–Albright Dystonia Scale[7]

- Tests: dystonia only
- Time to administer: 5 to 30 minutes

- Required training: no training
- Body regions: eyes, mouth, neck, trunk, upper extremities (right and left), and lower extremities (right and left)
- Scoring/grading:
  - 0 = absence of dystonia
  - 1 = slight, less than 10% of the time and no effect on function
  - 2 = mild, less than 50% of the time and does not interfere with function
  - 3 = moderate, more than 50% of the time and interferes with function or positioning
  - 4 = severe, more than 50% of the time or dystonia that prevents normal positioning or function
- Total score: add up scores for each of the body regions; total 0 to 32.

The HAT is the only one of the four discussed that assesses both spasticity and dystonia. The HAT is made up of seven different items that are scored as positive or negative based on the response to a specific movement. It was designed for children 4 to 19 years of age. A score of 0 means the movement or action is absent, and a score of 1 means the movement or action is positive or occurred. The seven different items include three for dystonia, two for spasticity, and two for rigidity. The dystonia measures include increased involuntary movements or postures of a limb with tactile stimulus of another body part, increased involuntary movements or postures with purposeful movements of another body part, and increased tone with movement of another body part. The two spasticity measures include velocity-dependent resistance to stretch and the presence of a spastic catch. The two rigidity measures include equal resistance to passive stretch during bidirectional movement of a joint and the maintenance of a limb position after passive movement. A total score of 0 to 7 is possible. If there are positive scores in more than one subcategory, then the patient is considered to have mixed tone.[8,9,2]

The Hypertonia Assessment[8,9]

- Tests: dystonia only
- Time to administer: 5 to 10 minutes
- Required training: no training
- Scoring:
  - 0 = movement or action is absent.
  - 1 = movement or action is present.
- Items to score:
- Dystonia items:
  - Increased involuntary movements or postures of a limb with tactile stimulus of another body part
  - Increased involuntary movements or postures with purposeful movements of another body part
  - Increased tone with movement of another body part

- Spasticity items
  - ○ Velocity-dependent resistance to stretch
  - ○ Presence of a spastic catch
- Rigidity items
  - ○ Equal resistance to passive stretch during bidirectional movement of a joint
  - ○ The maintenance of a limb position after passive movement
- Score: total 0 to 7; if positive scores in more than one subcategory, then the patient is considered to have mixed tone.

TREATMENT OPTIONS

Once a patient is found to have a hypertonic movement disorder and it has been subcategorized into spasticity or a mixed movement disorder including spasticity treatment, options can be considered. Treatment can include physical and occupational therapy, bracing, enteral medications (diazepam, baclofen, dantrolene, tizanidine, cannabinoids, clonidine, gabapentin, levodopa, trihexyphenidyl, tetrabenazine, atypical antipsychotics), botulinum toxin injections, neurolytic blocks, orthopedic surgery, or neurosurgery for movement disorders (selective dorsal rhizotomy [SDR], intrathecal baclofen pump [ITB], ventral dorsal rhizotomy [VDR], or deep brain stimulation [DBS]). Treatment may be with a single modality or through the combination of multiple different modalities.[1,10,2,3]

Treatment Modalities for Hypertonia

- Stretching
- Bracing or casting
- Physical or occupational therapy
- Enteral medications
- Botulinum toxin injections
- Neurolytic blocks (phenol, ethanol)
- Orthopedic surgery
- Neurosurgery (SDR, ITB, VDR, DBS)

CHEMONEUROLYSIS

Phenol

Phenol is an alcohol with proteolytic properties, and when injected at 5% to 7% onto a motor neuron, it causes chemical neurolysis, effectively denervating the target muscle distal to the injection site.[2] It is used for focal spasticity management. Phenol was first described for the use of spasticity in 1959 where it was given intrathecally, then in 1960 used for nerve blocks, and 1964 used for motor point blocks.[1,11] Nerve blocks to manage spasticity are typically focused on the motor point (intramuscular nerve), motor branches of nerves, or peripheral nerves.[11]

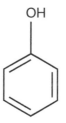

Figure 22.1 The molecular structure of phenol.

Common Nerve Targets for Phenol and the Distal Muscles Affected[2]

- Musculocutaneous nerve (elbow flexor group)
- Obturator nerve (hip adductors)
- Motor branches of the sciatic nerve (hamstrings)

Phenol is used at 5% to 7%. Phenol decreases spasticity by denaturing the epineurium of the target nerve resulting in a signal blockage. This effectively decreases the efferent input to the muscle and decreases the afferent impulses from the muscle spindle. If phenol is used on a nerve that also sends sensory information, the results will be numbness and tingling in the sensory distribution. Due to the mechanism being denaturation or the destruction of nerve tissue by protein necrosis, phenol should not be used near sensitive structures, sensory nerves, or vascular tissue.[1,11,12] The initial onset of phenol is nearly immediate, accounting 60% of the spasticity reduction, and the peak effect occurs at approximately 1 week following injections.[10] Another study found peak effect in 24 to 48 hours.[11] The duration of benefit following phenol injections is 4 to 12 months.[10] Another study found duration of benefit to be 2 to 6 months.[11] Another commonly cited benefit is the low cost of phenol.[2]

Accurate localization when using phenol is paramount due to the potential for destruction of unintended structures. Phenol does not readily diffuse when injected so accurate needle placement is critical. Localization is most commonly done through either electrostimulation or ultrasound (US). Phenol is most commonly done under general anesthesia due to the need for fine needle movements, accurate localization, pain from the injection itself, and the length of time needed to complete the procedure.[1,13,14] When phenol localization is done with both electrostimulation and US guidance, it was found that a lower dose was able to be used with equal effects.[15]

There is no dosing guideline for phenol; however, in children, it is typically recommended to stay below <30 mg/kg body weight. A 5% phenol solution contains 50 mg/mL and a 6% phenol solution contains 60 mg/mL. Therefore, the recommended dose of up to 0.5 mL/kg is considered safe.[1] In adults, a single treatment should not exceed 1 g, which is approximately 17 mL of 6% phenol.[2] Dosing can also be titrated to need, by doing a single motor point or multiple motor points, and phenol can be repeated as needed.[11] At higher doses, there is a risk of dysrhythmias and bradycardia.[1] Phenol has been gone away from by some physicians due to the variability of the results, potential side effects, and the procedural difficulty discussed above.[4] Phenol can safely be used in combination with botulinum toxins.[2]

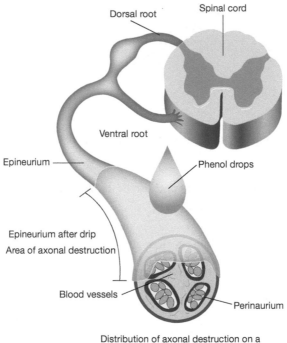

Distribution of axonal destruction on a
peripheral nerve after phenol application

Figure 22.2 Demonstration of phenol denaturing the epineurium of the target nerve resulting in a signal blockage.

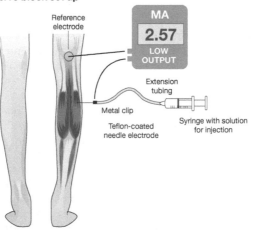

Figure 22.3 Accurate localization when using phenol is paramount due to the potential for destruction of unintended structures. Phenol does not readily diffuse when injected so accurate needle placement is critical. Localization is most commonly done through either electrostimulation or ultrasound. Here is a representation of localization using electrostimulation.

Phenol

- Mechanism: denaturation of epineurium resulting in denervation and distal signal blockade
- Target nerves: motor nerves
- Localization: electrostimulation or US
- Anesthesia. most commonly completed under general anesthesia
- Duration of procedure: 10 to 60 minutes
- Time to onset: minutes
- Duration of action: 4 to 12 months
- Concentration: 5% to 7%
- Dosing: up to 0.5 mL/kg (max of 30 mg/kg body weight)
  - 1 to 2 mL/nerve

Ethanol

Ethanol is another alcohol that has been used in place of phenol. When ethanol is used, it is usually 50% to 100% concentration and dosed at 5 to 10 mL per nerve. The mechanism, target nerves, localization technique, need for anesthesia, duration of procedure, time to onset, and duration of action of ethanol are similar to that of phenol.[1,16,17]

- Mechanism: denaturation of epineurium resulting in denervation and distal signal blockade
- Target nerves: motor nerves
- Localization: electrostimulation or US
- Anesthesia: most commonly completed under general anesthesia
- Duration of procedure: 10 to 60 minutes
- Time to onset: minutes
- Duration of action: 4 to 12 months
- Concentration: 50% to 100%
- Dosing: 5 to 10 mL/nerve

COMPLICATIONS

The most common complication or side effect of phenol is dysesthesias; this occurs when a sensory nerve has been injected. The literature reports that less than 5% of patients who receive phenol injections have associated dysesthesias.[1,2] Other literature reports the rate of dysesthesias to be 10% to 30%, more common with mixed motor and sensory nerves.[11] This is most common in areas where sensory nerves are in close proximity to motor nerves. Scarring at the injection site and surrounding tissues can also occur as well as muscle fibrosis.[2] There is also thought that if a nerve is repeatedly blocked with phenol or alcohol, the effect may be more permanent or that the injections will be decreasing effectiveness as scar tissue around the nerve increases.[1]

Table 22.2 Advantages and Disadvantages of Phenol or Ethanol

Advantages	Disadvantages
Price (low cost)	Risk of dysesthesias
Rapid onset of action	Risk of muscle fibrosis
Long duration of action	Need for patient sedation
Can be used on large muscle groups	Scarring at injection site
Can be repeated in less than 3 months	Pain with injection and electrostimulation for localization
Can be completed in combination with botulinum toxin	Increased time to complete procedure
	Complexity of procedure (skill)

Source: Elovic EP, Esquenazi A, Alter KE, Lin JL, Alfaro A, Kaelin DL. Chemodenervation and nerve blocks in the diagnosis and management of spasticity and muscle overactivity. *PM&R*. 2009;*1*(9):842–851. https://doi.org/10.1016/j.pmrj.2009.08.001; Gormley ME Jr, Krach LE, Piccini L. Spasticity management in the child with spastic quadriplegia. *Eur J Neurol*. 2001;*8*(Suppl 5):127–135. https://doi.org/10.1046/j.1468-1331.2001.00045.x

CASE REPORT

A 4-year-old female with spastic diplegic CP secondary to prematurity at 27 weeks' gestation and periventricular leukomalacia is a Gross Motor Function Classification System scale IV. She has minimal upper extremity involvement and good cognition.

The patient can take steps in a gait trainer with a pelvic support and has severe scissoring with contractures and some dystonic posturing. She has sustained clonus at her ankles and mild contractures with hip abduction 90° and popliteal angles 45°, and her ankles can be dorsiflexed to a neutral position. She can short sit independently without holding on to objects and creeps in a "bunny hop" fashion. She weighs 16 kilograms.

The patient has received physical and occupational therapy and is on oral baclofen, but she still has severe hypertonia. Her parents do not wish to pursue an SDR or ITB. The spasticity evaluation team recommended neurolytic blocks or chemodenervation.

Given this patient's age and distribution of spasticity and dystonia, the goal of treatment is to reduce her hypertonia and improve her ability to walk. Her scissoring, decreased step length, and plantar flexed feet while walking was felt to be interfering the most with her gait. To best adequately treat all of these areas, a combination of phenol neurolysis and botulinum toxin injections were felt best because of dosing limitations when treating multiple areas. Utilizing single event multilevel chemoneurolysis (SEMLC) and administering both types of spasticity-reducing injections would allow adequate dosing in the treatment areas in one treatment episode.

The scissoring or hip adductor hypertonia was felt to be best treated with phenol neurolysis of the obturator nerve because of its low-risk dysesthesias and relatively simpler location. The decreased step length and contractures were felt to be best treated initially with botulinum toxin injections to her hamstrings to reduce the risk of dysesthesias and muscle scarring from the potential need for repeat injections. Similarly, botulinum toxin injections to the plantar flexors (gastrocnemius/soleus) were felt to be appropriate. Phenol neurolysis could be used to treat her hamstring and plantar flexor hypertonia at a later time if she was not responding to botulinum toxin injections.

Treatment: The patient was sedated with general anesthesia, and while in a supine position, electrostimulation was used to find branches to the obturator nerve and the other muscles. Once located, each obturator nerve was injected with 2 mL of 6% phenol (total 4 mL, 0.25 mL/kg). Each medial hamstring and gastrocnemius/soleus complex were injected with 40 units of onabotulinumtoxin A (total 160 units, 10 U/kg).

One month later, the patient was able to walk independently for short community distances using a reverse walker and AFOs. She had no leg scissoring, an improved step length, and a plantigrade foot position. She required repeat injections approximately 5 months later and had similar improvement. She had no significant adverse events.

REFERENCES

1. Murphy KP, McMahon MA, Houtrow AJ. (eds.). *Pediatric Rehabilitation: Principles and Practice*. Springer Publishing Company; 2020:100–123.

2. Dy R, Roge D. Medical updates in management of hypertonia. *Phys Med Rehabil Clin N Am.* 2020;31(1):57–68. https://doi.org/10.1016/j.pmr.2019.09.010

3. Evans SH, Cameron MW, Burton JM. Hypertonia. *Curr Probl Pediatr Adolesc Health Care.* 2017;47(7):161–166. https://doi.org/10.1016/j.cppeds.2017.06.005

4. Deputy SR, Tilton AH. Treatment of disorders of tone and other considerations in pediatric movement disorders. *Neurother.* 2020;17(4):1713–1723. https://doi.org/10.1007/s13311-020-00984-6

5. Pandyan AD, Johnson GR, Price CI, Curless RH, Barnes MP, Rodgers H. (1999). A review of the properties and limitations of the Ashworth and modified Ashworth scales as measures of spasticity. *Clin Rehabil.* 1999;13(5):373–383. https://doi.org/10.1191/026921599677595404

6. Shu X, McConaghy C, Knight A. Validity and reliability of the modified Tardieu scale as a spasticity outcome measure of the upper limbs in adults with neurological conditions: a systematic review and narrative analysis. *BMJ Open.* 2021;11(12):e050711. https://doi.org/10.1136/bmjopen-2021-050711

7. Pavone L, Burton J, Gaebler-Spira D. Dystonia in childhood: clinical and objective measures and functional implications. *J Child Neurol.* 2013;28(3):340–350. https://doi.org/10.1177/0883073812444312

8. Jethwa A, Mink J, Macarthur C, Knights S, Fehlings T, Fehlings D. Development of the Hypertonia Assessment Tool (HAT): a discriminative tool for hypertonia in children. *Dev Med Child Neurol.* 2010;52(5):e83–e87. https://doi.org/10.1111/j.1469-8749.2009.03483.x.

9. Marsico P, Frontzek-Weps V, Balzer J, van Hedel HJ. Hypertonia assessment tool: reliability and validity in children with neuromotor disorders. *J Child Neurol.* 2017;32(1):132–138. https://doi.org/10.1177/0883073816671681

10. Zhang B, Darji N, Francisco GE, Li S. The time course of onset and peak effects of phenol neurolysis. *Am J Phys Med Rehabil.* 2021;100(3):266–270. https://doi.org/10.1097/PHM.0000000000001563

11. Escaldi S. Neurolysis: a brief review for a fading art. *Phys Med Rehabil Clin N Am.* 2018;*29*(3):519–527. https://doi.org/10.1016/j.pmr.2018.03.005

12. Gracies JM, Elovic E, McGuire J, Simpson D. (1997). Traditional pharmacological treatments for spasticity part I: local treatments. *Muscle Nerve Suppl.* 1997;*20*(S6):61–9

13. Elovic EP, Esquenazi A, Alter KE, Lin JL, Alfaro A, Kaelin DL. Chemodenervation and nerve blocks in the diagnosis and management of spasticity and muscle overactivity. *PM&R.* 2009;*1*(9):842–851. https://doi.org/10.1016/j.pmrj.2009.08.001

14. Gormley ME Jr, Krach LE, Piccini L. Spasticity management in the child with spastic quadriplegia. *Eur J Neurol.* 2001;*8*(Suppl 5):127–135. https://doi.org/10.1046/j.1468-1331.2001.00045.x

15. Matsumoto ME, Berry J, Yung H, Matsumoto M, Munin MC. Comparing electrical stimulation with and without ultrasound guidance for phenol neurolysis to the musculocutaneous nerve. *PM&R.* 2018;*10*(4):357–364. https://doi.org/10.1016/j.pmrj.2017.09.006

16. Kocabas H, Salli A, Demir AH, Ozerbil OM. Comparison of phenol and alcohol neurolysis of tibial nerve motor branches to the gastrocnemius muscle for treatment of spastic foot after stroke: a randomized controlled pilot study. *Eur J Phys Rehabil Med.* 2010;*6*(1):5–10.

17. Chua KS, Kong KH. Alcohol neurolysis of the sciatic nerve in the treatment of hemiplegic knee flexor spasticity: clinical outcomes. *Arch Phys Med Rehabil.* 2000;*81*(10):1432–1435. https://doi.org/10.1053/apmr.2000.9395

18. Barry MJ, VanSwearingen JM, Albright AL. Reliability and responsiveness of the Barry–Albright dystonia scale. *Dev Med Child Neurol.* 1999;*41*(6):404–411. https://doi.org/10.1017/s0012162299000870

23 Intrathecal Therapy for Spasticity

Michael Saulino, Reza Farid, and Andrea Perrone Toomer

INTRODUCTION

Intrathecal baclofen (ITB) therapy is a highly effective technique to reduce spastic hypertonia associated with the upper motor neuron syndrome (UMNS). This chapter describes the management of the newly implanted patient, the nature of chronic maintenance therapy, troubleshooting ITB therapy, and the procedures for managing ITB overdose and withdrawal. As of 2023, there are two manufacturers that have U.S. Food and Drug Administration (FDA) approval for chronic ITB infusion. These systems are the SynchroMed II system by Medtronic and the Prometra II system by Flowonix. With this recognition, the management principles are generally considered to be similar. Where appropriate, manufacturer-specific differences in technical application are discussed.[1]

DIAGNOSTIC APPROACH

Patient Selection

The first step in successful management in ITB is to select patients who will benefit the most from therapy. Spasticity can be measured by many methods (see Appendix), but there is no measure to determine how severely a patient's spasticity impacts them. Physicians should refrain from determining that a patient's spasticity is not "severe" enough to warrant intervention simply because the measured spasticity score did not meet or exceed the provider's predetermined level. Not all spasticity requires treatment, but when spasticity is problematic for the patient or their caregivers, treatment is warranted. ITB therapy can be considered for patients with severe, generalized spasticity who are not adequately managed with a combination of therapies, oral and injectable medications, and in whom more conservative treatment is not providing the desired benefit. ITB can be considered in all disease phases and should not be reserved for individuals who have failed other therapies or are in late stages of their disease process. Patients receiving ITB may still require other interventions, but the therapy has been shown to be cost-effective.[2-4,50]

Prior to initiating therapy, clear delineation of goals should be jointly agreed upon by the patient, their family, and their doctor. Common goals of spasticity management include decrease skeletal deformity and improve mobility, ease burden of care, improve quality of life (QOL), reduce feeling of stiffness or muscle pain, improve sleep and wellness, enhance self-image, inclusion, and participation, decrease complications, and enhance the acquisition of new skills.[5]

Common conditions presenting with spasticity are as follows:

- Cerebral palsy (CP)
- Spinal cord injury (SCI), complete and incomplete
- Brain injury, traumatic and nontraumatic
- Cerebrovascular accident/hemorrhage
- Multiple sclerosis (MS)

A variety of other conditions have been successfully treated with ITB but less is known about the effectiveness of the therapy for those conditions.

Intrathecal Baclofen Screening Dose

FDA approval for ITB included a requirement that patients receive a screening test dose prior to pump implant. The intrathecal injection of a screening dose, typically a 50 mcg bolus injection into the lumbar region, allows the clinician and the patient to appreciate the changes that they might expect after pump implant, assess for contractures, and uncover any underlying strength or weakness in the affected regions.[6] In the pediatric population, the use of a screening dose provides the additional opportunity to measure cerebrospinal fluid (CSF) pressure, ruling out occult hydrocephalus. On the other hand, some clinicians argue that the trial does not adequately predict long-term outcome, delays time to implant, and adds a risk of infection. When a patient requires anticoagulation, physicians need to balance the risk versus benefits of proceeding with an intrathecal screening dose with the need to hold anticoagulation prior to the injection. As reported in Boster et al., 70% of managing physicians routinely use a screening dose prior to implant.[51]

There is wide variability in how and where screening dose administration should occur. Weaning of oral medications prior to the screening dose is ideal but not always possible. The screening injection can be completed in any clinical setting where appropriate cardiopulmonary assessments can safely occur. Patients should receive a thorough baseline spasticity assessment prior to the injection and then serial examinations to assess response.

- A 50 mcg bolus injection into the lumbar region allows the clinician to evaluate the clinical response to ITB and quantify the reduction in spasticity.
- Baseline spasticity assessment can be compared to spasticity after administration of the ITB screening test dose.
- Objective reduction in spasticity can be assessed with exams such as Modified Ashworth Scale (MAS), joint range of motion (ROM), and strength.
- Assessment of gait speed, stability, and quality should be assessed in this ambulatory patient.
- The ITB screening test allows the patient to appreciate the changes that could be expected after pump implantation and initiation of therapy.

Adverse effects of an intrathecal screening dose include postinjection spinal headache, nausea, vomiting, drowsiness, sedation, hypotonia, dizziness, paresthesia, hypotension, and respiratory depression. Patients should not be released until their adverse symptoms have abated. Rarely, patients may need overnight observation.

TREATMENT OPTIONS

Intrathecal Baclofen Therapy Initiation

Once a patient has had a positive test of ITB dose, the patient can then proceed to implantation of the intrathecal delivery system. While the implantation procedure might be considered a relatively minor surgery, the patient population served by ITB therapy can be somewhat fragile. Special attention should be paid to the cardiac, pulmonary, and nutritional status of preoperative subjects. Patients should be clinically stable prior to surgery to minimize perioperative complications. Patients on chronic anticoagulation will need to discontinue medications in the days preceding the procedure.[6]

Various options for pump and catheter placement should be considered prior to the procedure. The size of the implanted pump should be determined based on the patient's body habitus and anticipated intrathecal dosing. The tip of the intrathecal catheter is routinely placed in the mid-lower thoracic region, particularly if reduction of lower extremity spasticity is the primary concern. More rostral tip placement can be attempted to improve upper extremity hypertonicity.[7–9]

Baclofen solution is typically placed in the reservoir intraoperatively with immediate commencement of intrathecal infusion. It is generally recommended to initiate therapy with the 500 mcg/mL concentration to provide maximum flexibility for dosing in the lower range without having to dilute the drug. The initial dosage of ITB is often determined by the patient's response from the test dose. A reasonable starting dose is 100% to 200% of the bolus dose divided over a 24-hour period. If a patient demonstrated prolonged or excessive hypotonia during the screening phase, it may be prudent to start at 50% of the bolus dose divided over a 24-hour period. Occasionally, it may be appropriate to start at even lower dose. Once therapy has been initiated, patients should be appropriately monitored until they demonstrate stable neurologic, respiratory, and cardiac function.

Dose adjustments can commence immediately after pump implantation. In general, 24 hours is a reasonable time to wait between each dosing adjustment to allow for the full effects of the ITB to be observed. Dose modifications are performed by "interrogating" the pump with a handheld programmer, programming the needed adjustments, and then updating the pump's dosing schedule. The programmer communicates with the pump via radiotelemetry. Various modes of administration include the following:

- Simple continuous (dose delivered continuously throughout 24-h cycle)
- Complex continuous (variable dose delivered continuously during 24-h cycle). This dosing mode allows for differential effects throughout the course of the day. For example, a patient may find it beneficial to be on a lower dose during the day (in order to minimize weakness and maximize functional mobility) and a higher dose during the night (in order to minimize nocturnal spontaneous spasms).
- Periodic bolus (regularly scheduled boluses of ITB within 24-h cycle). Periodic bolus dosing delivers several boluses rapidly over a few minutes with relatively

low delivery between the boluses. This mode of delivery may allow for greater distribution of drug with enhanced access to more cephalad spinal levels. This mode of delivery may be particularly beneficial for addressing upper extremity hypertonia.

These various modes of delivery are represented diagrammatically in Figure 23.1. In this example, the total daily dosing for the three modes of delivery is the same but the dose at any particular time is variable.

During the titration phase of ITB therapy, the amount of each intrathecal adjustment varies depending on patient tolerability. Non-ambulatory patients may tolerate dose adjustments of 20% of total daily dose, whereas others, especially ambulatory patients, will require lower titration increments (5%–10%). Adverse effects that may be seen during this phase of therapy include excessive hypotonia, changes in bowel[10,11] and bladder status,[12] and increased thromboembolic risk.[13,14] The frequency and size of dosing adjustments should be individualized based of the response to prior changes. Some patients tolerate rapid titration with daily dosing adjustments while others may require longer periods of observation and accommodation prior to undertaking further adjustments. While there is no evidence-based ideal titration frequency, dose adjustments 1 to 2 times weekly until optimal dose is achieved is reasonable and practical. While one of the goals of this therapy is elimination of oral spasticity medications, some patients may also benefit from some residual use of oral medications to address variable breakthrough spasms or to address upper extremity spasticity that is not addressed by ITB therapy. The titration phase of therapy could last 6 to 9 months after implantation.

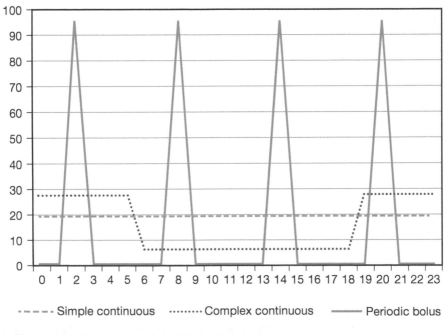

- - - - - Simple continuous   ········· Complex continuous   ——— Periodic bolus

Figure 23.1 Various modes of intrathecal delivery.

Since ITB has the capacity to affect a patient's active functional status, a rehabilitation program after implantation is appropriate. The setting, scope, and complexity of this program will vary depending upon the patient's individual goals as well as the availability of these services in a given region. Options for post-acute care include inpatient rehabilitation hospital, skilled nursing facility, long-term care hospital, home health, and outpatient therapy.[15] Issues that potentially require attention during this phase of therapy include incisional care, medical management (spinal headache, pain assessment, medication adjustment, dosing changes), mobility, self-care ability, and bowel/bladder function. Patients, especially ambulatory individuals, should be thoroughly counseled on the need for post-implant rehabilitation in order to maximize the benefits of ITB therapy.[16]

Intrathecal Baclofen Therapy Maintenance

Pump reservoir refills are a sterile, office-based, procedure that occurs every few weeks to months for the duration of treatment. The refill interval is the time required for the pump to dispense the volume of solution from a full reservoir to the low-reservoir volume. The refill interval will vary depending on the baclofen concentration and daily dose. Pump refills are scheduled to have sufficient residual reservoir volume prior to the alarm date to avoid associated symptoms of ITB withdrawal.[17] Pump refills are typically accomplished by palpating the pump and using a template to guide a needle into the reservoir chamber. In more challenging situations, such as morbid obesity or unusual pump position, fluoroscopy or ultrasound (US) can also be used to assist in guiding the needle through the access port into the reservoir chamber.[18,19] The remaining baclofen solution of the previous refill is aspirated and measured. It should correspond to the calculated volume by the pump programmer. The new baclofen solution is then instilled through the same needle. The needle tip must be reliably determined to be within the reservoir chamber. Inadvertent injection of an intrathecal solution into the subcutaneous tissue can result in serious adverse events,[20] such as swelling and baclofen withdrawal. During titration, some patients require ITB dose increases with a subsequent increase in refill frequency. Under these circumstances, a higher concentration of baclofen solution will extend the refill interval. When changing concentrations, it is imperative to program the pump correctly by incorporating a bridge bolus to compensate for the residual baclofen solution in the pump and catheter.[21] Failure to compensate for this residual solution can result in serious under- or overdosing. Traditionally, the therapeutic effect of ITB has been considered mostly closely linked to the dose administered.

Abrupt reduction or cessation of ITB delivery can result in withdrawal syndrome that can have serious, if not fatal, consequences. The severity of ITB withdrawal syndrome is not consistently related with dosing levels. Perhaps the most common symptomatic presentation is return of the patient's "baseline" degree of hypertonia. Additional characteristics of this syndrome can include pruritus, seizures, hallucinations, and autonomic dysreflexia. Some patients will demonstrate a life-threatening syndrome exemplified by exaggerated/rebound spasticity, fever, hemodynamic instability, and altered mental status. If not treated aggressively, this syndrome can progress to include rhabdomyolysis, elevated liver function test (LFT) levels, hepatic and renal failure, disseminated intravascular coagulation, multi-organ system failure, and rarely death.[22] Typically, the withdrawal symptoms will abate in several days though there are reports of prolonged ITB withdrawal syndrome.[23] Following recognition of ITB withdrawal, initial treatment includes supportive care, careful observation, and replacement of baclofen either via enteral or preferably through restoration of intrathecal delivery.[16] At present, there is no intravenous form of baclofen available although there is some investigative activity into this possibility.[24,25] There is no consistent oral to intrathecal conversion rate. Thus, oral baclofen administration may require frequent modification in order to attenuate the withdrawal syndrome. Adjunctive pharmacotherapy can also include administration of benzodiazepines (enteral or intravenous), tizanidine, dantrolene, or cyproheptadine.[16] Once the withdrawal syndrome has been modulated, then identification and correction of the delivery system malfunction. Troubleshooting intrathecal delivery systems is discussed in the following.

In contrast to withdrawal, which can occur despite vigilant attention, ITB overdose is generally due to human miscalculation during dosing adjustments or concentration changes.[26] Mechanical difficulties leading to overdosing are rare. Subdural encapsulation of the intrathecal catheter with subsequent rupture of the subdural pocket could lead to inadvertent excessive baclofen exposure.[27] The possibility of overinfusion by the pump itself can rarely occur with the recognition that this phenomenon is more likely with off-label agents than with baclofen.[28,29] Overdose can occur during catheter patency studies if the drug within the catheter is inadvertently injected into the subarachnoid space.[27] Additionally, if a catheter disruption is detected and the patient is undergoing restoration of intrathecal delivery, overdosing can occur if intrathecal delivery is resumed at the same dosing level prior to disruption. In this clinical scenario, patients should be started on dosing levels similar to levels initiated at pump implantation.[16]

Symptoms of baclofen overdose include profound hypotonia or flaccidity, hyporeflexia, respiratory depression, apnea, seizures, coma, autonomic instability, hallucinations, hypothermia, and cardiac rhythm abnormalities.

- Initial management of overdose is supportive and includes maintenance of airway, respiration, and circulation. Intubation and ventilatory support may be necessary.
- Secondary measures include reduction or temporary interruption of intrathecal delivery by pump reprogramming as well as cessation of concomitant medications that could contribute to central nervous system (CNS) depression.
- Additional measures for ITB overdose include CSF drainage via catheter access port (CAP) aspiration or lumbar puncture. Patients who are treated for baclofen overdose must be watched closely for rebound withdrawal once the pump is stopped and the drug load is decreased.[30]

COMPLICATIONS

Intrathecal Baclofen Troubleshooting

While ITB therapy is considered a reliable treatment for severe spasticity, the possibility of suboptimal therapy must always be considered in the management of patients. Troubleshooting is a means of optimizing ITB therapy. Suboptimal therapy includes those patients who present with hypertonia as well as those who appear hypotonic. Troubleshooting should be considered when a patient presents with either of these two scenarios. While we will focus on difficulties with drug delivery systems, it is important to recognize that some problems will be related to the patient's underlying condition. For patients with chronic, nonprogressive neurologic conditions (e.g.,

SCIs, stroke), ITB dosing should be relatively stable during the maintenance phase of therapy.[31] Individuals with progressive diseases (e.g., amyotrophic lateral sclerosis or MS) may require frequent evaluation and dose adjustments.[30,32] Comorbidities of neurologic disease can serve as noxious stimuli that act as triggers for increased spasticity (e.g., urinary tract infection, bladder distention, urolithiasis, etc.).[33] Additionally, several disorders have the capacity to mimic ITB underdosing/withdrawal, including sepsis, autonomic dysreflexia, neuroleptic malignant syndrome, and malignant hyperthermia.[22] If no patient-related cause for increased spasticity is discovered, an investigation into potential system malfunction should be undertaken.

Two initial techniques for investigation into potential pump malfunction include pump interrogation and checking the pump residual reservoir volume. The pump's active dosing parameters should match the previously prescribed dosing. If a programming error is detected, reversion to the appropriate dosing level may result in symptom reversal. The presence of an alarm condition or discovery of an unexpected "extra" residual volume in the reservoir suggest a pump-related malfunction. Alarm conditions generally occur due to either a low battery or low-reservoir volume. A low battery alarm condition will be noted at the end of battery life. Of note, the expected battery life is different among pump manufacturers.[34] A low-reservoir alarm will indicate that the pump has delivered nearly all of the contents of the reservoir and that the patient needs an immediate refill. Exposure of the Medtronic intrathecal delivery system to high magnetic fields (such as during an MRI scan) will result in a temporary cessation of drug delivery.[48] Rarely, there is a delayed restart of drug delivery that can be associated with underdosing/withdrawal phenomena. Detection of the rotor stall and restart can be assessed by inspection of the system's internal logs.[35] It is pertinent to note that intrathecal delivery systems from manufacturers other than Medtronic have different MRI recommendations.[36] Additionally, there are rare cases of rotor stall of the SynchroMed II system in the absence of magnetic field exposure.[29,37]

A combined diagnostic and therapeutic maneuver is to explore alternative delivery. A single ITB bolus dose comparable to or higher than the test dose (usually 50 to 100 mcg) can be programmed over 5 minutes and sequentially reevaluated over the next few hours. An alternative method of troubleshooting is a bolus administration (single or multiple) via lumbar puncture. Attainment of adequate spasticity control with ITB boluses administered by lumbar puncture in the absence of radiographic findings suggests the possibility of microtears.[38] Responding patients can be prescribed scheduled bolus doses to allay their symptoms until they experience a return to baseline or until a further workup can be completed.

Checking the residual volume within the pump reservoir is an appropriate undertaking. The low-reservoir alarm in the Medtronic system is based on programmed settings and is not a measurement of actual volume. Therefore, premature emptying of the pump reservoir will not trigger the low-reservoir alarm. There are rare reports of overinfusion, as manifested by symptoms of overdosing and a lower-than-expected reservoir residual volume.[39,40] Similarly, an increase in reservoir residual volume may suggest an abnormality of the pump rotor or a severely kinked catheter, resulting in underdosing or withdrawal. If there is any doubt as to the content of reservoir solution (such as drug concentration), then a new solution should be instilled. Similarly, if a low-reservoir alarm is detected, then a timely refill should be undertaken. The presence of a permanent rotor stall, unexplained rotor stalls, overinfusion, or low battery condition should prompt urgent replacement of the pump.

Catheter patency or malfunction may be suggested by the result of CAP aspiration. Diagnostic CAP aspiration may be performed after the pump is confirmed to be functioning through interrogation and pump reservoir volume verification. This procedure involves accessing a port that is in direct continuity with the catheter. If the distal end of the catheter lies within the subarachnoid space, CSF should be readily withdrawn through the catheter. Aspiration of only 2 to 3 mL is sufficient for determination of a normal aspiration since the volume of the catheter is typically less than 0.25 mL. Failure to aspirate fluid strongly suggests catheter disruption or occlusion. If partial catheter occlusion has occurred, aspiration may be difficult. If a complete kink/occlusion has occurred, minimal fluid would be obtained from CAP aspiration. If CSF cannot be aspirated, catheter revision or replacement is likely to be needed. Further diagnostic workup with scintigraphy may be necessary. If the catheter cannot be aspirated, consider the risks of overdose from drug in the catheter before proceeding with a catheter contrast study.

Imaging evaluation of the catheter typically begins with plain radiography with the understanding that some catheters are radiolucent.[19] A flat AP plate of the abdomen and lateral lumbar and thoracic spine series should be obtained in order to visualize all tubing, connectors, and entrance of the catheter into the spinal canal. A contrast study can be used to visualize the catheter and verify catheter tip location. Once the CAP and catheter have been cleared of the drug solution and CSF obtained, contrast medium can be injected and visualized fluoroscopically or with computed tomography (CT). If a CT study is undertaken, all portions of the pump and catheter should be visualized, which usually requires examination of the abdomen, lumbar spine, and thoracic spine. Extravasation of contrast out of the catheter can diagnose catheter breaks, catheter tip loculations, and catheter migration into the subdural or epidural spaces.[41] Contrast should not be injected if 2 to 3 mL of CSF cannot be easily aspirated, since this can potentially expose the patient to an ITB overdose from infusion of drug remaining in the catheter.[27] The CT myelogram also has the advantage of providing structural information relative to other organs that could be serving as noxious stimuli. A priming bolus must be programmed after a successful CAP aspiration to avoid subsequent underdose and potentially acute withdrawal. An added feature of the CT myelogram study is the capacity to add three-dimensional reconstruction to the imaging that may potentially improve detection of catheter malfunction.[42]

There are some nonradiologic techniques for diagnosing catheter disruption. Since spasticity is related to hyperreflexia, electrodiagnostic evaluation can detect hypertonia reduction in a more sensitive fashion compared to clinical examination. The H-reflex, the F-wave, and most commonly, the H/M ration have seen used to markers as markers of ITB delivery or dysfunction.[43] Some centers will repeat a traditional baclofen trial via lumbar puncture. If spasticity reduction is again obtained, catheter dysfunction is assumed and catheter replacement proceeds accordingly.[38] Lastly, detection of CSF pressure signatures at the point of the pump-to-catheter connection can theoretically confirm that the catheter tip is located within the intrathecal space, the catheter is intact and unobstructed, and the infusion system is capable of delivering the prescribed drug into the CSF. Conversely, failure to detect CSF pressure signatures suggests catheter malfunction. The results of early feasibility study suggest that a change in CSF pressure transmitted through the catheter fluid path may help detect intrathecal catheter complications.[44]

Other imaging techniques for diagnosis of catheter malfunction include radio-nuclide scintigraphy and MRI. Indium-111 DTPA can be injected into the pump reservoir and used as a tracer to determine the patency of the infusion system. After injection, serial sequential scanning occurs every 24 hours for 2 to 3 days. Normal studies should demonstrate an intact catheter and full ventriculogram. This technique can detect evidence of catheter occlusion, pump malfunctions, and large leaks. Disadvantages of this procedure include cost, the need for 2 to 3 days to confirm the abnormality and limited anatomic resolution, potentially high false-negative rate, need to do careful calculations to determine proper timing of imaging, and poor access by some centers to this technology. Indium-111 DTPA has not been tested or approved for delivery through intrathecal pumps.[45] MRI of the thoracic spine can demonstrate spinal hemorrhage, abscess, and other soft tissue abnormalities near the catheter tip. Rarely, granulomas can develop at the catheter tip, but these have only been pathologically confirmed with intrathecal opiate therapy for chronic pain. While rare, granulomas have the potential to cause serious neurologic injury from spinal cord compression. MRI of the catheter tip with gadolinium contrast is the diagnostic test of choice for granuloma detection.[46] It is vitally important to recognize that each manufacturer has a different protocol for patient evaluation following MRI.[47]

Summary

The efficacy of ITB therapy has been demonstrated for over 3 decades. Initially, patients with UMNS who demonstrated difficulties with passive function (such as positioning, hygiene, etc.) were the most common group referred for this therapy. More recently, patients with problematic active function (such as ambulation) have been referred and have successfully utilized this intervention. Both groups are best served by a dedicated medical, surgical, and rehabilitation team that is capable of managing all aspects of this therapy described in this chapter. As the sophistication of intrathecal delivery systems increases and newer agents become available, the requirement for a team-based approach will become even more paramount. If clinicians are interested in utilizing ITB therapy, they should develop a robust team environment to manage the routine, urgent, and emergent needs of their patient population.

Compliance and maintenance of clinic appointments is paramount to prevent baclofen withdrawal. All ITB patients and/or caregivers should be provided the daily dose, dosing schedule, and low-reservoir alarm date in writing at each appointment. Refill appointments should be scheduled while the patient is in the clinic, and any patient who misses a refill appointment must be rescheduled prior to the alarm date. Patient education is important along the process of ITB therapy from patient selection through long-term management, and continued education and communication prevents many urgent and emergent situations related to missed refill appointments.

CASE REPORT

A 52-year-old female presents 1 year after a stroke. She has right hemiplegic spasticity. She ambulates with a hemi-walker but complains of wrist, finger, thumb, and elbow flexion, forearm pronation, cramping in her calf and thigh, and unsteadiness of gait with toes clenching. Exam adds the presence of clonus at the calf in the gastrocsoleus complex and in posterior tibialis. A striatal toe is present when ambulating.

- Therapeutic options include removal of noxious stimuli, therapeutic modalities, oral medications, and consideration for chemodenervation and/or chemical neurolysis.
  - The required dose, duration, intensity, and frequency of therapeutic modalities are unknown.
  - Oral medications might provide benefit but may require high dosing with frequent use, raising the risk of adverse cognitive effects.
  - Toxin use may provide advantages in focal areas of spasticity, but recurring use is cost prohibitive and there is limited evidence of long-term benefits.
  - Chemical blocks with phenol and alcohol products are inexpensive but technically challenging and can only be completed in specific areas.
  - Surgical interventions are not practical and will produce weakness without addressing the underlying spasticity itself.

ITB can best address this patient's global spasticity, with the expectation of greatly reducing tone in the lower limb while potentially helping in the upper limb. ITB has been shown to be effective in patients with severe spasticity due to stroke and generally not affecting the non-hemiparetic side.[6,49]

After discussion regarding treatment options, an ITB screening test was performed to assess patient response to ITB therapy. The patient had a reduction in modified Ashworth scores in the right lower extremity following a 50 mcg screening test with a return to baseline level of spasticity at 4 hours. Considering the short duration of the response, it would be clinically appropriate to start the ITB dosing at 100 mcg/day.

- Had the response been more profound or longer lasting, it would be appropriate to start at 100% of the screening test dose and program 50 mcg/day.

After initiation of therapy, the ITB dosing was increased by 10% increments once to twice weekly until the patient experienced a reduction in tone. The patient reported adequate control of daytime spasticity but reported persistent spasms in the evening disrupting sleep. In this scenario, the use of complex continuous dosing allows for a higher dose of ITB during the problematic times of the day. Alternatively, using a flexible dosing program to deliver a bolus dose prior to bedtime might address problematic spasticity while minimizing the total daily dose.

The patient has successfully utilized ITB therapy for greater than 2 years. Her general medical condition has been largely uneventful. She occasionally notes a global increase in hypertonicity that is temporally associated with urinary tract infections. Today, she presents 1 month after a similar occurrence. She denied other symptoms. At the last visit, ITB dosing was increased 10%. The patient feels that there was little effect with this dosing adjustment. She does demonstrate increased spasticity on exam. The pump surgical sites appear intact. She is due for reservoir refill today.

First-Level Interventions

- Radiotelemetry interrogation of the pump system was undertaken. No electronic abnormalities were detected.
- Refill of pump reservoir was undertaken without a change in drug concentration. Actual aspirated volume from pump reservoir was within 0.5 cc of predicted volume.

- Pump was reprogrammed with a 10% increase in dosing and conversion from simple continuous delivery to periodic bolus delivery
- Patient was given a prescription for plain films of the abdomen and AP/lateral thoracic and lumbar spine films to be obtained if no change in symptom complex continues.

Second-Level Interventions

- Plain radiography demonstrated no apparent intrathecal catheter. Review of patient records finds that patient's catheter is a brand-specific version that is radiolucent.
- A CAP aspiration is attempted. No fluid is obtained despite multiple attempts.

Third-Level Interventions

- The patient underwent repeat ITB trialing via lumbar puncture. Procedure is executed with fluoroscopic guidance to avoid inadvertent damage to the intrathecal catheter. Patient experiences a reduction in tone similar to her initial ITB trial.
- The patient undergoes nuclear medicine cisternography with 500 μCr of In-111 placed into the pump reservoir. Sequential imaging demonstrates no radionucleotide beyond the pump/catheter interface.

Outcomes

- Patient was referred to neurosurgery for catheter revision.
- Exploration of the pump pocket demonstrates fraying of the pump catheter connector section.
- Patient underwent proximal revision of the catheter.
- Dosing was reset to initial dosage of 100 mcg/day, simple continuous.
- Patient underwent re-titration of ITB dose to prior effective levels over the next several months with appropriate dosage increases of 10% to 20% each visit.

APPENDIX

1. Modified Ashworth Scale
   - 0 No increase in muscle tone
   - 1 Slight increase in muscle tone, manifested by a catch and release or by minimal resistance at the end of the ROM when the affected part(s) is moved in flexion or extension
   - 1+ Slight increase in muscle tone, manifested by a catch, followed by minimal resistance throughout the remainder (less than half) of the ROM
   - 2 More marked increase in muscle tone through most of the ROM, but affected part(s) easily moved
   - 3 Considerable increase in muscle tone; passive movement difficult
   - 4 Affected part(s) rigid in flexion or extension
2. Tardieu Scale
   - a. Measures quality and angle of the muscle reaction to stretch

     i. Quality
       0   No resistance throughout passive movement
       1   Slight resistance throughout with no clear catch at a precise angle
       2   Clear catch at a precise angle followed by release
       3   Fatigable clonus (<10 secs) occurring at a precise angle
       4   Unfatigable clonus (>10 secs) occurring at a precise angle
       5   Joint immobile
     ii. Velocity
       V1   Stretch of the muscle at a slow speed
       V2   Stretch of muscle at the speed of gravity
       V3   Stretch of muscle at a speed > gravity
     iii. Angle
       R1   Point of first resistance upon rapid stretch (V2 or V3)
       R2   Point of terminal resistance with slow stretch (V1)

3. Penn Spasm Scale
  a. Frequency of spasticity
     1   No spasm
     2   Spasm induced only by stimulation
     3   Infrequent occurring less than once per hour
     4   Spontaneous spasms occurring more than once per hour
     5   Spontaneous spasms occurring more than 10 times per hour
  b. Severity of spasticity
     1   Mild
     2   Moderate
     3   Severe

4. Pediatric Evaluation of Disability Inventory
  a. https://www.pearsonclinical.com.au/products/view/165

5. Patient Reporting Impact of Spasticity Measure
  a. https://journals.lww.com/jnpt/fulltext/2005/12000/the_patient_reported_
     impact_of_spasticity_measure.56.aspx

6. Canadian Occupational Performance Measure
  a. https://www.thecopm.ca/

7. Burke–Fahn–Marsden Dystonia Rating Scale
  a. https://pubmed.ncbi.nlm.nih.gov/3966004/

8. Barry–Albright Dystonia Scale
  a. https://pubmed.ncbi.nlm.nih.gov/10400175/

9. Movement Disorder Childhood Rating Scale
  a. https://eprovide.mapi-trust.org/instruments/movement-disorder
     -childhood-rating-scale-revised-4–18-yrs
  b. https://eprovide.mapi-trust.org/instruments/movement-disorder
     -childhood-rating-scale-0–3-yrs

10. Dyskinesia Impairment Scale
  a. https://www.aacpdm.org/UserFiles/file/Dyskinesia-Impairment-Scale-
     Scoring.pdf

11. Global Impression of Change
  a. https://en.wikipedia.org/wiki/Clinical_Global_Impression

12. Numeric Pain Scale
  a. https://www.sralab.org/rehabilitation-measures/numeric-pain-rating-scale

REFERENCES

1. Meng E, Hoang T. MEMS-enabled implantable drug infusion pumps for laboratory animal research, preclinical, and clinical applications. *Adv Drug Deliv Rev.* 2012;64(14):1628–1638. https://doi.org/10.1016/j.addr.2012.08.006

2. Bensmail D, Ward AB, Wissel J, et al. Cost-effectiveness modeling of intrathecal baclofen therapy versus other interventions for disabling spasticity. *Neurorehabil Neural Repair.* 2009;23(6):546–552. https://doi.org/10.1177/1545968308328724

3. de Lissovoy G, Matza LS, Green H, et al. Cost-effectiveness of intrathecal baclofen therapy for the treatment of severe spasticity associated with cerebral palsy. *J Child Neurol.* 2007;22(1):49–59. https://doi.org/10.1177/0883073807299976. PMID: 17608306

4. Hoving MA, Evers SM, Ament AJ, van Raak EP, Vles JS; Dutch Study Group on Child Spasticity. Intrathecal baclofen therapy in children with intractable spastic cerebral palsy: a cost-effectiveness analysis. *Dev Med Child Neurol.* 2008;50(6):450–5. https://doi.org/10.1111/j.1469-8749.2008.02059.x. Epub 2008 Apr 14. PMID: 18422682.

5. Molnar GE. Rehabilitation in cerebral palsy. *West J Med.* 1991;154(5):569–572. https://doi.org/10.1177/1545968308328724. Epub 2009 Feb 19. PMID: 19228818.

6. Creamer M, Cloud G, Kossmehl P, et al. Effect of intrathecal baclofen on pain and quality of life in poststroke spasticity: a randomized trial (SISTERS). *Stroke.* 2018;49(9):2129–2137. https://doi.org/10.1161/STROKEAHA.118.022255

7. Narouze S, Benzon HT, Provenzano D, et al. Interventional spine and pain procedures in patients on antiplatelet and anticoagulant medications (second edition): guidelines from the american society of regional anesthesia and pain medicine, the european society of regional anaesthesia and pain therapy, the american academy of pain medicine, the international neuromodulation society, the north american neuromodulation society, and the world institute of pain. *Reg Anesth Pain Med.* 2018;43(3):225–262. https://doi.org/10.1097/AAP.0000000000000700

8. Burns AS, Meythaler JM. Intrathecal baclofen in tetraplegia of spinal origin: efficacy for upper extremity hypertonia. *Spinal Cord.* 2001;39(8):413–419. https://doi.org/10.1038/sj.sc.3101178

9. Motta F, Stignani C, Antonello CE. Upper limb function after intrathecal baclofen treatment in children with cerebral palsy. *J Pediatr Orthop.* 2008;28(1):91–96. https://doi.org/10.1097/BPO.0b013e31815b4dbc

10. Jacobs NW, Maas EM, Brusse-Keizer M, et al. Effectiveness and safety of cervical catheter tip placement in intrathecal baclofen treatment of spasticity: a systematic review. *J Rehabil Med.* 2021;53(7):jrm00215-2857. https://doi.org/10.2340/16501977-2857

11. Kofler M, Matzak H, Saltuari L. The impact of intrathecal baclofen on gastrointestinal function. *Brain Inj.* 2002;16(9):825–836. https://doi.org/10.1080/02699050210128898

12. Morant A, Noe E, Boyer J, et al. Paralytic ileus: a complication after intrathecal baclofen therapy. *Brain Inj.* 2006;20(13–14):1451–1454. https://doi.org/10.1080/02699050601082016

13. Vaidyanathan S, Soni BM, Oo T, et al. Bladder stones—red herring for resurgence of spasticity in a spinal cord injury patient with implantation of Medtronic Synchromed pump for intrathecal delivery of baclofen—a case report. *BMC Urol.* 2003;3:3. https://doi.org/10.1186/1471-2490-3-3

14. Carda S, Cazzaniga M, Taiana C, et al. Intrathecal baclofen bolus complicated by deep vein thrombosis and pulmonary embolism. A case report. *Eur J Phys Rehabil Med* 2008;44(1):87–88.

15. Murphy NA. Deep venous thrombosis as a result of hypotonia secondary to intrathecal baclofen therapy: a case report. *Arch Phys Med Rehabil.* 2002;83(9):1311–1312. https://doi.org/10.1053/apmr.2002.34270

16. Lam Wai Shun P, Bottari C, Dubé S, et al. Factors influencing clinicians' referral or admission decisions for post-acute stroke or traumatic brain injury rehabilitation: a scoping review. *PM R.* 2021.

17. Saulino M, Anderson DJ, Doble J, et al. Best practices for intrathecal baclofen therapy: troubleshooting. *Neuromodulation.* 2016;19(6):632–641. https://doi.org/10.1111/ner.12467

18. Rigoli G, Terrini G, Cordioli Z. Intrathecal baclofen withdrawal syndrome caused by low residual volume in the pump reservoir: a report of 2 cases. *Arch Phys Med Rehabil.* 2004;85(12):2064–2066. https://doi.org/10.1016/j.apmr.2004.02.020

19. Maneyapanda MB, Chang Chien GC, Mattie R, et al. Ultrasound guidance for technically challenging intrathecal baclofen pump refill: three cases and procedure description. *Am J Phys Med Rehabil.* 2016;95(9).692–7. https://doi.org/10.1097/PHM.0000000000000495

20. Miracle AC, Fox MA, Ayyangar RN, et al. Imaging Evaluation of Intrathecal Baclofen Pump-Catheter Systems. *AJNR Am J Neuroradiol.* 2011;32(7):1158–64. https://doi.org/10.3174/ajnr.A2211

21. Coyne PJ, Hansen LA, Laird J, et al. Massive hydromorphone dose delivered subcutaneously instead of intrathecally: guidelines for prevention and management of opioid, local anesthetic, and clonidine overdose. *J Pain Symptom Manage.* 2004;28(3):273–276. http://doi.org/10.1016/j.jpainsymman.2003.11.011

22. Elovic E, Kirshblum SC. Managing spasticity in spinal cord injury: safe administration of bridge boluses during intrathecal baclofen pump refills. *J Spinal Cord Med.* 2003;26(1):2–4. http://doi.org/10.1080/10790268.2003.11753652

23. Coffey RJ, Edgar TS, Francisco GE, et al. Abrupt withdrawal from intrathecal baclofen: recognition and management of a potentially life-threatening syndrome. *Arch Phys Med Rehabil.* 2002;83(6):735–741. http://doi.org/10.1053/apmr.2002.32820

24. Hansen CR, Gooch JL, Such-Neibar T. Prolonged, severe intrathecal baclofen withdrawal syndrome: a case report. *Arch Phys Med Rehabil.* 2007;88(11):1468–1471. http://doi.org/10.1016/j.apmr.2007.07.021

25. Schmitz NS, Krach LE, Coles LD, et al. A Randomized dose escalation study of intravenous baclofen in healthy volunteers: clinical tolerance and pharmacokinetics. *PM & R.* 2017;9(8):743–750. http://doi.org/10.1016/j.pmrj.2016.11.002

26. Agarwal SK, Kriel RL, Cloyd JC, et al. A Pilot Study Assessing pharmacokinetics and tolerability of oral and intravenous baclofen in healthy adult volunteers. *J Child Neurol.* 2015;30(1):37–41. http://doi.org/10.1177/0883073814535504

27. Dalton C, Keenan E, Stevenson V. A novel cause of intrathecal baclofen overdosage: lessons to be learnt. *Clin Rehabil.* 2008;22(2):188–190. http://doi.org/10.1177/0269215507081962

28. Lew SM, Psaty EL, Abbott R. An unusual cause of overdose after baclofen pump implantation: case report. *Neurosurgery.* 2005;56(3):E624; discussion E624.

29. Sauter K, Kaufman HH, Bloomfield SM, et al. Treatment of high-dose intrathecal morphine overdose. *J Neurosurg.* 1994;81(1):143–146. http://doi.org/10.3171/jns.1994.81.1.0143

30. Sgouros S, Charalambides C, Matsota P, et al. Malfunction of SynchroMed II baclofen pump delivers a near-lethal baclofen overdose. *Pediatr Neurosurg.* 2010;46(1):62–65. http://doi.org/10.1159/000315319

31. Bethoux F, Boulis N, McClelland 3rd S, et al. Use of intrathecal baclofen for treatment of severe spasticity in selected patients with motor neuron disease. *Neurorehabil Neural Repair.* 2013;27(9):828–833. http://doi.org/10.1177/1545968313496325

32. Heetla HW, Staal MJ, Kliphuis C, et al. The incidence and management of tolerance in intrathecal baclofen therapy. *Spinal Cord.* 2009;47(10):751–6. http://doi.org/10.1038/sc.2009.34

33. Erwin A, Gudesblatt M, Bethoux F, et al. Intrathecal baclofen in multiple sclerosis: too little, too late? *Mult Scler.* 2011;17(5):623–629. http://doi.org/10.1177/1352458510395056

34. Vaidyanathan S, Soni BM, Oo T, et al. Delayed complications of discontinuation of intrathecal baclofen therapy: resurgence of dyssynergic voiding, which triggered off autonomic dysreflexia and hydronephrosis. *Spinal Cord.* 2004;42(10):598–602. http://doi.org/10.1038/sj.sc.3101631

35. Manchikanti L, Kaye AD, Falco FJE, et al. *Intrathecal Drug Delivery Systems. Essentials of Interventional Techniques in Managing Chronic Pain.* Springer International Publishing; 2018:671.

36. Kosturakis A, Gebhardt R. SynchroMed II intrathecal pump memory errors due to repeated magnetic resonance imaging. *Pain Physician.* 2012;15(6):475–477.

37. Sayed D, Chakravarthy K, Amirdelfan K, et al. A Comprehensive practice guideline for magnetic resonance imaging compatibility in implanted neuromodulation devices. *Neuromodulation.* 2020;23(7):893–911. http://doi.org/10.1111/ner.13233

38. Galica R, Hayek SM, Veizi IE, et al. Sudden intrathecal drug delivery device motor stalls: a case series. *Reg Anesth Pain Med.* 2016;41(2):135–139. http://doi.org/10.1097/AAP.0000000000000368

39. Whelan A, Patterson E, Montgomery K, et al. Baclofen boluses via lumbar puncture for diagnosing loss of intrathecal baclofen efficacy: a case series. *PM R.* 2021;13(11):1309–1311. http://doi.org/10.1002/pmrj.12523

40. Maino P, Koetsier E, Perez RS. Fentanyl overdose caused by malfunction of synchromed ii intrathecal pump: two case reports. *Reg Anesth Pain Med.* 2014;39(5):434-7. http://doi.org/10.1097/AAP.0000000000000132

41. Wesemann K, Coffey RJ, Wallace MS, et al. Clinical accuracy and safety using the synchromed ii intrathecal drug infusion pump. *Reg Anesth Pain Med.* 2014;39(4):341–346. http://doi.org/10.1097/AAP.0000000000000107

42. Turner MS. Assessing syndromes of catheter malfunction with SynchroMed infusion systems: the value of spiral computed tomography with contrast injection. *PM R.* 2010;2(8):757–766. http://doi.org/10.1016/j.pmrj.2010.05.011

43. Delhaas EM, van der Lugt A. Low-dose computed tomography with two- and three-dimensional postprocessing as an alternative to plain radiography for intrathecal catheter visualization: a phantom pilot study. *Neuromodulation.* 2019;22(7):818–822. http://doi.org/10.1111/ner.12966

44. Stokic DS, Yablon SA. Neurophysiological basis and clinical applications of the H-reflex as an adjunct for evaluating response to intrathecal baclofen for spasticity. *Acta Neurochir Suppl.* 2007;97(Pt 1):231–241. http://doi.org/10.1007/978-3-211-33079-1_32

45. Saulino M, Turner M, Miesel K, et al. Can cerebrospinal fluid pressure detect catheter complications in patients who experience loss of effectiveness with intrathecal baclofen therapy? *Neuromodulation.* 2016;20(2):187–197. http://doi.org/10.1111/ner.12471

46. Delhaas EM, van Assema DME, Fröberg AC, et al. Isotopic scintigraphy in intrathecal drug delivery failure: a single-institution case series. *Neuromodulation.* 2021;24(7):1190–1198. http://doi.org/10.1111/ner.13275

47. Deer TR, Prager J, Levy R, et al. Polyanalgesic Consensus Conference--2012: consensus on diagnosis, detection, and treatment of catheter-tip granulomas (inflammatory masses). *Neuromodulation.* 2012;15(5):483–95; discussion 496. http://doi.org/10.1111/j.1525-1403.2012.00449

48. De Andres J, Villanueva V, Palmisani S, et al. The safety of magnetic resonance imaging in patients with programmable implanted intrathecal drug delivery systems: a 3-year prospective study. *Anesth Analg.* 2011;112(5):1124–1129.

49. Creamer M, Cloud G, Kossmehl P, et al. Effect of intrathecal baclofen on pain and quality of life in poststroke spasticity: a randomized trial (SISTERS). *Stroke.* 2018;49(9):2129–2137. http://doi.org/10.1213/ANE.0b013e318210d017

50. Saulino M, Guillemette S, Leier J, et al. Medical cost impact of intrathecal baclofen therapy for severe spasticity. *Neuromodulation.* 2015;18(2):141–9; discussion 149. https://doi.org/10.1111/ner.12220

51. Boster AL, Bennett SE, Bilsky GS, et al. Best practices for intrathecal baclofen therapy: screening test. *Neuromodulation.* 2016;19(6):616–622.

24 Multiple Sclerosis-Related Spasticity

Ahmed Z. Obeidat and Nicholas C. Ketchum

INTRODUCTION

Multiple sclerosis (MS) is a common cause of neurologic disability in young adults. MS is an immune-mediated, neurodegenerative disease of the central nervous system (CNS).[1,2] Millions of people are living with MS worldwide, and while treatable, the disease remains incurable.[2]

Epidemiology

MS can affect people throughout their life span; however, the peak incidence is between 20 to 40 years. MS is at least twice as common in women as men, and prevalence increases with latitude northern to the equator. In the United States, nearly one million people live with MS, with higher prevalence in northern regions.[3] MS can affect all races and ethnicities but is more common in Caucasians compared to non-Caucasians, but it can be more severe and is increasing in incidence in African Americans and Hispanic populations.[2,4] Incidence of spasticity in the setting of MS is variable, with reported ranges between 40% and 80%.[5]

Clinical Course

The most common clinical course is characterized by a relapsing pattern of clinical symptoms and neurologic attacks, which may or may not improve over time. Some patients who start the disease with a relapsing clinical course advance to a stage characterized by a slow progression of symptoms and neurologic disability with no or little clearly defined relapses, while others may continue to have relapse or MRI activity during progression. This latter stage is referred to as secondary progressive MS (SPMS) and can be further classified into active SPMS or inactive SPMS. A smaller proportion of patients (approximately 15%) will have a progressive-from-onset-disease course with no clearly defined relapses, a subtype referred to as primary progressive MS (PPMS).[6]

Etiology

The exact cause(s) of MS remains unknown and etiology is considered multifactorial. A common understanding of MS pathogenesis includes the interaction between genetics, the immune system, and environmental factors. The HLA-DRB1*15:01 allele is considered the strongest risk factor for MS development.[7-9] However, viral-related factors such as those related to the Epstein-Barr Virus (EBV) are considered strong and intriguing components of the disease pathogenesis. Interestingly, the history of EBV exposure is nearly universal in MS patients, and studies support a causal association with EBV exposure preceding disease development. However, it remains under investigation whether EBV's role is in the initiation of the disease process or the initiation and progression of MS.[8] Low serum vitamin D levels have been implicated as an important risk factor for the development of MS.[7] Other risk factors include a westernized diet, obesity, smoking, low sunlight exposure, and other environmental toxins.

Diagnosis

There is no single laboratory or other test to diagnose MS. The diagnosis is clinical and is based on consensus criteria that continue to be updated over time. The most current diagnostic criteria are the revised 2017 McDonald criteria.[10] Importantly, modern criteria allow for earlier diagnosis of MS. The median time from symptom onset to diagnosis is 4.6 months using the 2017 criteria compared to 20 months using the 1983 Poser criteria. A shorter diagnosis time allows for earlier treatment initiation and better clinical outcomes.[11] The diagnosis of MS includes a combination of clinical history, neurologic exam, MRI, and cerebrospinal fluid (CSF) analysis.

Treatment

The treatment of MS has evolved and can be considered in at least four parts:

- Acute treatment of the relapses
  - Corticosteroids, adrenocorticotropic hormone, plasma exchange or immune adsorption, and rehabilitation[12]
- Disease modification, with goals of reducing relapses, MRI activity, and disability progression
  - More than nine distinct groups of disease-modifying therapies (based on the proposed mechanism of action) have various clinical and radiological effectiveness and distinct safety profiles.[13]
- Symptom management
  - Spasticity, neurogenic bladder, weakness, imbalance, pain, attention difficulties, and fatigue[14,15]
- Management of comorbidities
  - Depression, anxiety, metabolic disease, and aging-associated conditions[16]

Compared to the other common causes of the upper motor neuron syndrome (UMNS) that can lead to spasticity, MS is unique in the fact that it can be progressive where the other conditions are neurologically static. MS is also unique in the fact that it can lead to spinal-origin or cerebral-origin spasticity, which means that the clinical presentation can be quite variable. These facts make proper assessment and management of spasticity in patients with MS uniquely challenging.

DIAGNOSTIC APPROACH

History and Physical

The assessment of spasticity in patients with MS is done similarly to other etiologies of the condition:

- **History:** Make sure to include caregivers and, when possible, engage a patient's therapist as they have clinical experience with how the patient's spasticity affects their passive and active function.
- **Exam:** Using Gracies' 5-step approach is helpful to guide the assessment of the patient.[17] Elements of a physical exam include the following assessments:
  - Passive range of motion (ROM)
  - Assessment of resistance to passive movement/spasticity:
    - Tardieu Scale
    - Ashworth Scale (AS)/Modified Ashworth Scale (MAS)
  - Active ROM
  - Rapid alternating movement
  - Assessment of function
    - If the patient is able to ambulate, assess ambulation with and (if safe) without assistive devices or bracing.
  - Manual muscle testing

Clinical Tools

There are tools specific to MS that can help assess a patient's spasticity, the impact that spasticity has on their function, and ways to help tailor goal setting. These scales are also frequently used as common outcome measures in clinical trials that assess therapies for MS. The Kurtzke Expanded Disease Severity Scale (EDSS) is one of the most widely used scales used to assess the global functioning of patients with MS (Table 24.1).[18,19] The EDSS can also be used to delineate when treatment options should be considered. As an example, in a recent review, authors recommended referral to a spasticity specialist once a patient reached a score of 4 on the EDSS rather than 6.5, which is the current recommendation.[20]

The Multiple Sclerosis Functional Composite (MSFC) Scale is another commonly used scale. It is comprised of three domains: timed 25-foot walk, 9-hole peg, and the Paced Auditory Serial Addition Test (PASAT-3).[19,21] This composite measure attempts to capture the function of the upper and lower extremities, as well as cognitive function. The 88-item Multiple Sclerosis Spasticity Scale (MSSS-88) is an 88-item questionnaire designed specifically for patients with MS that assesses the global impact of spasticity on a patient's symptoms, physical functioning, emotional health, and social functioning. Each item assesses how much a patient's spasticity has bothered them in the past 2 weeks, from 1 (not bothered at all) to 4 (extremely bothered).[22]

TREATMENT OPTIONS

We briefly discuss treatment options specifically as they pertain to spasticity in MS. Each category of treatment is discussed in more detail elsewhere in this text.

Therapy, Physical Modalities

A recent meta-analysis showed some evidence that outpatient therapy programs, including stretching, balance activities, strengthening, endurance, and walking, made a significant improvement in spasticity.[23] Electrical stimulation (e-stim), in the form of transcutaneous electrical stimulation (TENS) or functional electrical stimulation (FES), were recommended as adjunct treatments by the same meta-analysis.[23]

Table 24.1 Kurtzke Expanded Disease Severity Scale (EDSS)

0.0	Normal exam
1.0	No disability, minimal signs in one functional system (FS)
1.5	No disability, minimal signs in more than one FS
2.0	Minimal disability in one FS
2.5	Minimal disability in two FS
3.0	Moderate disability in one FS, or mild disability in three or four FS
3.5	Fully ambulatory but with moderate disability in one FS
4.0	Fully ambulatory without aid, self-sufficient, but relatively severe disability in one FS, able to walk without assistive device or rest >500 m
4.5	Fully ambulatory without aid, able to work a full day, may otherwise have some limitation of full activity or require minimal assistance, able to walk without assistive device or rest >300 m
5.0	Able to walk without assistive device or rest ~200 m, impairment of full daily activities
5.5	Able to walk without assistive device or rest for ~100 m
6.0	Intermittent or unilateral constant assistive device use required to walk 100 m
6.5	Constant bilateral assistive device use required to walk ~20 m
7.0	Unable to walk >5 m even with assistive device, propels wheelchair, able to transfer independently
7.5	Unable to take more than a few steps, able to propel wheelchair, needs assist with transfers
8.0	Unable to propel wheelchair, but able to be up in chair most of the day, may be able to perform self-cares
8.5	Restricted to bed much of the day, some use of arms
9.0	Needs total assist with mobility and self-cares, can communicate and eat
9.5	Needs total assist with mobility, self-cares, communication, and feeding
10.0	Death due to MS

Source: From Kurtzke JF. Rating neurologic impairment in multiple sclerosis: an expanded disability status scale (EDSS). *Neurology*. 1983;33(11):1444–1452. https://doi.org/10.1212/wnl.33.11.1444

Extracorporeal shock wave therapy (ESWT) has been researched over the past several years for its use in spasticity. It is a noninvasive modality that delivers high pressure to the desired area of treatment. ESWT may reduce spasticity by several mechanisms, including possible effects of promoting nitric oxide (NO) synthesis and NO-induced angiogenesis, modulating muscle spindle activity, and inhibiting stretch reflexes.[24] Radial shock wave therapy (RSWT) is a form of ESWT and has been increasing in popularity for treatment of spasticity. RSWT delivers pressure waves via a pneumatically propelled bullet inside a tube, striking a metal applicator. RSWT is more cost-effective and has less need for local anesthesia as compared to ESWT.[25] In MS specifically, a recent study demonstrated that four weekly treatments of RSWT reduced pain and MAS of plantar flexors; however, this effect was noted to be short-lived.[26]

Oral Medications

A recent publication by Otero-Romero et al. reviews the evidence for oral antispasmodic medications specific to their use in MS.[27] Here we briefly overview some of these common medications used for the treatment of spasticity in MS.

Diazepam

Diazepam is a benzodiazepine that facilitates release of gamma-aminobutyric acid (GABA) from the GABA-A receptor.[28] Dosages range between 2 and 30 mg and has long been used for spinal origin spasticity, including MS.[27]

Baclofen

Baclofen is a GABA-B agonist that modulates spasticity through inhibition of mono- and polysynaptic reflexes.[28] It is commonly a first-line medication used for treatment of spasticity in MS. Dosing ranges between 15 and 100 mg/day, divided in 2 to 4 doses. It has been shown to improve spasticity and decrease clonus in MS.[27]

Tizanidine

Tizanidine is a centrally acting alpha-2 agonist that facilitates presynaptic interneuronal inhibition in the spinal cord.[29] Dosing ranges between 2 and 36 mg/day, typically divided in 2 to 3 doses. Tizanidine has been shown to reduce spasticity and reduce spasms and clonus in MS, with studies showing a similar effect compared to baclofen and diazepam.[27]

Dantrolene

Dantrolene is an oral muscle relaxant with a peripherally acting mechanism, influencing calcium release from the sarcoplasmic reticulum by binding to the ryanodine receptor.[28] Given this peripheral mechanism, there may be less risk of sedation as is seen in other antispasmodic medications. Doses range from 25 to 400 mg/day.[27]

Cannabinoids

Cannabinoids have been demonstrated to be effective for the treatment of MS-related spasticity, particularly nabiximols, an extract of delta-9-tetrahydrocannabinol (THC) and cannabidiol (CBD). This is available in Canada, Europe, and many other countries (not the United States) as an add-on treatment for treatment of spasticity in MS when first-line treatments are not effective.[27] A small study also suggested that it may improve some walking parameters.[30,31]

Botulinum Toxin Injections

Botulinum toxin (BoNT) injections are used for spasticity management by temporarily blocking acetylcholine release of spastic muscles in a focal manner. Onset of action is several days following the injections and duration of available formulations is generally 3 months. A recent study demonstrated that in patients with MS, BoNT reduce the MAS of the injected muscle groups by an average of one point and may be helpful for reaching active functional goals.[32]

Intrathecal Baclofen

Intrathecal baclofen (ITB) is indicated for patients with severe spasticity in the setting of MS.[33] ITB is delivered through a surgically implanted pump and catheter, directly delivering baclofen near GABA-B receptors in the spinal cord. This allows for a significantly lower dose to be administered as compared to oral baclofen, bypassing the blood–brain barrier, and fewer side effects of somnolence as is commonly seen in oral baclofen use. ITB has been shown to be effective and safe in the setting of severe spasticity secondary to MS.[34,35] A recent review suggests that in addition to reducing spasticity as measured by the MAS, it may also maintain or improve walking in ambulatory patients with MS.[36]

COMPLICATIONS

The risks of sedation and constipation must be taken into consideration when using oral baclofen.[37] Tizanidine and dantrolene may lead to hepatic dysfunction, so liver function should be monitored when using these medications.[27] Given the coincidence of neurogenic bladder in MS, care must be taken to coordinate the timing and dosage of injections with providers who may be providing bladder BoNT, or other indications.[38] Given ITB involves surgery and an implanted device, surgical risk and potential for device failure must be taken into account; however, this risk has been suggested to be low, with a 90% device survival rate over the course of one registry.[39] As with any treatment for spasticity, risk of hypotonia and unmasking underlying weakness must be considered, especially with ambulatory patients with risk of fall.

CASE REPORT

JP is a 56-year-old female who was diagnosed with primary progressive MS. Her initial symptoms were numbness and tingling in her right lower extremity, followed by the onset of spasms and weakness. She noted a constant stiffness in her right leg with associated frequent curling of her toes. She reported several falls over the past few months. She enjoyed walking for exercise and her new symptoms made this more difficult. She also reported significant fatigue, which she associated with the onset of her MS. On physical exam, she was noted to have excessive right plantar flexion, toe flexion, and ankle inversion, with mild right hip circumduction to help clear her right lower extremity. There was excessive right knee extension in stance. Her upper extremities were normal without abnormal posturing. A sensory exam revealed a mild reduction of light touch throughout her right lower extremity. Manual muscle testing revealed a Medical Research Council (MRC) grade of 5/5 in both upper extremities, with lower extremity strength as shown in Table 24.2, MRC grade of lower extremities. Spasticity was assessed using the MAS, as seen in Table 24.3.

Table 24.2 Medical Research Council Muscle Strength Grade in Bilateral Lower Extremities – Initial Visit

Muscle Group	Right	Left
Hip flexors	5	5
Hip abductors	5	5
Knee extensors	5	5
Knee flexors	4	5
Ankle dorsiflexors	4	5
Ankle plantar flexors	5	5

The patient's goals included fewer spasms and more stability with ambulation. She was subsequently provided with a prescription for physical therapy. She completed outpatient therapy and was instructed on a home exercise program. Her balance and timed 25-minute walk test improved but she continued to note that her toes would curl, she would drag her foot on occasion, and she had painful spasms that occurred particularly at night. A discussion of treatment options was had with the patient and her significant other. Given focal spasticity and concerns of fatigue, onabotulinumtoxinA (ONA) was recommended. Once insurance authorization was obtained, she was treated with 300 units of ONA in the right lower extremity as outlined in Table 24.4. Electromyography (EMG), e-stim, and ultrasound (US) guidance were all utilized for guidance.

Table 24.3 Assessment of Spasticity – Modified Ashworth Scale – Initial Visit

Muscle Group	Right	Left
Hip flexors	0	0
Hip adductors	0	0
Knee extensors	1	0
Knee flexors	1	0
Ankle plantar flexors	2	0
Ankle invertors	1	0
Toe flexors	1	0

Table 24.4 ONA Injection #1

Muscle Group	Dose (Units)	Sites
Gastrocnemius, medial head	75	3
Soleus	75	3
Posterior tibialis	50	2
Flexor digitorum longus	50	2
Flexor hallucis longus	50	2

Table 24.5 Medical Research Council Muscle Strength Grade in Bilateral Lower Extremities – Year 2

Muscle Group	Right	Left
Hip flexors	4	4
Hip abductors	4	4
Knee extensors	3	3
Knee flexors	3	3
Ankle dorsiflexors	3	3
Ankle plantar flexors	4	4

The patient followed up at 6 weeks post injections. She reported consistent compliance with her home exercise program, improvement of stiffness and spasms, and fewer falls. She denied any excessive weakness or other side effects following the injections. This treatment regimen worked well, and she returned for reevaluation and re-treatment approximately every 12 weeks.

Two years later, the patient's MS continued to progress. She now has spastic paraparesis, which limits her ambulation to only being able to walk short distances with a wheeled walker. The patient also needs assistance with toileting, bathing, and lower extremity dressing from a caregiver. Her current strength and spasticity exam are as follows:

Spasticity is assessed using the MAS (Table 24.3). Her hip adduction impacts her mobility, her transfers, and her ability to stand as well as perineal care and dressing. She has been receiving ONA 600 units as outlined in Table 24.7, with a good reduction of her spasticity, improved ability to transfer, less difficulty with her activities of daily living (ADLs), and less caregiver burden.

She was on a stable regimen for approximately 3 years and then started to have further progression of her MS, including lower extremity weakness and onset of upper extremity weakness and spasticity. Functionally, she now requires the assistance of a caregiver for transfers and needs significant assistance for toileting, perineal care, and lower extremity dressing. The patient's decrease in ambulatory ability has led

Table 24.6 Assessment of Spasticity - Modified Ashworth Scale – Year 2

Muscle Group	Right	Left
Hip flexors	2	1
Hip adductors	2	2
Knee extensors	2	2
Knee flexors	3	2
Ankle plantar flexors	3	2
Ankle invertors	3	2
Toe flexors	3	2

Table 24.7 ONA Injection Year 2

Muscle Group	Dose (Units)	Sites
Right adductor longus	75	3
Right gastrocnemius, medial head	75	3
Right soleus	100	3
Right posterior tibialis	75	2
Right flexor digitorum longus	50	2
Right flexor hallucis longus	75	2
Left adductor longus	50	2
Left soleus	50	2
Left flexor digitorum longus	50	2

Table 24.8 ONA Injection Year 5

Muscle Group	Dose (Units)	Sites
Right flexor digitorum longus	100	4
Right flexor hallucis longus	100	4

her to rely on a power wheelchair for mobility. She also has difficulty with urinary incontinence, which was diagnosed as overactive bladder (OAB) by her urologist. The urologist recommends treatment of OAB with ONA. Given that the patient is already receiving 600 units of ONA for spasticity of her lower extremities, the decision is made to discuss ITB therapy.

After much discussion, she consents to a test dose of ITB, which leads to a dramatic reduction of her spasticity. She is referred to neurosurgery, who ultimately proceeds with the implantation of an ITB pump. After implant, she is transferred to acute inpatient rehabilitation for work on transfers, upper extremity ADLs, and ITB dose titration. She is ultimately titrated to a dose of 250 mcg/day ITB with excellent control of her spasticity globally. Given her excellent control of generalized spasticity from her ITB pump, she is initially able to defer ONA injections altogether. She eventually develops focal areas of problematic spasticity in her right toe flexors, which makes footwear difficult to don, impedes her ability to keep her foot placed on the footplate of her power wheelchair, and causes uncomfortable spasms. The patient's ITB dose is increased to help combat these issues, but the higher doses lead to a larger decrease in spasticity than desired. The previous ITB dose retained enough spasticity in the patient that she was able to assist in transfers and the patient prefers this. As such, she opted for focal treatment of her problematic right lower extremity with ONA. Since her goals are more for passive rather than active function, the targeted problematic muscles are able to be treated more aggressively.

REFERENCES

1. Ropper AH, Samuels MA, Klein JP, Prasad, S. *Adams and Victor's Principles of Neurology.* New York: McGraw-Hill Medical Pub; 2020.

2. Ward M, Goldman MD. Epidemiology and pathophysiology of multiple sclerosis. *Continuum (Minneapolis Minn).* 2022;28(4):988–1005. https://doi.org/10.1212/CON.0000000000001136

3. Wallin MT, Culpepper WJ, Campbell JD, et al. The prevalence of MS in the United States: a population-based estimate using health claims data. *Neurology.* 2019;92(10):e1029–e1040. http://doi.org/10.1212/WNL.0000000000007035

4. Amezcua L, McCauley JL. Race and ethnicity on MS presentation and disease course. *Mult Scler J.* 2020;26(5):561–567. http://doi.org/10.1177/1352458519887328

5. Francisco GE, Bandari DS, Bavikatte G, et al. High clinician-and patient-reported satisfaction with individualized onabotulinumtoxinA treatment for spasticity across several etiologies from the ASPIRE study. *Toxicon: X,* 2020;7:100040. http://doi.org/10.1016/j.toxcx.2020.100040

6. Klineova S, Lublin FD. Clinical course of multiple sclerosis. *Cold Spring Harb Perspect Med.* 2018;8(9):a028928. http://doi.org/10.1101/cshperspect.a028928

7. Marcucci SB, Obeidat AZ. EBNA1, EBNA2, and EBNA3 link Epstein-Barr virus and hypovitaminosis D in multiple sclerosis pathogenesis. *J Neuroimmunol.* 2020;339:577116. https://doi.org/10.1016/j.jneuroim.2019.577116

8. Lanz TV, Brewer RC, Ho PP, et al. Clonally expanded B cells in multiple sclerosis bind EBV EBNA1 and GlialCAM. *Nature.* 2022;603(7900):321–327. https://doi.org/10.1038/s41586-022-04432-7

9. Bjornevik K, Cortese M, Healy BC, et al. Longitudinal analysis reveals high prevalence of Epstein-Barr virus associated with multiple sclerosis. *Science.* 2022;375(6578):296–301. https://doi.org/10.1126/science.abj8222

10. Thompson AJ, Banwell BL, Barkhof F, et al. Diagnosis of multiple sclerosis: revisions of the Mcdonald criteria. *Lancet Neurol.* 2018;17 (2):162–173. https://doi.org/10.1016/S1474-4422(17)30470-2

11. Tintore M, Cobo-Calvo A, Carbonell P, et al. Effect of changes in MS diagnostic criteria over 25 years on time to treatment and prognosis in patients with clinically isolated syndrome. *Neurology.* 2021;97(17):e1641–e1652. https://doi.org/ 10.1212/WNL.0000000000012726

12. Repovic P. Management of multiple sclerosis relapses. *Continuum (Minneapolis Minn.).* 2019;25(3):655–669. https://doi.org/10.1212/CON.0000000000000739

13. Yang JH, Rempe T, Whitmire N, Dunn-Pirio A, Graves JS. Therapeutic advances in multiple sclerosis. *Front Neurol.* 2022;13:824926. https://doi.org/10.3389/fneur.2022.824926

14. Spain R. Approach to symptom management in multiple sclerosis with a focus on wellness. *Continuum (Minneap Minn.).* 2022;28(4):1052–1082. https://doi.org/10.1212/CON.0000000000001140

15. Newsome SD, Thrower B, Hendin B, Danese S, Patterson J, Chinnapongse R. Symptom burden, management and treatment goals of people with MS spasticity: results from SEEN-MSS, a large-scale, self-reported survey. *Mult Scler Relat Disorder.* 2022;68:104376. https://doi.org/10.1016/j.msard.2022.104376

16. Ostolaza A, Corroza J, Ayuso T. Multiple sclerosis and aging: comorbidity and treatment challenges. *Mult Scler Relat Disords.* 2021;50:102815. https://doi.org/10.1016/j.msard.2021.102815

17. Gracies JM, Bayle N, Vinti M, et al. Five-step clinical assessment in spastic paresis. *Eur Phys Rehabil Med.* 2010;46(3):411–421.

18. Kurtzke JF. Rating neurologic impairment in multiple sclerosis: an expanded disability status scale (EDSS). *Neurology.* 1983;33(11):1444–1452. https://doi.org/10.1212/wnl.33.11.1444

19. Meyer-Moock S, Feng YS, Maeurer M, Dippel FW, Kohlmann T. Systematic literature review and validity evaluation of the Expanded Disability Status Scale (EDSS) and the Multiple Sclerosis Functional Composite (MSFC) in patients with multiple sclerosis. *BMC Neurol.* 2014;14:58. https://doi.org/10.1186/1471-2377-14-58. PMID: 24666846; PMCID: PMC3986942.

20. Erwin A, Gudesblatt M, Bethoux F, et al. Intrathecal baclofen in multiple sclerosis: too little, too late? *Multiple Sclerosis Journal.* 2011;17(5):623–629. https://doi.org/10.1177/1352458510395056

21. Cutter GR, Baier ML, Rudick RA, et al. Development of a multiple sclerosis functional composite as a clinical trial outcome measure. *Brain.* 1999;122 (Pt 5):871–882. https://doi.org/10.1093/brain/122.5.871. PMID: 10355672.)

22. Hobart JC, Riazi A, Thompson J, et al. Getting the measure of spasticity in multiple sclerosis: the multiple sclerosis spasticity scale (msss-88). *Brain.* 2006;129(1):224–234. https://doi.org/10.1093/brain/awh675

23. Etoom M, Khraiwesh Y, Lena F, et al. Effectiveness of physiotherapy interventions on spasticity in people with multiple sclerosis: a systematic review and meta-analysis. *Am J Phys Medrehabil.* 2018;97(11):793–807. https://doi.org/10.1097/PHM.0000000000000970.

24. Santamato A, Notarnicola A, Panza F, et al. SBOTE study: extracorporeal shock wave therapy versus electrical stimulation after botulinum toxin type A injection for post-stroke spasticity–a prospective randomized trial. *Ultrasound Mede Biol.* 2013;39(2):283–291.

25. Gonkova MI, Ilieva EM, Ferriero G, Chavdarov I. Effect of radial shock wave therapy on muscle spasticity in children with cerebral palsy. *Int J Rehabil Res.* 2013;36(3):284–290. https://doi.org/10.1097/MRR.0b013e328360e51d.

26. Marinelli L, Mori L, Solaro C, et al. Effect of radial shock wave therapy on pain and muscle hypertonia: a double-blind study in patients with multiple sclerosis. *Mul Scler J.* 2015;21(5):622–629.https://doi.org/10.1177/1352458514549566.

27. Otero-Romero S, Sastre-Garriga J, Comi G, et al. Pharmacological management of spasticity in multiple sclerosis: systematic review and consensus paper. *Mult Scler J.* 2016;22(11):1386–1396. https://doi.org/10.1177/1352458516643600.

28. Meythaler JM. Pharmacologic management of spasticity: oral medications. In: Brashear A, Elie Elovic. *Spasticity: Diagnosis and Management. Demos;* 2016.

29. Ghanavatian S, Derian A. Tizanidine. [Updated 2022 Sep 5]. In: StatPearls [Internet]. Treasure Island (FL): StatPearls Publishing; 2022. https://www.ncbi.nlm.nih.gov/books/NBK519505/, accessed 1/23/2023

30. Coghe G, Pau M, Corona F. *et al.* Walking improvements with nabiximols in patients with multiple sclerosis. *J Neurol.* 2015;262:2472–2477. https://doi.org/10.1007/s00415-015-7866-5.

31. Chan A, Silván CV. Evidence-based management of multiple sclerosis spasticity with nabiximols oromucosal spray in clinical practice: a 10-year recap. *Neurodegenerdis Manag.* 2022;12(3):141–154. https://doi.org/10.2217/nmt-2022-0002.

32. Baccouche I, Bensmail D, Leblong E, et al. Goal-setting in multiple sclerosis-related spasticity treated with botulinum toxin: the gaseptox study. *Toxins.* 2022;14(9):582. https://doi.org/10.3390/toxins14090582.

33. Lioresal (baclofen intrathecal) package insert. Amneal Pharmaceuticals, 2023.

34. Sammaraiee Y, Yardley M, Keenan L, Buchanan K, Stevenson V, Farrell, R. Intrathecal baclofen for multiple sclerosis related spasticity: a twenty-year experience. *Mult Scler Relat Disord.* 2019;27:95–100. https://doi.org/10.1016/j.msard.2018.10.009.

35. Natale M, D'Oria S, Nero VV, Squillante E, Gentile M, Rotondo M. Long-term effects of intrathecal baclofen in multiple sclerosis. *Clin Neurol Neurosurg.* 2016;143:121–125. https://doi.org/10.1016/j.clineuro.2016.02.016.

36. Lee HP, Win T, Balakrishnan S. The impact of intrathecal baclofen on the ability to walk: a systematic review. *Clin Rehabili.* 2022;37(4);462–477. https://doi.org/10.1177/02692155221135827.

37. Ghanavatian S, Derian A. Baclofen. In *StatPearls* [Internet]. StatPearls Publishing; 2021. Accessed 1/23/23.

38. Botox (onabotulinumtoxinA) package insert. AbbVie, Inc. 2022.

39. Konrad PE, Huffman JM, Stearns LM, Plunkett RJ, Grigsby EJ, Stromberg EK, Roediger MP, et al. Intrathecal drug delivery systems (idds): the implantable systems performance registry (ispr). *Neuromodulation: J Int Neuromodulation Soc.* 2016;19(8):848–856. https://doi.org/10.1111/ner.12524.

25 The Combo Meal: Combined Treatments for Spasticity Management

John McGuire

INTRODUCTION

Patients with focal spasticity can normally be managed with a single treatment. This is rarely the case in patients with generalized spasticity. Patients with multisegmental or generalized disabling spasticity typically require a combination of treatments to manage their spasticity.[1] Despite being considered standard of care by most experienced clinicians, there is a lack of controlled studies on how oral medications, chemodenervation with botulinum neurotoxins (BoNT), chemical neurolysis with phenol or alcohol, intrathecal baclofen (ITB), and orthopedic surgery are used together. Typically, the least invasive treatments are started initially, and if ineffective, they can be combined with more invasive treatments as needed. A combination of these treatments may have a synergistic therapeutic benefit to managing for patients with disabling spasticity.[2]

DIAGNOSTIC APPROACH

Prior to initiating any treatment, establishing appropriate patient-specific goals and a thorough physical examination is critical for successful outcomes. Whether the goals are to provide symptomatic relief and improve passive function or active function, they must be clearly identified and agreed upon by the patient, caregiver, therapist, and physician. A focused medical and neurologic examination of the patient is needed to identify and treat any potential causes of increased spasticity such as pressure sores, constipation, fractures, deep venous thrombosis, or infections. Whether injectable, surgical, or medical treatments are used, they should be combined with the appropriate physical and occupational therapy and home exercise program to be most effective.[3] Each treatment has potential strengths and weaknesses so an optimal treatment plan should maximize the benefits of each while minimizing the risks. This chapter reviews potential combinations of treatments to optimally manage patients with multisegmental or generalized disabling spasticity.

TREATMENT OPTIONS

Oral Medications and Botulinum Toxin

Oral medications and BoNT are probably the most combined treatments for patients with multisegmental or generalized spasticity. In a prospective observational multicenter study, Equenazi et.al. (2012) reported 34% of the 487 patients treated with BoNT and/or phenol were also taking oral antispasticity medications. Because of dosing limitations, not all problematic muscles can be managed with BoNT and/or phenol in patients with generalized spasticity. Especially patients with pain and/or difficulty sleeping are often best treated with a combined treatment of BoNT and oral antispasticity medication. Typically, a higher dose in the evening may improve sleep and reduce the daytime drowsiness commonly associated with oral antispasticity medications. Also, a lower dose of baclofen, tizanidine, dantrolene, and/or gabapentin used together maybe more effective and better tolerated than a higher dose of one alone.

Chemodenervation and Chemical Neurolysis

Chemodenervation with BoNT and chemical neurolysis with phenol or alcohol injections can be combined to effectively manage patients with multifocal or multisegmental spasticity.[3] In the Patient Registry of Outcomes in Spasticity Care (PROS) study of 487 patients with stroke or traumatic brain injury (TBI) who were treated with BoNT and/or phenol, only 9 patients were managed with both BoNT and phenol. The reason cited was that not all injectors were comfortable doing phenol or phenol was not available at each center. When used in combination, phenol is typically used for larger more proximal muscles and BoNT for neck, trunk, and distal extremity muscles.

Oral Medication and Intrathecal Baclofen

When oral medications fail to manage a patient's disabling spasticity, they may be a candidate for ITB pump. Once an ITB pump is placed, a patient can usually be weaned off their oral medications. Eighty percent of our patients were taking oral medications prior to ITB, and 10% were taking oral medications after their pump was placed (Figure 25.1).

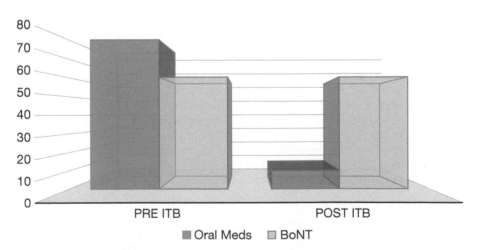

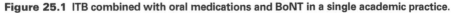

Figure 25.1 ITB combined with oral medications and BoNT in a single academic practice.

Botulinum Neurotoxin and Intrathecal Baclofen

When an ITB pump does not adequately manage a patient's generalized disabling spasticity, the addition of BoNT may be needed to optimize a patient's treatment. In our practice, 60% of our patients who have baclofen pumps were treated with BoNT injections before pump placement and 60% continued to need BoNT injections after their pumps were placed (Figure 25.1). In non-ambulators or non-standers, 90% of the BoNT was injected into arm or neck muscles. In patients who were able to use their legs for standing, transfers, or ambulation, 50% of the BoNT was injected into arm and neck muscles and 50% was injected into leg muscles.

The Full Combo Platter: Intrathecal Baclofen, Botulinum Neurotoxins, Oral Medications, Phenol, and Orthopedic Procedure

In some cases, all of the typically available treatment modalities may be needed to be utilized to adequately manage a single patient's spasticity. This highlights the fact that spasticity management is not linear in nature; we do not move on from one treatment modality to the next and leave the prior modality behind. An individualized approach must be taken for each patient and a unique treatment paradigm utilized in each case.

COMPLICATIONS

The risks of each individual treatment modality must be considered before implementing it for a patient. Additionally, one must consider potential additive effects of multiple concomitant spasticity treatments in the same patient. Also, when implementing a combination of treatments in a single patient, timing of initiation or titration may become important. For example, if changing the dose of an oral medication at the same time as making an ITB pump adjustment, it may be challenging to discern which change is responsible for the observed outcome. As such, utilizing a "one change at a time" approach may simplify these complex situations.

CASE REPORTS

The cases below highlight how combining treatments can be used safely and effectively to manage disabling multifocal and generalized spasticity. Combined spasticity treatments are generally well tolerated and more effective than one treatment alone. The strengths of each treatment can synergize to maximize patient benefits. Typically, the least invasive treatments are started first and then combined with additional treatments as needed. More studies are needed to better understand how to use these treatments together more effectively.

Case #1: A 68-year-old female with history of hypertension and diabetes admitted to inpatient rehabilitation 6 days after a right MCA stroke complicated by spastic left hemiparesis. Her initial rehab was limited by difficulty with sleeping and increased tone and pain of her left shoulder and hip adductors, left knee flexors, and left ankle plantar flexors and inverters. The increased spasticity of her left lower extremity made it difficult for her to stand, transfer, and ambulate. The increased spasticity of her left upper extremity made reaching, dressing, and hygiene more difficult. She was started a 5 mg of oral baclofen at night with the goal of improved sleep and reduced spasticity. After three nights, her dose was increased to 10 mg that helped with her sleep but only minimal reduction of her spasticity. She was also started on gabapentin 100 mg BID to help with her left arm and leg pain. She had minimal reduction of her shoulder and knee pain and felt the medications were making her tired, so her gabapentin was changed to 100 mg at night. Over the next 2 weeks, she was able to tolerate an increased dose of baclofen to 10 mg in the AM and 20 mg in the PM and gabapentin 100 mg in the AM and afternoon and 300 mg at night. Her sleep improved but she continued to be limited by pain and left arm and leg spasticity. Physical examination revealed 3/5 to 4/5 left upper and lower extremity strength with a Modified Ashworth Score (MAS) of 2 to 3 of her left shoulder abductors, hip abductors, knee flexors, and ankle plantar flexors. She underwent a diagnostic anesthetic block (DAB) of her left arm and leg. Two milliliters of a 50/50 mixture of 1% lidocaine and 0.5% bupivacaine were injected into her left gracilis, posterior tibialis, pectoralis major, and latissimus dorsi muscles. After the DAB, she had reduced pain and improved active and passive range of motion (ROM) of her left shoulder, knee, and ankle and improved standing and ambulation. The injections also improved her ability to participate in therapy and sleep. The benefits of the injections lasted for 2 to 3 days. One month after stroke, she continued to take her baclofen and gabapentin and she was injected with 400 units of onabotulinumtoxinA (ONA) to her left arm and leg (Table 25.1). Two weeks post injections, she had reduced spasticity, reduced pain, and improved active and passive ROM of her left arm and leg; upper extremity dressing and hygiene were easier; and she also had improved endurance with walking and going up and down the stairs. The benefits of the injections lasted for 2 months with no increased weakness. Over the next year, every 3 to 4 months, she was treated with an increased doses of ONA to her left arm and left leg. Because she was able to tolerate higher doses of ONA, she was able to reduce her oral medications (Table 25.2). One year after stroke, she was sleeping well and had minimal to no complaints of left arm or leg pain. She was modified independent with her activities of daily living (ADLs) and she ambulated with a straight cane. This case highlights how oral medications and BoNT can be used in combination to successfully manage a patient's after stroke pain and spasticity.

Case #2: A 22-year-old gentleman with spastic paraparesis after a gunshot wound to his back with resultant T8 complete spinal cord injury (SCI). Three months post injury, he was limited by severe hip flexor, hip adductor, and knee flexor and extensor spasms and bilateral ankle clonus that interfered with his bowel program, intermittent catheterization program, as well as lower extremity dressing and slide board transfers. He was not interested in any surgery at this time and did not want to pursue a baclofen pump at this time. After a positive response to a DAB, he was treated with 6% phenol to both hip adductors and medial hamstrings and abobotulinumtoxinA (ABO) to bilateral iliopsoas, sartorius, rectus femoris, and soleus muscles (Table 25.3). Immediately after that, he had markedly reduced hip adductor spasticity and knee flexor spasms. After 1 to 2 weeks, he had significant relief of bilateral lower extremity spasms and improved lower extremity dressing and slide board transfers. These hip and knee flexor spasms no longer interfered with his bowel and bladder programs. The benefits of the injections lasted for 3 months. This case highlights how BoNT and phenol can effectively be used in combination in a patient with multifocal or multisegmental spasticity.

Case #3: A 28-year-old gentleman with a C5 incomplete SCI and severe spastic quadriparesis. Despite taking 120 mg/day of oral baclofen, 16 mg/day of tizanidine, and 2,400 mg/day of gabapentin, he continued to be limited by severe upper and

Table 25.1 Case #1: Onabotulinum Toxin A: Injection #1, 30 Days After Stroke

Muscle	Dilution (mL: 100 units)	Dose	# Sites	Technique
Left Upper Extremity				
Pectoralis Major	2:1	50 units	2	EMG
Latissimus Dorsi	2:1	50 units	2	EMG
Brachialis	2:1	30 units	2	EMG
Brachioradialis	2:1	20 units	1	EMG
Pronator Teres	2:1	25 units	1	EMG
Flexor Carpi Radialis	2:1	30 units	2	EMG
Flexor Carpi Ulnaris	2:1	20 units	1	EMG
Left Lower Extremity				
Gracilis	2:1	50 units	2	EMG
Med Gastroc	4:1	50 units	3	EMG
Lat Gastroc	2:1	25units	1	EMG
Post Tib	4:1	50 units	3	EMG
Total Units Administered		**400 units**		
Total Units Discarded = 0 Units				

Case #1: Oral Medications 30 Days After Stroke	
Medication	**Dose**
Baclofen	10 mg AM, 20 mg PM
Gabapentin	100 mg AM, 100 mg noon, 300 mg PM

lower extremity spasticity. After a successful intrathecal trial of 50 mcg of baclofen, he had a baclofen pump placed. For 6 months, his dose of ITB gradually increased to 400 mcg/day with 50 mcg boluses every 6 hours. His upper and lower extremity spasticity were dramatically reduced, and his dressing, hygiene, bowel, and bladder programs were much easier to perform. He was weaned off his oral baclofen, but he continued to take gabapentin 300 mg TID for nerve pain and tizanidine 2 to 4 mg at night PRN for occasional lower extremity spasms.

Case #4: A 49-year-old gentleman with spastic left hemiparesis after a right parietal intracerebral hemorrhage with disabling left arm and leg spasticity. He was initially treated with 400 units of ONA to his lower extremity and 200 units ONA injected into his upper extremity. His spasticity continued to be problematic, and after a successful trial of 50 mcg of ITB, he had an ITB pump placed. Over 3 to 4 months, his ITB dose was increased to 800 mcg/day. Higher doses of ITB caused increased leg weakness. He continued to be limited by left arm, neck, and toe flexor spasticity. His upper extremity and neck muscles were treated with 500 units of ONA and 100 units of ONA for his toe flexor spasticity. The combined treatment helped reduce his

Table 25.2 Case #1: Botox Injection 4, 1 Year After Stroke

Muscle	Dilution (mL: 100 Units)	Dose	# Sites	Technique
Left Upper Extremity				
Levator Scapulae	4:1	25 units	2	EMG
Pectoralis Major	4:1	75 units	3	EMG
Latissimus Dorsi	4:1	75 units	3	EMG
Teres Major	4:1	25 units	2	EMG
Brachialis	4:1	50 units	4	EMG
Brachioradialis	4:1	25 units	2	EMG
Pronator teres	4:1	25 units	2	EMG
Flexor Carpi Radialis	4:1	30 units	2	EMG
Flexor Carpi Ulnaris	4:1	20 units	2	EMG
Flexor Digitorum Profundus	4:1	50 units	4	EMG
Left Lower Extremity				
Gracilis	4:1	50 units	2	EMG
Med Gastroc	4:1	75 units	3	EMG
Lat Gastroc	4:1	25 units	1	EMG
Post Tib	4:1	50 units	3	EMG/e-stim
Total Units Administered		**600 units**		
Total Units Discarded = 0 Units				

Case #1: Oral Medications 1 Year After Stroke	
Medication	**Dose**
Baclofen	10 mg PM
Gabapentin	200 mg PM

spasticity, improve his active and passive ROM, and improve his arm and leg function with improved gait stability and endurance.

Case #5: A 52-year-old woman with spastic quadriparesis from MS. She was unable to tolerate oral spasticity medications, and after a successful trial of 25 mcg of ITB, she had an ITB pump placed. Her lower extremity spasticity was managed with 60 mcg of ITB. Higher doses of ITB were not tolerated as they decreased her spasticity such that it unmasked weakness in her lower extremities. Thus, at her optimal ITB dose, she continued to have difficulty with grasping her walker with her right hand because of finger flexor spasticity. She had 100 units of incobotulinumtoxinA (INA) divided between her right flexor pollicis longus and flexor digitorum superficialis and profundus. After the INA, she was able to grasp her walker and ambulate without physical assistance. These cases demonstrate how BoNT and ITB can effectively be used in combination to manage a patient with multifocal or multisegmental disabling spasticity.

Table 25.3a Case #2: Dysport Injection #1

Muscle	Dilution (mL: 100 units)	Dose	# Sites	Technique
Right Lower Extremity				
Iliopsoas	1:1	200 units	4	EMG
Sartorius	1:1	150 units	3	EMG
Rectus Femoris	1:1	200 units	4	EMG
Soleus	1:1	200 units	4	EMG
Right Lower Extremity				
Iliopsoas	1:1	200 units	4	EMG
Sartorius	1:1	150 units	3	EMG
Rectus Femoris	1:1	200 units	4	EMG
Soleus	1:1	200 units	4	EMG
Total Units Administered		**1,500 units**		
Total Units Discarded = 0 Units				

Table 25.3b Case #2: Phenol Injection #1

Motor Nerve	%	Dose	Sites	Technique
Right Obturator	6%	2 mL	2	E-stim
Right Medial Hamstring	6%	2 mL	2	E-stim
Left Obturator	6%	2 mL	2	E-stim
Left Medial Hamstring	1:1	2 mL	2	E-stim
Total Administered		8 mL		

Case #6: A 35-year-old gentleman with anoxic brain injury who is limited with increased tone of both upper and lower extremities. He initially had an ITB pump placed that helped reduce spasticity in both lower extremities and trunk muscles. Optimal dosing of ITB was flex programming, 657.3 mcg/day, divided into four scheduled periodic boluses of 100 mcg every 6 hours and a basal rate of 10.4 mcg/hr (Table 25.4). He did not tolerate higher doses of ITB, and he continued to be limited by increased tone of both upper extremities and his neck muscles. He also had pain and difficulty sleeping that was treated with gabapentin 300 mg TID. He had severe spasticity (MAS 4) of his shoulder adductors and elbow flexors that interfered with dressing and hygiene. He was treated with phenol injection to both elbow flexors and pectoralis major muscles and BoNT injections to both wrist and finger flexors and neck muscles (Table 25.4). After the injections, he had improved active and passive ROM and improved dressing, toileting, and hygiene. He was also limited by severe bilateral ankle plantar flexor contractures. He subsequently underwent bilateral split anterior tendon transfer (SPLATT) and tendo Achilles lengthening (TAL) that helped improve his standing, transfers, and mobility. This case highlights how ITB, BoNT, oral medications, phenol, and orthopedic procedures can effectively be used in combination to manage a patient with generalized disabling spasticity.

Table 25.4a Case #6: Incobotulinum Toxin A Injection #6

Muscle	Dilution (mL: 100 units)	Dose	# Sites	Technique
Neck				
Right Splenius Capitis	2:1	20 units	1	EMG
Right Splenius Cervicis	2:1	20 units	1	EMG
Right Levator Scapulae	2:1	40 units	2	EMG
Left Splenius Capitis	2:1	20 units	1	EMG
Left Splenius Cervicis	2:1	20 units	1	EMG
Left Levator Scapulae	2:1	40 units	2	EMG
Right Upper Extremity				
Brachioradialis	4:1	20 units	1	EMG
Pronator Teres	2:1	20 units	1	EMG
Flexor Carpi Radialis	4:1	40 units	2	EMG
Flexor Carpi Ulnaris	4:1	40 units	2	EMG
Flexor Digitorum Superficialis	4:1	40 units	2	EMG
Flexor Digitorum Profundus	4:1	40 units	2	EMG
Flexor Pollicis Longus	4:1	20 units	1	EMG/e-stim
Left Upper Extremity				
Brachioradialis	4:1	20 units	1	EMG
Pronator Teres	2:1	20 units	1	EMG
Flexor Carpi Radialis	4:1	40 units	2	EMG
Flexor Carpi Ulnaris	4:1	40 units	2	EMG
Flexor Digitorum Superficialis	4:1	40 units	2	EMG
Flexor Digitorum Profundus	4:1	40 units	2	EMG
Flexor Pollicis Longus	4:1	20 units	1	EMG/e-stim
Total Units Administered		**600 units**		
Total Units Discarded = 0 Units				

Table 25.4b Case #6: Oral Medications

Medication	Dose
Gabapentin	300 mg TID

Table 25.4c Case #6: Phenol Injection #4

Motor Nerve	%	Dose	Sites	Technique
Right Pectoralis Major	6%	2 mL	2	E-stim
Right Musculocutaneous	6%	2 mL	2	E-stim
Left Pectoralis Major	6%	2 mL	2	E-stim
Left Musculocutaneous	1:1	2 mL	2	E-stim
Total Administered		8 mL		

Table 25.4d Case #6: Oral Medications

Medication	Dose
Gabapentin	300 mg TID

Table 25.4e Case #6: Intrathecal Baclofen

Program	Bolus Schedule	Daily Dose (mcg/day)	Basal Rate (mcg/hr)	Concentration (mcg/mL)
Flex	100 mcg @ 0600 100 mcg @ 1200 100 mcg @ 1800 100 mcg @ 2355	657.3	10.5	2,000

REFERENCES

1. Biering-Soerensen B, Stevenson V, Bensmail D, et al. European expert consensus on improving patient selection for the management of disabling spasticity with intrathecal baclofen and/or botulinum toxin type A. *J Rehabil Med.* 2022;54:jrm00241. https://doi.org/10.2340/16501977-2877

2. Saulino M, Ivanhoe CB, McGuire JR, RidleyB, Shilt JS, Boster AL. Best practices for intrathecal baclofen therapy: patient selection. *Neuromodulation.* 2016;19(6):607–615. https://doi.org/10.1111/ner.12447

3. Esquenazi A, Mayer N, Lee S, et al. Patient registry of outcomes in spasticity care. *Am J Phys Med Rehabil.* 2012;91(9):729–746. https://doi.org/10.1097/PHM.0b013e31824fa9ca

Index